ADVANCES IN SURGERY®
VOLUME 17

ADVANCES IN SURGERY®

VOLUMES 1–12 (out of print)

VOLUME 13

VOLUME 14

VOLUME 15

VOLUME 16

ADVANCES *in*
SURGERY®

EDITOR

G. THOMAS SHIRES
Cornell University Medical College
New York, New York

ASSOCIATE EDITORS

JOHN L. CAMERON
Johns Hopkins Hospital
Baltimore, Maryland

GEORGE L. JORDAN, JR.
Baylor College of Medicine
Houston, Texas

LLOYD D. MACLEAN
Royal Victoria Hospital
Montreal, Canada

JOHN MANNICK
Harvard Medical School
Boston, Massachusetts

RONALD K. TOMPKINS
UCLA Center for the Health Sciences
Los Angeles, California

CLAUDE E. WELCH
Massachusetts General Hospital
Boston, Massachusetts

VOLUME 17 • 1984

YEAR BOOK MEDICAL PUBLISHERS • INC.
CHICAGO

Library of Congress Catalog Card Number: 65-29931

International Standard Serial Number: 0065-3411

International Standard Book Number 0-8151-5705-3

Table of Contents

Total Parenteral Nutrition in Surgical Patients

MURRAY F. BRENNAN, M.D., F.A.C.S., AND GLENN
D. HOROWITZ, M.D.

*Department of Surgery, Memorial Sloan-Kettering Cancer Center,
New York, New York*

TOTAL PARENTERAL NUTRITION (TPN) in the surgical patient is
now an accepted method of clinical support. In the last year,
few major advances have been made; several areas, however,
have received emphasis. Vigorous study and research are continuing to improve methods of access, the formulation of appropriate vitamin and trace metal requirements, the understanding of energy and substrate needs in different conditions, the
evaluation by sophisticated metabolic studies of the efficacy of
various regimens being employed, clinical trials to identify
both survival benefit and decrease in morbidity, and preliminary studies critically examining the value of various defined
amino acid solutions.

TPN is being applied more frequently to the nutritional support of surgical patients unable to ingest, absorb, or digest via
the gastrointestinal (GI) tract. No longer must the hospitalized
surgical patient who is unable to eat suffer the ravages of prolonged starvation.

In the last few years, the exact role of parenteral nutrition
in surgical care has been more accurately defined. It is now
clear that scientifically rigorous clinical studies needed to
prove the merits of TPN in the surgical patient are unlikely to
be performed. Studies that involve malnourished patients re-

1

0065-3411/84/0017-0001-0036-$04.00

ceiving no nutritional support are no longer ethically acceptable. Consequently, many conclusions must be based on retrospective studies or studies that rely heavily on inference. Fortunately, many groups working in applied clinical research are defining biologic benefits and disadvantages that will assist in the decision as to which patients should or should not receive TPN.

This chapter reviews briefly the present status of TPN in surgical patients. The term "surgical patient" as used herein will refer to any patient undergoing surgical operation or being managed by a surgeon and with a disease historically considered the province of the surgeon. The present review addresses venous access, what is known of energy need evaluation, the role of special solutions for organ failure, and the increasing use of enhanced branched chain amino acid (BCAA) formulations. Also provided are some comments on requirements and the recent results of intravenous (IV) nutritional support with respect to the outcome of surgical diseases.

Venous Access

Central venous access is moving in several directions. The use of Silastic "permanent" (i.e., long-term) cuffed catheters is now an established practice in many institutions.[1, 2] These catheters are used for central venous access in patients whose peripheral venous system has been exhausted by the use of sclerosing drugs and in patients who require prolonged courses of TPN, often at home. The conventional, percutaneously placed, polyvinylchloride (PVC) catheters continue to be widely used, but documentation of the high frequency of subclinical venous thrombosis is increasing.[3] In studies employing contrast venography, rates of venous occlusion or partial thrombosis approximate the 25% first suggested by autopsy studies.[4] However, it appears that only 5% of patients with this type of central IV lines have a degree of venous occlusion sufficient to warrant removal.[5] While vigorous studies of the prevalence of thrombosis with Silastic catheters have not been conducted, evidence from animal studies suggests that the diminished thrombogenicity is real.[6] Meanwhile, reports demonstrating a reduction of thrombosis with PVC catheters in the clinical setting utilizing a continuous infusion of heparin (3,000 units/L)[7] or intermittent heparin bolus (5,000 units every 6 hours)[8] have appeared recently. Heparin-bonded catheters inserted prior to cardiopulmonary bypass have prevented catheter-adherent thrombus formation.[9] In retrospective and concurrent but not randomized studies, reduced catheter infection rates and reduced mechanical problems have been found when the Silastic catheter is compared to the PVC catheters.[10]

In many patients with a scarcity of access sites, the appearance of fever no longer mandates removal of every central line. This is not meant to minimize the potential of the catheter as the source of fever, but only to indicate that in patients in whom access is difficult and fever common (e.g., the immunosuppressed patient or the cancer patient), the solitary access site need not invariably be relinquished. In cancer patients we have used the catheter exchange technique without harm to the patient.

In a recent comparison of our sequential experience after instituting a catheter exchange policy, we found the percentage of catheters removed because they were a suspected source for sepsis declined from 36% to 14%, with an increasingly high yield of culture-positive catheters when removed (Tables 1 and 2).[11]

Because of the frequent need for central venous access, both for infusion and for venous blood sampling, many patients are receiving two Silastic catheters placed either adjacently or at remote entry sites.[12] As the development of double lumen catheters has advanced, newer catheters demonstrate improved technical features that allow easier placement than some of the earlier models.[13]

Efforts are now directed at perfecting techniques whereby such catheters can be placed percutaneously in a manner similar to that used for placing the noncuffed PVC subclavian catheter. Reports demonstrating the placement of such catheters as a bedside procedure have now been published[14] and a prospective randomized study comparing percutaneous Silastic cuffed catheter placement to PVC percutaneous placement has been completed.[15] That study suggested no advantage of the simpler PVC catheter over the Hickman catheter.

The progress with long-term central venous catheters has markedly diminished the need for various other forms of access, such as arteriovenous shunts or grafts.[16]

TABLE 1.—OUTCOME OF 94 CATHETER EXCHANGES

REASON FOR EXCHANGE	End of Treatment	REASONS FOR REMOVAL				TOTAL
		Thrombosis	Accidental Removal	Death	Suspected Sepsis	
Fever (not catheter related)	17	3	4	14	17	55
Initiation	8	0	1	7	1	17
Mechanical problems	4	1	1	2	3	11
Reposition	3	0	1	2	1	7
Leaking	1	0	1	0	2	4
Total	33	4	8	25	24	94

TABLE 2.—EFFECT OF CATHETER EXCHANGE ON CATHETER REMOVAL
FOR SUSPECTED SEPSIS

	1975–77		1978–81	
	No.	(%)	No.	(%)
Catheters used for TPN	105	(100)	252	(100)
Catheters removed for suspected sepsis	38/105	(36)	35/252	(14)
Catheters exchanged for fever	0/105	(0)	55/252	(22)
Catheters removed for suspected sepsis and subsequently incriminated as a source	8/38	(21)	11/35	(31)

Assessment of Requirements

Conventional assessment of the need for nutritional support has relied heavily on assessment of weight loss, serum albumin, anergy, and micronutrient and vitamin levels. Once an indication has been established for TPN, quantitative energy need is usually replaced empirically.

Laboratory assessment of the protein-calorie malnourished patient has been used to predict operative complications and mortality following major abdominal procedures.[17] After statistical analysis of preoperative conventional nutritional parameters in 121 elective surgical patients and postoperative outcome, a predictive model (the prognostic nutritional index [PNI]) was retrospectively developed relating the risk of operative morbidity and mortality to baseline nutritional status[17]:

$$PNI\ (\%) = 158 - 16.6\ (Alb) - 0.78\ (TSF) - 0.20\ (TFN) - 5.8\ (DH)$$

where Alb is serum albumin in gm/dl, TSF is triceps skin fold in mm, TFN is serum transferrin levels in mg/dl, and DH is cutaneous delayed hypersensitivity reactivity to any of three recall antigens (mumps, SK-SD, *Candida*), graded as 0 (nonreactive), 1 (<5 mm induration), or 2 (≥5 mm induration).

When the PNI was applied prospectively to a group of preoperative patients the model was able to select a subset of patients with an increased risk of morbidity and mortality from surgical procedures. This was then confirmed by a study showing that adequate perioperative TPN could significantly reduce the morbidity and mortality in patients at risk according to the PNI.[17]

Recently Baker et al. suggested that clinical diagnosis of protein-calorie malnutrition was reproducible and correlated very well with standard laboratory measurements of nutritional status.[18] The disagreement among the observers (19%) regarding the nutritional category of their surgical patients was surprisingly similar to the percentage of patients in Mullen's group not treated preoperatively with TPN, but whose PNI would indicate, and subsequent operative fate would validate, that they were at more risk than was clinically apparent.[17] There appears to be a subset of preoperative patients about to undergo operative procedures with a defined morbidity and mortality that may benefit from perioperative TPN.

Body Weight and Energy Stores

Energy is stored in the form of fat, protein, or glycogen, and a change in these components usually causes a change in body weight. However, since water is a large and rather labile component of body weight and contributes nothing to energy stores, a change in body weight is not a simple change in energy stores.

Body water can be measured by isotope dilution techniques[19] and the remainder of the weight difference at two time points could be ascribed to additions or deletions in energy or lean body stores. The dilemma now becomes what proportion of nonwater weight change is due to fat, protein, or glycogen.

A change in energy stores is simply the difference between energy intake and energy output. The earliest work in direct calorimetry in humans was directed at demonstrating that man, like all other living organisms and chemical reactions, obeyed the first law of thermodynamics. Atwater and Benedict[20] showed clearly that chemical energy ingested was identical to the total amount of energy dissipated and excreted. The equations for basal metabolic rate and body surface area were derived from much of this pioneering work.[21]

The unit of energy used in studies of energy balance in biologic systems is the kilocalorie (kcal). The kilocalorie is defined as the amount of heat necessary to raise the temperature of water 1 C, from 15 C to 16 C. The energy supplied in food can be determined by burning a quantity of material in a bomb calorimeter. The energy can be measured directly by recording the temperature change of the water bath that is encircling the bomb calorimeter or indirectly by determining the amount of oxygen used in burning the food.

The same methods are used to measure the heat liberated by the animal body. Energy can be measured directly by placing the animal in a calorimeter or indirectly by measuring the amounts of oxygen consumed and carbon dioxide produced and converting these values to calories. From the respiratory quotient (RQ), which is the ratio of the volume of carbon dioxide produced to the volume of oxygen consumed during an interval of time, a rough indication of the type of substrate metabolized is obtained. For carbohydrates, RQ will equal 1, as evidenced by the equation:

$$C_6H_{12}O_6 + 6O_2 \rightarrow 6CO_2 + 6H_2O$$

$$RQ = \frac{6 \text{ vol } CO_2}{6 \text{ vol } O_2} = 1.00$$

In the oxidation of fat, however, oxygen is required for the β-oxidation of carbon, so RQ will be less than 1. For example:

$$\text{Palmitate} + 23O_2 \rightarrow 16CO_2 + 16H_2O$$

$$RQ = \frac{102 \text{ vol } CO_2}{145 \text{ vol } O_2} = 0.703$$

Food fats that are composed chiefly of palmitic, oleic, and stearic acids give a quotient of 0.706. On the other hand, lipogenesis will yield an RQ greater than 1.

$$4.5 \text{ Glucose} + 4O_2 \rightarrow 1 \text{ palmitate} + 11CO_2 + 11H_2O$$
$$RQ = 2.75$$

Other substrates are listed in Table 3.[22]

It is more difficult to calculate the RQ of the combustion of protein in the body because some oxygen and carbon of the constituent amino acids remain combined with nitrogen and are excreted as nitrogenous wastes (mainly urea) in the urine and feces.

The metabolism of a single substrate does not occur in the whole organism. Cells can oxidize multiple substrates concurrently and can convert glucose into fat and glycogen. Hence an RQ derived from gas analysis cannot provide exact information concerning the metabolic pool. Factors other than oxidative processes can affect the value of the RQ. These processes not

TABLE 3.—RESPIRATORY
QUOTIENT CALCULATED FROM
CHEMICAL EQUATIONS FOR
OXIDATION

Glycerol	0.86
Glyceric aldehyde	1.00
β-Hydroxybutyric acid	0.89
Acetoacetic acid	1.00
Acetone	0.75
Lactate	1.00
Pyruvate	1.20
Ethyl alcohol	0.667

related to energy need have been summarized by Richardson[22]; some are listed below.

Increase RQ:

Hyperventilation

Acid formation

Lactic acids (exercise, convulsions, asphyxia, epineph-rine)

Keto acids (diabetes, carbohydrate starvation)

Decrease RQ:

Hypoventilation

Acid removal (vomiting, nasogastric aspiration, excretion of free acid)

Alkalosis produced by alkali therapy

Thus, the RQ should not be regarded as an exact indicator of specific metabolic processes but as a result of all the changes in the body that require oxygen and lead to pulmonary excretion of carbon dioxide.

The daily energy expenditure of an individual consists of the resting energy expenditure (REE) and the expenditure associated with physical activity. The REE includes the basal metabolic rate (BMR) and the thermal effect resulting from food intake and nonshivering thermogenesis in response to temperature alterations in the environment.

BMR is a carefully controlled measurement that must be performed at least 12 hours postprandially in a thermoneutral environment with the subject supine for at least 30 minutes and completely at ease mentally and physically. The BMR is the sum of the metabolic processes necessary for maintenance of cellular and organ function. By interpreting in vitro tissue slice oxygen consumption, the liver, brain, heart, and kidney, which together represent 5%–6% of the body weight, account for 60%–70% of the BMR. In contrast, skeletal muscle, which makes up 40% of the body weight, accounts for only 16%–30% of the resting metabolism.[23] Protein synthesis and the Na-K pump coupling systems may be responsible for two thirds or more of the BMR. The BMR is primarily regulated by thyroid hormone, and it has been suggested that the mode of action of this hormone may be by regulating sodium transport in thyroid-sensitive tissues.[24]

The ingestion of food increases energy expenditure and is described as the "specific dynamic action" of food. The thermal effect is closely related to the caloric content and composition of the meal. Protein ingestion produces the greatest metabolic response, and this has been attributed to the relatively high metabolic cost of peptide bond synthesis in the absorbed amino acids.[25] Similar effects are seen with bolus injection or constant IV infusion of diets. It has been shown that infusing amino acids will increase energy expenditure by 10% over 24 hours in normal subjects and postoperative patients, whereas glucose and lipid infusions have little effect.[26] However, increased energy expenditure is noted when carbohydrates are given in excess of caloric requirements, whether orally or IV.[27, 28]

For proper management of some patients it may be important to estimate their energy expenditure. Indirect calorimetry facilities are rarely available now that routine methods for the measurement of thyroid hormone exist. Commercially available "metabolic carts" can be used to measure oxygen consumption and carbon dioxide production at the bedside. The REE can be estimated from the formula: $REE = 3.94 \times VO_2 + 1.11 \times V CO_2$. The REE can then be adjusted for protein metabolism by measuring the urinary nitrogen in grams per day. The adjusted metabolic expenditure (AME) equals the $REE - 2.17 \times$ urinary nitrogen.

Since gas exchange analysis is not always feasible, a useful method of predicting REE remains the Harris-Benedict equation:

$$REE \text{ (for males)} = 66.4230 + 13.7516\ W + 5.0033\ H - 6.7750\ A$$
$$REE \text{ (for females)} = 655.0955 + 9.6534\ W + 1.8496\ H - 4.6756\ A$$

where W is weight in kilograms, H is height in centimeters, and A is age in years

These formulas describe normal man in the postabsorptive, supine setting reasonably well; however, in the clinical setting, one must overestimate the energy expenditure by 10%–25% to account for ambulation, normal postoperative wound healing, and other effects of disease. Multiple trauma and sepsis further increase energy expenditure. Estimating energy expenditure and providing adequate substrate replacement are important in preserving lean body mass, and if nitrogen intake is adequate, nitrogen balance is a function of energy intake.[28]

Excess carbohydrate intake, however, may be deleterious to some patients. Patients with respiratory dysfunction should be monitored closely, as high glucose loads lead to increased carbon dioxide production, which cannot be cleared adequately and may lead to further respiratory depression.[29] Finally, the production of fatty infiltration of the liver may be related to excess energy intake, especially common in patients on long-term TPN.[30, 31]

Energy Requirements

The potential energy reserves of a healthy man weighing 70 kg (154 lb) consist of approximately 140,000 kcal stored as fat, 25,000 kcal stored as metabolizable protein, 500 kcal stored as liver glycogen, and 800 kcal stored as muscle glycogen.[32] The minimum caloric requirement in a normal adult maintained at complete bed rest is 20 kcal/kg/day.

Approximately 30–45 kcal/kg/day is required for normal activity in a healthy individual. A hospitalized patient at rest may need 80% of this amount; however, with surgical conditions, such as burns and sepsis, the caloric requirement may increase by more than 200%.

Most tissues of the body normally obtain their energy from glucose, the intermediate products of carbohydrate and protein metabolism, free fatty acids, and ketone bodies. The brain, red blood cell (RBC) mass, bone marrow, and renal medulla metabolize glucose preferentially. The brain oxidizes 140–180 gm of glucose per day (500–600 kcal). The remaining obligate glucose utilizers oxidize approximately one-half that amount.

In the fed state, the body uses glucose as its main energy

source, while excess carbohydrates and fat are converted to tri-
glycerides in the adipose stores. Glucose is metabolized via the
Embden-Myerhof pathway to pyruvic acid. Two moles of ATP
are generated per 1 mole of glucose. These reactions occur in
the absence of oxygen and represent anaerobic oxidation. During aerobic glycolysis the ATP production is 19 times greater.
Thus, the net production per mole of glucose metabolized is 38
moles. The RBCs lack mitochondria and the enzymes for the
Krebs cycle and thus metabolize glucose to lactate only.

Elevated blood glucose concentrations stimulate the pancreas
to secrete insulin. Insulin is intimately involved in all the metabolic processes of the body related to substrate availability,
utilization, and mobilization in conditions of feasting, fasting,
and stress. Insulin is the principal anabolic hormone leading to
glucose and fat storage as well as uptake of amino acids by
skeletal muscle when the circulating insulin concentrations are
high. The lack of insulin, or conditions in which the action of
insulin is opposed by catecholamines, glucagon, or cortisol, are
associated with elevations of blood glucose, free fatty acids, and
amino acids.

Insulin lowers the levels of blood amino acids, in particular
the BCAAs, enhances the incorporation of amino acids into protein, and suppresses synthesis of hepatic enzymes involved in
gluconeogenesis. Insulin stimulates the transport of glucose
across the cell membrane of cardiac and skeletal muscle, fat
cells, and fibroblasts. Glucose entry into the brain and liver are
not dependent on insulin. In the hepatocyte as well as in muscle, insulin promotes glycogen synthetase activity, causing glycogen deposition. Insulin also enhances fat synthesis and inhibits fat mobilization. It promotes glucose entry into the
adipocyte and is a potent inhibitor of lipolysis, preventing free
fatty acid release from triglyceride stores.

EFFECTS OF STARVATION

During starvation the caloric requirements are met by cata-
bolizing the body's energy reserves.[33] Hepatic and muscle glycogen could maintain the blood glucose for several hours and
provide approximately 12 hours of calories to meet basal energy requirements if fat stores were unavailable.

Triglyceride is the most abundant and readily available

stored energy and fat contains little intracellular or extracellular water, so 1 gm of stored fat yields 8 kcal. Fat is a good storage substrate and loss of fat is associated with little detriment. Protein has a low caloric value (4 kcal/gm) and in hydrated storage form yields less than 1 kcal/gram of muscle tissue. As fat cannot be converted to glucose, protein is catabolized and converted by hepatic gluconeogenesis to glucose for brain oxidation.

Although gluconeogenesis from glycerol released in hydrolysis of triglyceride is possible, the amount produced is small: 12 gm of glucose from 100 gm of fat. The major source of glucose during fasting is the gluconeogenic amino acids, in particular alanine and glutamine. Protein catabolism in fasting man causes an increase in urinary nitrogen losses of as much as 15–20 gm of nitrogen per day. A close correlation exists between the amino acids released from muscle and those taken up by the liver.[34] Peripheral nerves, erythrocytes, leukocytes, and the renal medulla also use glucose but convert it to pyruvate and lactate. These are then transaminated in the muscle, principally to alanine. Although less than 10% of muscle is alanine, its output exceeds that of all other amino acids during fasting and accounts for 30%–40% of the total amino acid released across the muscle bed.[35] All other tissues use either free fatty acids or ketone bodies for their caloric needs, thereby sparing body protein.

With prolonged fasting the brain adapts to utilizing increased quantities of the water soluble β-hydroxybutryrate and acetoacetate byproducts of free fatty acid metabolism in the liver. Glucose requirements are decreased, thereby sparing the rapid dissolution of muscle. This is reflected by a reduction of total urinary nitrogen to 3–4 gm/day. In this manner a fast can be prolonged, as fat becomes the predominant caloric source for the entire body.

Insulin decreases as circulating glucose falls during starvation, while glucagon rises. The low level of insulin also enhances lipolysis and the production of glycerol and free fatty acids. Simultaneously, glucagon acts on the liver to stimulate gluconeogenesis and on the fat stores to mobilize free fatty acids.

It is clear, then, that available energy stores are limited and that we can predict the consequences of complete fasting under varying conditions[33] (Table 4). The majority of surgical patients, however, do not undergo absolute starvation but rather a modified fast while in the hospital. The addition of small quantities of glucose can drastically decrease the amount of urinary nitrogen losses and the amount of lean tissue dissolution.[36, 37]

Very few, if any, surgical patients can escape the placement of an IV catheter. The infusion of 140–150 gm of glucose as 3 L of 5% dextrose is common. In effect, this provides all obligate glucose users with their energy requirements in the unstressed state. Urinary nitrogen losses will be markedly reduced and death from starvation postponed or prevented.

Problems arise, however, when stress is superimposed. This may be infection, operation, chemotherapy, or any one of the many stresses surgical patients undergo. The onset of such stress increases overall metabolic demand for all substrates and often introduces new obligate glucose uses, such as a healing wound. In addition, metabolic abnormalities occur that can impair or interfere with utilization of substrate (Table 5).

The response of the patient with trauma, operation, sepsis, or some other injury results in a variable response to the administration of exogenous nutrient (Table 6).

Requirements for Additives to TPN

Considerable progress has been made in determining the micronutrient and vitamin requirements in TPN.

TRACE METAL REQUIREMENTS

Trace metal deficiency syndromes are potential iatrogenic diseases created by trace metal–free IV nutrition.[38] At a recent conference, the American Medical Association Subcommittee on Trace Metals reviewed the available literature on the use of supplementary trace metals in TPN. Its findings suggest that routine supplementation with zinc and copper should be a part of any well-managed IV nutritional support regimen. While deficits in these trace elements cannot be demonstrated in the plasma until 2 or 3 weeks of parenteral nutrition have been completed without such additives, it would seem most appro-

TABLE 4.—BODY ENERGY STORES: DEPLETION TIMES FOR VARYING CLINICAL SITUATIONS

	NITROGEN LOSS (gm/day)	EQUIVALENT PROTEIN LOSS (gm/day)	EQUIVALENT LEAN TISSUE LOSS (gm/day)	DAYS TO LOSE 50% OF TOTAL	
				Muscle Mass	Body Cell Mass
Acute fasting	10	63	280	41	69
Chronic fasting	3	19	84	137	232
Sepsis/major injury	20	125	560	21	34
Month of prior starvation and then sepsis	15	94	420	16	35

TABLE 5.—NUTRITIONAL AND METABOLIC
CONSEQUENCES OF STARVATION AND INJURY

CONSEQUENCE	STARVATION	INJURY
Anorexia	+	+
Weight	↓	↓
Basal metabolic rate	↓	↑
Blood glucose	↓	↑
Blood lactate	±	↑
Serum insulin	↓	↓
Plasma glucagon	↑	↑
Total plasma amino acids	↓	↑
Urinary nitrogen excretion	↓	↑
Glucose tolerance	↓	↓
Whole-body glucose turnover rate	↓	↑
Whole-body glucose recycling (%)	↑	±
Whole-body glucose recycling rate	±	↑
Whole-body protein turnover	↓	↑
Whole-body protein synthesis	↓	↑
Whole-body protein catabolism	±	↑
Gluconeogenesis from alanine	↑	↑

The ↑ indicates a significant increase, ↓ a significant decrease, and ± either no change or a nonsignificant trend. For anorexia, + denotes its presence.

TABLE 6.—METABOLIC RESPONSE TO TOTAL
PARENTERAL NUTRITION DURING STARVATION AND
INJURY

RESPONSE	STARVATION	INJURY
Weight	↑	↑
Blood glucose	↑	↑
Serum insulin	↑	↑
Insulin glucose ratio	±	↓
Plasma glucagon	↓	±
Plasma amino acid	↑	↑
Urinary nitrogen excretion	↑	↑
Nitrogen balance	+	±
Whole-body glucose turnover	NK	↑
Whole-body glucose recycling (%)	NK	±
Whole-body glucose recycling rate	NK	↑
Whole-body protein turnover	↓	↑
Whole-body protein synthesis	↓	↑
Whole-body protein catabolism	↓	↓
Gluconeogenesis from amino acids	↓	↓

*The ↑ indicates an increase, ↓ a decrease, + positive, ± no change, and NK = not known.

priate to begin supplementation from the time that IV nutritional support with amino acids and glucose begins.[39]

It has been suggested that certain patients are more likely to become zinc deficient than others. These include patients with cirrhosis, patients with severe diarrhea or GI fistulas,[40, 41] and patients with multiple injuries,[42] inflammatory bowel disease, pancreatic insufficiency, and chronic uremia. Patients who are in positive zinc balance often show improved insulin secretion and nitrogen metabolism. Caution must be exercised with zinc supplementation since the metal is competitive with copper, and signs of copper deficiency may be brought out with excessive zinc intake.

Manganese, which has long been known to create a significant deficiency syndrome in animals, continues to be recommended as an additive to TPN solutions. Evidence for manganese deficiency in man, however, is lacking.

Although rare, the association of glucose intolerance and chromium deficiency now appears to be accepted. Chromium is not a component of any known metalloenzyme, but rather seems to function as a glucose tolerance factor which is important in the binding of insulin to receptor sites in cells. Consequently, most regimens for long-term patients now contain chromium supplementation. Progress in this area has been hampered by the lack of good plasma or blood assays for chromium. Clinical manifestations of chromium deficiency have been reported in several patients on long-term TPN. Symptoms included glucose intolerance, peripheral neuropathy, and metabolic encephalopathy.

Selenium deficiency states have been identified in populations receiving TPN in a country where the known selenium intake and plasma selenium is one third of that commonly seen in the United States. The symptoms of myalgia and muscle tenderness responded to IV selenium therapy. The lack of readily available plasma, blood, or tissue assays for selenium has hampered progress in this area. It is clear that extremely low levels of selenium occur in patients on long-term parenteral nutrition. While the normal plasma concentrations in adults in the United States are approximately 100–140 ng/ml, levels as low as 10 ng/ml have been seen in patients receiving TPN for 3–5 years. Shorter courses of TPN (7–18 months) are associated with falls in plasma selenium levels of 30%–50%. Interestingly, despite these remarkably low levels, the clinical syndromes thought to be associated with selenium deficiency have not been identified.[44, 45] It may be that in areas where inherent selenium deficiency exists, such as New Zealand and China, prolonged deficiency over many years predisposes to the development of identifiable clinical syndromes.[44, 45]

Currently available amino acid solutions do not contain significant quantities of selenium, and available preparations for supplementation are limited.[46] It appears that the vehicle in which the selenium is added is important, with considerable loss of available selenium occurring when selenium is added to solutions that are stored under refrigerated conditions. With a supplemental dose of 50 µg/day of selenite, the low plasma levels of the long-term home TPN patient can be restored to normal within 14 days, provided the selenite is added directly to the solution immediately prior to infusion (M. E. Shils, unpublished observations). Other groups have used from 50 to 150 µg/day, based on estimated daily requirements.

Iodine is commonly added to the available trace metal supplementation regimens and is safe, but little evidence has been found for creation of an iodine deficiency syndrome when supplementation is lacking. The availability of iodine, which may be absorbed by the cutaneous application of iodine antiseptic solutions, perhaps minimizes this potential problem.

Rare instances have been identified that give strong support to the ability of the other trace metal deficiency syndromes to exist in patients receiving long-term parenteral nutrition. The strongest evidence may be for molybdenum. Molybdenum deficiency is associated with a defect in xanthine metabolism and, while rare, should be considered when the syndrome of headaches, night blindness, irritability, lethargy, and coma, in the presence of abnormal metabolism of sulfur amino acids (methionine and cysteine) and abnormal purine degradation, is not responsive to more conventional restoration of abnormalities of fluid or electrolyte metabolism.[47] Other trace metal deficiencies have been identified but have not yet reached clinical significance.

The question of whether or not to supplement patients with iron has long been debated in the United States but has been standard practice in Europe for many years. The normal daily loss of iron by an adult male is small, and menstruation is often arrested in the severely ill adult female. The most significant ongoing source of loss of iron is phlebotomy. As 0.34% of hemoglobin is iron, a 100-cc blood sample can result in a loss of approximately 50 mg of iron. Such a degree of phlebotomy is not at all unusual in the seriously ill patient on TPN.

In a prospective study, we evaluated the ability of small quantities of iron added to the TPN solution to diminish the need for transfusion to maintain hematocrit. At a dose of 25–87.5 mg/week in daily additives to the TPN solution, we have not seen any untoward effects in 1,000 patient-days of treatment.[48] Current recommendations for trace metal supplementation are summarized in Table 7.

REQUIREMENTS FOR CALCIUM, MAGNESIUM, AND PHOSPHORUS

In a prospective study of calcium and phosphorus metabolism in patients receiving TPN, we demonstrated the frequency of hypercalciuria and the association of hypercalciuria with calcium intake.[49] A positive calcium balance was achieved at 10–15 mEq of calcium intake per day. The role of the IV load of sulfate contained in some amino acid solutions as a factor contributing to hypercalciuria is now being investigated.[50]

A positive phosphorus balance was achieved with intake of approximately 15 mmoles/day.[49] Magnesium balance can be maintained with intakes of approximately 15 mEq/day.

VITAMINS

Conventional supplementation of TPN solutions with vitamins is now firmly established. Debate and experimental eval-

TABLE 7.—CURRENT DAILY
REQUIREMENTS OF TRACE METALS

METAL (FORM)	REQUIREMENT	
Zinc ($ZnCl_2$)	5.00	mg
Copper ($CuSO_4 \cdot 5H_2O$)	1.43	mg
Manganese* ($Mn_2(SO_4)_2$)	0.49	mg
Iodine (Mn I)	0.556	mg
Chromium ($Cr_2(SO_4)_3 \cdot 15H_2O$)	0.016	mg
*Selenium (SeO_3)	50–120	μg

*Not established as essential in man.

uation are currently confined to only one or two components of any multivitamin preparation. This is true of vitamin D. The long-term bone abnormalities that occur in patients on home TPN have been linked to excessive vitamin D intake. While in short-term patients little change can be shown in abnormalities of alkaline phosphatase, serum calcium, serum phosphorus, or in the active metabolites of vitamin D (25 hydroxyvitamin D and 1,25 dihydroxyvitamin D), it would seem prudent to suspect a possible causal role for vitamin D in the development of bone disease in patients receiving TPN for 6 months or longer. Our own studies in short-term patients have suggested that no difference in levels of serum calcium, alkaline phosphatase, or vitamin D metabolites can be demonstrated whether the patient receives 200 units or 400 units a day as IV vitamin D. In an earlier study we had shown a biologically insignificant yet statistically significant rise in serum calcium when vitamin D intake was doubled from 1,000 IU/week to 2,000 IU/week.[51]

Vitamin K supplementation in patients on TPN has received minimal study. In elderly patients it has been estimated that the daily requirements are approximately 0.1 mg. This can be added directly to the solution, but is uncommonly done. More commonly, any abnormality of the prothrombin index is treated with intermittent injections of 10 mg of vitamin K. A currently acceptable regimen for vitamin supplementation without vitamin K is shown in Table 8.

ESSENTIAL FATTY ACID DEFICIENCY

Numerous papers have addressed the issue of essential fatty acid deficiency during fat-free TPN.

It is now clear that essential fatty acid deficiency prior to the use of TPN is extraordinarily uncommon.[52] Provision of 3.2% or more of total calories as IV fat will prevent essential fatty acid deficiency. If 15% of total calories are provided as oral fat, again essential fatty acid deficiency is prevented. Any lesser amount of fat in the diet will delay and diminish the rate of occurrence of essential fatty acid deficiency but will not prevent it. It would appear that sufficient linoleic acid is contained in 1,000 ml of 10% soybean oil emulsion to prevent essential fatty acid deficiency.

Perhaps more important than the development of essential

TABLE 8.—Recommended
Daily Vitamin Intake*

VITAMIN	DOSAGE
A	3,300 IU
D	200 IU†
E	10 IU†
C	100 mg
B1 (Thiamine)	3 mg
B2 (Riboflavin)	3.6 mg
B3 (Dexpanthenol)	15 mg
B5 (Niacin)	40 mg
B6 (Pyridoxine)	4 mg
B7 (Biotin)	60 µg
B9 (Folate)	0.4 mg†
B12	5 µg

*Provided by one ampule of
MVI-12 a day (available from USV
Labs, Tuckahoe, NY).
†Dosage still under evaluation.

fatty acid deficiency is the role of fat as an alternative substrate. Numerous studies have examined the relative efficacy of fat emulsions as a caloric source rather than merely as an agent for prevention of essential fatty acid deficiency. In the severely burned patient, nitrogen sparing apparently was obtained in relation to the amount of calories delivered as glucose.[53] Other studies in less stressed individuals have suggested that if adequate nitrogen is present, a glucose-based regimen and a fat-based regimen are equally efficacious. The most recent study of Kinney et al. has demonstrated that with 300 mg of nitrogen per kilogram per day, glucose and fat regimens or glucose alone as the energy source are equally effective in preserving nitrogen balance.[54] This argues for the judicious use of fat-based regimens in patients thought to have impaired tolerance to high carbohydrate loads, particularly patients requiring ventilatory or respiratory support.[55] Evidently, substituting large quantities of fat for carbohydrate in most patients cannot be justified on a scientific basis but may be justified on the basis of cost; the less expensive glucose-based regimens would be favored, reserving IV fat for the prevention of essential fatty acid deficiency.

The controversy as to whether linolenic acid is an essential fatty acid in man has not yet been resolved. This issue was raised because one commercially available fat preparation did not contain linolenic acid. A single case report has suggested that linolenic acid deficiency does exist, but widespread confirmation has not been provided mainly because of the unavailability of reliable linolenic acid assays.[56] It has been suggested that the deficiency of linolenic acid reported in the single case may have been due to selenium or choline deficiency.[57, 58] The judicious course appears to be the use of preparations that contain both linoleic and linolenic acid, but a strong argument for the inclusion of linolenic acid cannot yet be made.

TPN in Disease States

LIVER FAILURE

Hepatic function is critical in overall metabolism and in a surgeon's ability to provide nutritional support. The liver may clear up to 75% of the carbohydrate and amino acid load presented to it in one passage through its sinusoids, processing substrates in response to a complex series of hormonal and substrate-mediated signals. Liver failure disturbs gluconeogenesis, lipogenesis, and protein synthesis in a number of ways. In addition to defects in detoxification, there are alterations in levels of various micronutrients, such as trace elements, folate, and vitamin A.

The goals of nutritional support for patients with hepatic failure should include maintenance of adequate nutrition, enhancement of hepatic recovery and regeneration, and the prevention and/or amelioration of encephalopathy. In many circumstances trade-offs may be necessary. For example, adequate amounts of protein for the prevention of malnutrition may result in worsened CNS dysfunction. Consequently, specific goals must be established for each patient.[59]

The etiology of hepatic encephalopathy is as yet unknown. There are two major hypotheses. The toxic hypothesis holds that various toxins, most obviously ammonia but also the mercaptans, methanethiols, phenols, and short chain fatty acids, are responsible for the symptoms of hepatic coma.[60] The second theory suggests that derangements in CNS neurotransmitters are responsible for hepatic encephalopathy.

The mechanism by which ammonia might produce hepatic

coma is not clear. Numerous investigations have failed to implicate ammonia interference in energy production.[61, 62] Peripheral measurements of ammonia have not correlated well with the degree of encephalopathy.

The neurotransmitter hypothesis may be more useful in determining appropriate nutritional support. Studies of serotonin, dopamine, norepinephrine, and false transmitters (including β-hydroxyphenylethylamines, such as octopamine) have received much attention.

It is generally accepted that there are derangements in amino acid plasma concentrations in hepatic disease.[63] The classic amino acid pattern in patients with cirrhosis includes decreased levels of BCAA and elevated concentrations of the aromatic and sulfur-containing amino acids. The former are very responsive to the various hormonal derangements in hepatic dysfunction and the latter are generally regulated by the liver.[64, 65] Although total tryptophan is decreased, free tryptophan is variously elevated, and in acute encephalopathy it is greatly elevated. The reason for this increase is a marked increase of nonesterified fatty acids, which displace tryptophan from albumin. This pattern differs in acute encephalopathic hepatic necrosis, in which all amino acids are elevated with the exception of BCAA levels, which are normal. Intermediate patterns exist in a continuum according to the severity of hepatic dysfunction. Amino acids that are highly dependent on the liver for regulation of plasma concentration tend to be elevated with minor disturbances in hepatic function. These include phenylalanine, methionine, tyrosine, aspartate, and glutamate. Others such as serine, lysine, and threonine, are regulated by the liver only to a small degree and are elevated only with severe impairment of hepatic function.[66]

The plasma amino acid patterns are important in hepatic encephalopathy not for their actual concentrations, but for their mechanisms of regulating transport across the blood-brain barrier. The neutral amino acids (phenylalanine, tyrosine, methionine, histidine, and tryptophan) all compete with the BCAAs for entry into the CNS via a single carrier system. The lowered BCAA levels favor aromatic amino acid uptake and synthesis of serotonin, phenylethylamines, tyramine, and octopamine, which are neuromodulators.[65] Faraj et al.[66] have recently confirmed that as coma deepens, norepinephrine levels in certain

regions of the brain decrease and levels of indoleamines, serotonin, and the metabolites increase.

It is postulated that infusion of BCAA should decrease aromatic amino acid uptake in the CNS and ameliorate the symptoms of hepatic encephalopathy. Isolated reports seem to confirm this.[67]

RENAL INSUFFICIENCY

The problem of nutritional support of the patient who has
renal insufficiency without frank renal failure is common. Patients often have impaired ability to clear the waste products
of nitrogen metabolism. As a result, their blood urea nitrogen
(BUN) level rises. Except in patients in high output failure, the
limits to nutritional support are usually the limits imposed by
the amount of fluid that can be given to the patient. Once the
insensible losses of 500–1,000 ml are compensated, one is limited by the amount of urine being made. Fortunately, most patients do make urine and so some allowances can be made. An
alternative in the patient requiring dialysis is to liberalize the
fluid intake and thereby the ability to nutritionally support the
patient, taking care of any excesses of fluid intake by dialysis.
Clearly any nitrogen that is given to the patient will, in the
absence of sufficient nonprotein calories, merely be burned for
energy. It is therefore important that the patient receive a high
intake of nonprotein calories. Many studies have shown that
nitrogen balance can be improved in both the normal subject
and the patient with oliguric renal failure by the use of defined
amino acid mixtures. Jeejeebhoy[68] has shown that in patients
receiving 55 kcal/day, a positive nitrogen balance of 0.8 gm/kg/
day could be obtained with a defined amino acid mixture, compared to a nitrogen balance of 0.4 gm/kg/day when a casein
hydrolysate was employed. It is therefore clear that catabolism
can be decreased with the use of high-quality amino acid protein in conjunction with high nonprotein caloric support.

For a long time it has been known that essential amino acids, once provided, can be utilized to synthesize nonessential
amino acids by the use of available urea.[69] This was initially
proposed as a mechanism of decreasing azotemia. It can be
shown that there is urea incorporation into liver and muscle
protein when essential amino acids are given. Increased pro-

tein synthesis is, however, best obtained by a balance of essential amino acids and nonessential amino acids.

Studies by Bergstrom et al. suggested that in patients with renal insufficiency, optimum nitrogen balance was obtained with 2.65 gm/day of essential amino acids and 2.7 gm/day of nonessential amino acids for a total of approximately 33 gm of protein daily.[70] Despite the theoretical attractiveness of using essential amino acids alone, it seems that the uremic patient will do as well with a balance of approximately 50% each of nonessential and essential amino acids.

It should be emphasized that amino acids are lost during hemodialysis if patients are not supported with IV amino acids (Table 9). Approximately 8 gm of amino acids are lost in a single dialysis.[71] If patients are continued on a TPN regimen during dialysis, then the loss to the dialysate increases slightly, the major losses being all those amino acids that are infused. The net balance is greatly in favor of the patients being infused with amino acids (see Table 9). It is interesting to hypothesize the very significant deficit that must be incurred at hemodialysis.

The earliest studies of nutritional support for the patient in acute renal failure were those of Dudrick et al.[72] Using balanced quantities of essential amino acids and hypertonic glucose in 10 patients with acute or chronic renal failure following surgical complications, Dudrick et al. achieved weight gain, wound healing, and positive nitrogen balance without major changes in urea nitrogen. This was further evidence of the ability to replicate the findings of Giordano, using oral amino acids by the use of IV essential amino acids. Many subsequent stud-

TABLE 9.—AMINO ACID LOSSES DURING DIALYSIS

	PLASMA TOTAL AMINO ACIDS (%)	AMINO ACIDS LOST IN DIALYSATE
Without supplementation	33	8.2 ± 3.1 gm
With supplementation [400 ml Aminosyn 10%* (39.5 gm amino acids) and 400 ml Dextrose 50%]	20	12.6 ± 3.6 gm

*Abbott Laboratories, North Chicago, Ill.

ies have confirmed these observations. There has been a positive nitrogen balance and a concomitant decrease in BUN, serum phosphate, and serum potassium levels.[73]

Such uncontrolled studies were followed by prospective randomized studies examining the effect of IV administration of essential amino acids in glucose to patients suffering from acute renal failure.[74-76] In one study, 53 patients with a clear-cut episode leading to the development of acute renal failure and with prior known normal renal function were included in a trial. All patients had creatinine levels above 3 mg/dl, with a ratio of BUN to creatinine less than 20:1. In this study hypertonic glucose was compared to hypertonic glucose plus a renal failure solution, which was identical except for the addition of essential amino acids (isoleucine, leucine, lysine, methionine, phenylalanine, threonine, tryptophan, and valine). The groups were matched for age, sex, initial renal function, and etiology of renal failure (Table 10). Recovery from polyuric renal failure was particularly helped by use of the renal failure solution— 14 of 18 patients recovered, whereas only 7 of 16 patients who received glucose alone recovered (P = 0.05). Approximately half of the patients underwent dialysis at some time during treatment with the test solutions. Survival of patients requiring dialysis was significantly poorer than survival of patients not requiring dialysis. It should be emphasized that in nondialyzed patients, overall survival was high and the type of solution given did not significantly improve the recovery rate. These findings suggest that patients who need dialysis should receive nutritional support. Whether nutritional support must be in the form of a specialized solution is not answered by such a study, and considering the amount of amino acids that will be removed by dialysis, it is possible that equally efficacious results might be obtained by conventional nutritional regimens in patients who need dialysis.

In the study by Leonard et al., 11 patients received L essential amino acids and dextrose while 11 patients received dextrose alone following the development of acute renal failure.[76] Survival rates between the two groups were not different (55% and 56%, respectively). There was no difference in mean duration of renal failure among those surviving the acute renal failure, whether or not they received the solution containing amino acids. These patients were all treated with dialysis, as

TABLE 10.—ACUTE RENAL FAILURE (ARF): COMPARISON OF ESSENTIAL AMINO ACIDS
AND GLUCOSE WITH GLUCOSE ALONE AS NUTRITIONAL SUPPORT

	RECOVERED FROM ARF	DISCHARGED FROM HOSPITAL	SURVIVAL WITH DIALYSIS	SURVIVAL WITHOUT DIALYSIS
Essential amino acids + glucose ($n = 28$)	21/28 (75%)	61%	11/17 (65%)	10/11 (91%)
Glucose alone ($n = 25$)	11/25 (44%)*	40%	2/11 (18%)*	9/14 (64%)†

*$P < 0.05$
†P = NS.
Table modified from Abel et al.[74] Reproduced by permission.

they represented the group most likely to benefit in terms of survival in the study by Abel et al.[74] It appears, therefore, that patients who have acute renal failure and who require nutritional support for survival should receive amino acids and dextrose. At present, nutritional support with essential amino acids alone does not appear to be markedly more efficacious than a balanced solution of essential and nonessential amino acids.

Such an opinion is not supported uniformly. Essential amino acid solutions cost approximately 25% more than conventional solutions. Furthermore, Freund and Fischer came to an opposite conclusion based on a retrospective analysis of patients who received a balanced solution of nonessential and essential amino acids compared with patients who received essential amino acids alone.[77]

CARDIAC SURGICAL PATIENTS

A randomized study of 44 malnourished patients compared 20 who received immediate postoperative TPN and 24 who did not receive such treatment. The 5 days of nutritional support had no notable effect on the morbidity or mortality of the malnourished cardiac patients. Although preoperative malnutrition has been identified as a bad prognostic factor in cardiac patients as well as in many others, no effect of postoperative nutritional support was identified in this study when these patients were compared with a third nonmalnourished group of similar patients.[78]

Use of Branched Chain Amino Acid Solutions

Numerous studies have examined the use of BCAA solutions. Meguid et al. suggested that a BCAA solution provides a more positive nitrogen balance in patients receiving parenteral nutrition. However, in subsequent studies from the same laboratory this observation was not confirmed; instead, it was suggested that the effect of the enriched solution depended on the quantity of leucine in the solutions.[79] The same study found that administration of enriched leucine solutions led to decreased 3-methylhistidine excretion. In our studies on patients receiving enriched BCAA solutions following total cystectomy with equal quantities of glucose (Table 11), whole-body protein turnover studies demonstrated that conventional quantities (22% BCAA) were more efficacious in preserving synthesis, but only with increased catabolism and an increased whole-body protein turnover. The 45% BCAA solutions seemed to be poorly balanced and limited by the quantity of available leucine. When one examines forearm flux or amino acids in this particular model, the low leucine, high valine, and high isoleucine solution is less effective in retaining muscle amino acids than the more balanced (22% BCAA) solution.

Kern and colleagues have continued to use BCAA-enriched solutions extensively in stressed patients. They have demonstrated decreases in the postoperative catabolism when the solutions are infused.[80]

The exact composition of all these solutions needs careful documentation for accurate comparison. Recently it was shown that a solution with approximately 50% nonessential amino acids provides greater nitrogen sparing than a solution with 25% nonessential amino acids.[81]

A prospective blinded trial of the effects of BCAA-enriched TPN solution compared to the standard TPN solution in nonseptic, noncirrhotic patients following surgical operation or trauma has been conducted.[82] In this study with isonitrogenous

TABLE 11.—PROTEIN TURNOVER (Q), SYNTHESIS (S), AND
CATABOLISM (C) IN PATIENTS RECEIVING POSTOPERATIVE GLUCOSE
AND AMINO ACID SOLUTIONS*

GROUP	Q	C	S
0% BCAA ($n = 5$)	2.15 ± 0.05	2.15 ± 0.05	1.62 ± 0.03
22% BCAA ($n = 5$)	3.28 ± 0.14†	1.84 ± 0.12†	1.90 ± 0.17†
45% BCAA ($n = 5$)	2.85 ± 0.08†‡	1.32 ± 0.12†‡	1.37 ± 0.13†‡

*BCAA, branched chain amino acids. Numbers in table are in gm protein · kg^{-1} · day.
†$P < .05$, compared to 0% BCAA.
‡$P < .05$, compared to 22% BCAA.

and isocaloric input, urinary nitrogen excretion was lower on day 3 in the high BCAA group (50% BCAA), not different on day 6, and lower in the standard TPN group on the day of injury or operation (Table 12). The authors argue that nitrogen balance was achieved earlier with the BCAA-enriched solution. The authors also argue that because 3-methylhistidine excretion did not change, the nitrogen retention reflected improved protein synthesis. This is an unproved extrapolation of the data.

A number of studies have suggested a beneficial effect from infusion of BCAA-enriched solutions in liver failure.[83, 84]

The Role of Insulin as a Postoperative Anabolic Agent

Previous studies by Hinton et al.[85] using high quantities of glucose and insulin in the burned patient demonstrated some protein sparing as indicated by decreased urinary nitrogen losses. These studies have been reported occasionally in varying conditions. Recently, Inculet et al. reported on the influence of insulin during posttraumatic protein catabolism in patients receiving TPN. In six nondiabetic patients, urinary nitrogen losses were significantly elevated in the postoperative period; these losses were suppressed by the addition of an insulin infusion.[86] Examination of the efflux of amino acids from forearm musculature showed an increase in the posttraumatic period that could be markedly decreased by the infusion of insulin. Earlier studies on the infusion of insulin directly into the forearm musculature had shown the marked anabolic effect that

TABLE 12.—COMPARISON OF BCAA-ENRICHED TPN SOLUTION WITH STANDARD TPN
SOLUTION ADMINISTERED POST INJURY

	NITROGEN INTAKE (gm/day)	GLUCOSE INTAKE (cal/kg/day)	NITROGEN EXCRETION (gm/day)	$^3CH_3$ HISTIDINE (μg/day)
50% BCAA ($n = 7$)				
day 0	2.6 ± 0.5	237 ± 132	11 ± 8.6	255 ± 197
3	10.8 ± 1.9	671 ± 153	8 ± 4	181 ± 82
6	12.5 ± 0.8	761 ± 103	8 ± 4	151 ± 53
15.5% BCAA ($n = 8$)				
day 0	3.1 ± 0.8	243 ± 59	6 ± 4*	195 ± 155
3	10.6 ± 1.4	591 ± 79	13 ± 4*	176 ± 80
6	12.6 ± 1.2	685 ± 80	11 ± 5	165 ± 97

*$P < .05$, compared to 50% BCAA.
Table from Cerra et al.[82] Reproduced by permission.

insulin had on amino acid release from human forearm musculature.

Selective insulin deficiency during fasting has demonstrated marked increase in plasma leucine in the short term and less significant increases in prolonged fasting (> 48 hours). By the use of tracer technology it has been suggested that the main effect of this insulin deficiency is a decrease in protein synthesis whereby in short-term fasting, insulin deficiency results in decreased protein synthesis almost exclusively, whereas after 48 hours of fasting, both increased protein breakdown and decreased protein synthesis are associated with the lowered availability of insulin.[86, 87]

With continuing studies of this nature, we may be able to make some sensible recommendations on the value of insulin as an anabolic hormone—a subject that has been studied for 15 years.

The Use of 3-Methylhistidine

Many studies have relied on the rate of urinary excretion of 3-methylhistidine to indicate skeletal muscle degradation. Recent studies suggest that skeletal muscle contributes only 25% of the total urinary 3-methylhistidine excretion each day.[88] These studies, done on the adult female rat, also suggested that GI muscle provides approximately 10% of this excretion. Actin, the major source of 3-methylhistidine, appears to turn over more slowly than many other proteins within muscle. The identity of the remaining 3-methylhistidine excreted in the urine is not yet known. By the use of radioactively labeled 3-methylhistidine, it appears that there are other pools that turn over rapidly.

The problem has been compounded by the suggestion that cancer patients have a marked diminution in net release of 3-methylhistidine from hind limb muscle, as demonstrated by plasma assays for 3-methylhistidine.[89] Cancer patients, however, do not have markedly different release from other similarly depleted noncancerous controls. Certainly in the acutely ill patients, who are often well nourished, there is an increase in 3-methylhistidine excretion from the hind limb compared to depleted controls. However, the variance of the studies is close to the limits of the assay and is compounded by the variable diet that some controls have received. It appears that 3-methylhistidine release can be suppressed by the use of nutritional support,[90] and the argument has been made that selected patient populations such as cancer patients are less able to respond by diminution in 3-methylhistidine release than other patients when nutritional support is offered.[89]

Clinical Trials Other Than Organ Failure

Many of the clinical trials of the value of nutritional support were conducted in the oncologic patient. The initial studies with small numbers showed little effect of the routine use of TPN in all patients undergoing oncologic therapy.

Recently, a prospective randomized study examining the benefits of preoperative TPN in patients undergoing surgery for GI malignancy has been published. This positive study showed a decrease in mortality and morbidity (Table 13) in patients receiving preoperative parenteral nutrition.[91] Similar studies on TPN in other disease states are lacking, although strong evidence from less rigorously controlled observations has suggested the value of TPN in patients with inflammatory bowel disease, neonatal diarrhea, and burns.

Strong support for the use of TPN has been suggested by retrospective studies of patients with GI fistulas, and TPN is clearly of value when the problem is uncomplicated malnutrition due to the short bowel syndrome.[92]

Given the advances in nutritional support and the extensive knowledge of the deficits that accompany starvation, it is hard

TABLE 13.—PREOPERATIVE PARENTERAL FEEDING IN
PATIENTS WITH GASTROINTESTINAL CARCINOMA

	CONTROL (%) (N = 59)	PREOPERATIVE TPN* (%) (N = 66)
Preoperative malnutrition	38	41
Major complications	32	16†
Postoperative mortality	19	5†
Pneumonia	39	30
Wound infection	25	21

*TPN, total parenteral nutrition.
†$P < .05$.

to conceive of an ethically justified trial that would involve withholding nutritional support by the IV route in otherwise nutritionally depleted patients purely to establish the worthiness of TPN. In patients who are not currently malnourished but merely undergoing courses of therapy or treatment for short-lasting illness, such studies may still be justifiable. These studies would look at the ability of nutritional support to improve response or cure rates rather than to salvage patients who are nutritional derelicts.

REFERENCES

1. Hickman R.O., Buckner C.D., Clift R.A., et al.: A modified right atrial catheter for access to the venous system in marrow transplant recipients. *Surg. Gynecol. Obstet.* 148:871, 1979.
2. Daly J.M., Lawson M., Speir A., et al.: Angio access in cancer patients. *Curr. Probl. Surg.* 5:1, 1981.
3. Brennan M.F.: Total parenteral nutrition in the cancer patient. *N. Engl. J. Med.* 305:375–383, 1981.
4. Ryan J.A., Abel R.M., Abbot W.M.: Catheter complications in total parenteral nutrition: A prospective study of 200 consecutive patients. *N. Engl. J. Med.* 290:757–61, 1974.
5. Burt M.E., Dunnick N.R., Krudy A.G., et al.: Prospective evaluation of subclavian vein thrombosis during total parenteral nutrition by contrast venography, abstracted. *Clin. Res.* 29:264, 1981.
6. Welch G.W., McKeel D.W. Jr., Silverstein P., et al.: The role of catheter composition in the development of thrombophlebitis. *Surg. Gynecol. Obstet.* 138:421–4, 1974.
7. Fabri P.J., Mirtallo J.M., Rubero R.L.: Incidence and prevention of thrombosis of the subclavian vein during TPN. *Surg. Gynecol. Obstet.* 155:238–240, 1982.
8. Brismar B., Hardstedt C., Jacobson S., et al.: Reduction of catheter associated thrombosis in parenteral nutrition by IV heparin therapy. *Arch. Surg.* 117:1196–1199, 1982.
9. Hoar P.F., Wilson R.M., Mangano D.T., et al.: Heparin bonding reduces thrombogenicity of pulmonary arterial catheters. *N. Engl. J. Med.* 305:993–995, 1981.
10. Mitchell A., Atkins S., Royle G.T., et al.: Reduced catheter sepsis and prolonged catheter life using a tunnelled silicone rubber catheter for total parenteral nutrition. *Br. J. Surg.* 69:420–422, 1982.
11. Maher M.M., Henderson D.K., Brennan M.F.: Central venous catheter exchange in cancer patients during total parenteral nutrition. *J. Natl. Intrav. Ther. Assoc.* 5:54–60, 1982.
12. Raaf J.H.: Two broviac catheters for intensive long-term support of cancer patients. *Surg. Gynecol. Obstet.,* to be published.
13. Raaf J.H.: Vascular access in cancer patients via "double" broviac and dual lumen Silastic, right atrial catheters, abstracted.

14. Kirkemo A.K., Johnston M.R.: Percutaneous subclavian vein placement of the Hickman catheter. *Surgery* 91:349–351, 1982.
15. Wagman L.W., Kirkemo A.A., Johnston M.R.: Venous access: A prospective randomized trial of Hickman versus PVC subclavian catheters, unpublished manuscript.
16. Raaf J.H.: Vascular access grafts for chemotherapy use in forty patients at the M.D. Anderson Hospital. *Ann. Surg.* 190:614, 1979.
17. Mullen J.L., Buzby G.P., Matthews D.C., et al.: Reduction of operative morbidity and mortality by combined preoperative and postoperative nutritional support. *Ann. Surg.* 192:604–13, 1980.
18. Baker J.P., Detsky A.S., Wesson D.E., et al.: Nutritional assessment: A comparison of clinical judgment and objective measurements. *N. Engl. J. Med.* 306:969–72, 1982.
19. Halliday D., Millor A.G.: Precise measurement of total body water using quantities of deutrium oxide. *Biomed. Mass Spectrom.* 4:82, 1977.
20. Atwater W.O., Benedict F.G.: Experiments on the metabolism of matter and energy in the human body. *U.S. Dept. Agr. Off. Exp. Sta. Bull.* 136:1, 1903.
21. Harris J.A., Benedict F.G.: *A Biometric Study of Basal Metabolism in Man.* Washington, D.C., *Carnegie Institute of Washington publication* no. 297, 1919.
22. Richardson H.B.: The respiratory quotient. *Physiol. Rev.* 9:61, 1929.
23. Grande F.: Energy expenditure of organ and tissues, in *Assessment of Energy Metabolism in Health and Disease.* Columbus, Ohio, Ross Laboratories, 1980, pp. 88–92.
24. Edelman I.S.: Transition from the poikilotherm to the homeotherm: Possible role of sodium transport and thyroid hormone. *Fed. Proc.* 35:2180–84, 1976.
25. Kleiber M.: *The Fire of Life.* Huntington, N.Y., R.E. Kreiger Publishing Co., 1975.
26. Elwyn D.H., Kinney J.M., Jeevanandam M., et al.: Influence of increasing carbohydrate intake on glucose kinetics in injured man. *Ann. Surg.* 191:117–21, 1979.
27. Danforth E., Horton E.S., O'Connell M., et al.: Dietary-induced alterations in thyroid hormone metabolism during over-nutrition. *J. Clin. Invest.* 64:1336–47, 1979.
28. Elwyn D.H., Gump F.E., Munro H.N., et al.: Changes in nitrogen balance of depleted patients with increasing infusion of glucose. *Am. J. Clin. Nutr.* 32:1597–1611, 1979.
29. Hunker F.D.: Metabolic and nutritional evaluation of patients supported with mechanical ventilation. *Crit. Care Med.* 8:628–32, 1980.
30. Lowry S.F., Brennan M.F.: Abnormal liver function during parenteral nutrition relation to infusion excess. *J. Surg. Res.* 26:300–07, 1979.
31. Wagman L.D., Burt M.E., Brennan M.F.: The impact of total parenteral nutrition on liver function tests in patients with cancer. *Cancer* 49:1249–1256, 1982.
32. Cahill G.F.: Starvation in man. *N. Engl. J. Med.* 282:668–675, 1970.
33. Brennan M.F.: Uncomplicated starvation versus cancer cachexia. *Cancer Res.* 27:2359–2364, 1977.

34. Marliss E.B., Aoki T.T., Pozefsky T.: Muscle and splanchnic glutamine and glutamate metabolism in post-absorptive and starved man. *J. Clin. Invest.* 50:814, 1971.
35. Felig P., Pozefsky T., Cahill G.F.: Alanine: Key role in gluconeogenesis. *Science* 167:1003, 1970.
36. Gamble J.L.: Physiology information gained from studies on the life-raft ration. *Harvey Lect.* 42:247, 1947.
37. O'Connell R.C., Morgan A.P., Aoki T.T., et al.: Nitrogen conservation in starvation: Graded response to intravenous glucose. *J. Clin. Endocrinol. Metab.* 39:555, 1974.
38. Lowry S.F., Goodgame J.T., Smith J.C., et al.: Abnormalities of zinc and copper during total parenteral nutrition. *Ann. Surg.* 189:120–128, 1979.
39. Lowry S.F., Smith J.C., Brennan M.F.: Zinc and copper replacement during total parenteral nutrition. *Am. J. Clin. Nutr.* 34:1853–1860, 1981.
40. Walker B.E., Dawson J.B., Kelleher J., et al.: Plasma and urinary zinc in patients with malabsorption syndromes or hepatic cirrhosis. *Gut* 14:943–948, 1973.
41. Hallbook T., Hedelin H.: Zinc metabolism and surgical trauma. *Br. J. Surg.* 64:271, 1977.
42. Lindeman R.D., Bottomley R.G., Cornelison R.L., et al.: Influence of acute tissue injury on zinc metabolism in man. *J. Lab. Clin. Med.* 79:452, 1972.
43. Van Rij A.M., Thomson C.D., McKenzie J.M., et al.: Selenium deficiency in total parenteral nutrition. *Am. J. Clin. Nutr.* 32:2076–85, 1979.
44. Van Rij A.M., McKenzie J.M., Robison M.F., et al.: Selenium and total parenteral nutrition. *JPEN* 3:235–239, 1979.
45. Johnson R.A., Baker S.S., Fallon J.T., et al.: An accidental case of cardiomyopathy and selenium deficiency. *N. Engl. J. Med.* 304:1210–1212, 1981.
46. Smith J.L., Goos S.M.: Selenium in total parenteral nutrition: Intake levels. *JPEN* 4:23–26, 1980.
47. Abumrad N.N., Scheider A.J., Steel D.R., et al.: Amino acid intolerance during prolonged total parenteral nutrition reversed by molybdate therapy. *Am. J. Clin. Nutr.* 34:2551–2559, 1981.
48. Norton J.A., Peters M.L., Wesley R., et al.: Iron supplementation in total parenteral nutrition: A prospective study, unpublished manuscript.
49. Sloan G.M., White D.E., Brennan M.F.: Calcium and phosphorus metabolism during total parenteral nutrition. *Ann. Surg.* 197:1–6, 1983.
50. Cole D.E.C., Zlotkin S.H.: Increased sulfate as an etiological factor in the hypercalciuria associated with total parenteral nutrition. Am. J. Clin. Nutr. 37:108–113, 1983.
51. Kirkemo A.K., Burt M.E., Brennan M.F.: Serum vitamin level maintenance in cancer patients on total parenteral nutrition. *Am. J. Clin. Nutr.* 35:1003–1009, 1982.
52. Barr L.H., Dunn G.D., Brennan M.F.: Essential fatty acid deficiency during total parenteral nutrition. *Ann. Surg.* 193:304–311, 1981.
53. Long J.M., Wilmore D.W., Mason A.D., et al.: Effect of carbohydrate and fat intake on nitrogen excretion during intravenous feeding. *Ann. Surg.* 185:417–422, 1977.
54. Nordenstrom J., Askanazi J., Martin P.E., et al.: Protein and energy bal-

ances during total parenteral nutrition. *Surg. Forum* 33:96–98, 1982.

55. Askanazi J., Nordenstrom J., Rosenbaum S.H., et al.: Nitrogen for the patient with respiratory failure; Glucose vs fat. *Anesthesiology* 54:373–377, 1981.

56. Holman R.T., Johnson S.B., Hatch T.F.: A case of human linolenic acid deficiency involving neurological abnormalities. *Am. J. Clin. Nutr.* 35:617–23, 1982.

57. Meng H.C.: A case of human linolenic acid deficiency involving neurological abnormalities. *Am. J. Clin. Nutr.* 37:157–159, 1983.

58. Burt M.E., Hanin I., Brennan M.F.: Choline deficiency associated with total parenteral nutrition. *Lancet* 2:638–639, 1980.

59. Fischer J.: Panel report on nutritional support of patients with liver, renal and digestive disease. *Am. J. Clin. Nutr.* 34:1235–1245, 1981.

60. Zieve F.J., Zieve L., Doizaki W.M., et al.: Synergism between ammonia and fatty acids in the production of coma: Implication for hepatic coma. *J. Pharm. Exp. Ther.* 191:10–16, 1974.

61. Fischer J.E.: Portasystemic encephalopathy, in Wright R., Alberti K.G., Karran S., et al: (eds.): *Liver and Biliary Diseases.* Philadelphia, W.B. Saunders Co., 1979, pp. 973–1001.

62. Hindfeldt B., Plum F., Duffy T.E.: Effect of acute ammonia intoxication on cerebral metabolism in rats with portacaval shunts. *J. Clin. Invest.* 59:386–396, 1977.

63. Fischer J.E.: Amino acids in hepatic coma. *Dig. Dis. Sci.* 27:97–102, 1982.

64. Iber F.L., Rosen H., Levenson S.M., et al.: The plasma amino acids in patients with liver failure. *J. Lab. Clin. Med.* 50:417–425, 1977.

65. Rosen H.M., Yoshimura N., Hodgman J.M., et al.: Plasma amino acids patterns in hepatic encephalopathy of differing etiology. *Gastroenterology* 77:438–487, 1977.

66. Faraj B.A., Camp V.M., Ansley J.D., et al.: Evidence for central hypertyraminemia in hepatic encephalopathy. *J. Clin. Invest.* 67:395–402, 1981.

67. Fischer J.E., Rosen H.M., Ebeid A.M., et al.: The effect of normalization of plasma amino acids on hepatic encephalopathy in man. *Surgery* 80:77–91, 1976.

68. Jeejeebhoy K.N.: Nutritional support of the azotemic. *Urol. Clin. North Am.* 1:345–356, 1974.

69. Giordano C.: Use of exogenous and endogenous urea for protein synthesis in normal and uremic subjects. *J. Lab. Clin. Med.* 62:231–246, 1963.

70. Bergstrom J., Furst P., Josephson B.: Factors affecting the nitrogen balance in chronic uremic patients receiving essential amino acids intravenously or by mouth. *Nutr. Metab.* 14(suppl.):162–170, 1972.

71. Wolfson M., Jones M.R., Kopple J.D.: Amino acid losses during hemodialysis with infusions of amino acids and glucose. *Kidney Int.* 21:500–506, 1982.

72. Dudrick S.J., Steiger E., Long J.M.: Renal failure in surgical patients: Treatment with intravenous essential amino acids and hypertonic glucose. *Surgery* 68:180–186, 1970.

73. Wilkiemeyer R.M., Boyce W.H., Harrison L.H.: Intravenous hyperalimentation: A useful adjunct in surgery of the azotemic patients. *J. Urol.* 111:93–95, 1974.

74. Abel R.M., Beck C.H., Abbott W.M.: Acute renal failure treatment with intravenous amino acids and glucose. *N. Engl. J. Med.* 288:695–699, 1973.

75. Abel R.M., Shih V.E., Abbott W.M., et al.: Amino acid metabolism in acute renal failure: Influence of intravenous essential L-amino acid hyperalimentation therapy. *Ann. Surg.* 180:350–354, 1974.

76. Leonard C.D., Luke R.G., Sieger R.R.: Parenteral essential amino acids in acute renal failure. *Urology* 6:154–157, 1975.

77. Freund H., Fischer J.E.: Comparative study of parenteral nutrition in renal failure using essential and non-essential amino acid containing solutions. *Surg. Gynecol. Obstet.* 151:652–656, 1980.

78. Abel R.M., Fischer J.E., Buckley M.J., et al.: Malnutrition in cardiac surgical patients. *Arch. Surg.* 111: 45–50, 1976.

79. Meguid M.M., Landel A., Lo C.C., et al.: The mechanism of enhanced N excretion in postoperative receiving branched chain amino acid enriched solutions. *Surg. Forum,* Volume 3, 1982.

80. Kern K.A., Bower R.H., Atamian S., et al.: The effect of a new branched chain-enriched amino acid solution on postoperative catabolism. *Surgery* 92:780–885, 1982.

81. Jiang Z.-M., Chen T.-Y., Zhu-Yu, et al.: The role of nonessential amino acids in postoperative protein sparing therapy. *Chinese Med. J.* 95:257–260, 1982.

82. Cerra F.B., Upson D., Angelico R., et al.: Branched chains support postoperative protein synthesis. *Surgery* 92:192–199, 1982.

83. Marchesini G., Zoli M., Dondi C., et al.: Anticatabolic effect of branched chain amino acid-enriched solutions in patients with liver cirrhosis. *Hepatology* 2:420–425, 1982.

84. Herlin P.M., Gimmon Z., James H., et al.: Effects of branched chain amino acids after total hepatectomy. *Surg. Forum* 33:101–103, 1982.

85. Hinton S.P., Allison S.P., Littlejohn S.: Injury and glucose to reduce catabolic response to injury in burned patients. *Lancet* 1:767, 1971.

86. Inculet R.I., Finley R.J., Pace R.F., et al.: Influence of insulin on posttraumatic protein catabolism during steady state parenteral nutrition in man. *Surg. Forum* 33:94–95, 1982.

87. Miller B.M., Abumrad N.N.: Disparate effects of insulin in fasting on protein turnover in the conscious dog. *Surg. Forum* 33:87–89, 1982.

88. Millward D.J., Bates P.C., Grimble G.K., et al.: Quantitative importance of non-skeletal muscle sources of N^t-methylhistidine in urine. *Biochem. J.* 190:225–228, 1980.

89. Lundholm K., Bennegard K., Eden E., et al.: Efflux of 3-methylhistidine from the leg in cancer patients who exerience weight loss. *Cancer Res.* 42:4807–4811, 1982.

90. Burt M.E., Stein T.P., Brennan M.F.: A controlled randomized trial evaluating the effects of enteral and parenteral nutrition on protein metabolism in man. *J. Surg. Res.* 34:303, 1983.

91. Mueller J.M., Brenner U., Dienst C., et al.: Preoperative parenteral feeding in patients with gastrointestinal carcinoma. *Lancet* 1:68–71, 1982.
92. Dietl M.: Management of gastrointestinal fistulas, in Dietl M. (ed.): *Nutrition in Clinical Surgery*. Baltimore, Williams & Wilkins Co., 1980, pp. 173–176.

Management of Trauma to the Spleen

ROGER SHERMAN, M.D., F.A.C.P.

Department of Surgery, Emory University Medical School, Atlanta, Georgia

Perspective

SOME TIME DURING the second century after the birth of Christ, Galen, while contemplating the organs of animals, was confused and perplexed by the functions of the spleen. He called it the *mysterii pleni organon,* the organ filled with mystery.

Tracing the gradual evolution of present-day measures in the management of patients with trauma to the spleen through history is a fascinating study of a host of misconceptions concerning the structure and functions of this enigmatic organ. Four of the many unfounded concepts of splenic structure and function have played definitive roles in the formulation of management of trauma to the spleen for hundreds of years.

The first major misconception began before the birth of Christ, with Aristotle. Aristotle assumed that the spleen was not necessary for the maintenance of existence.[1] This assumption was the origin of the notion that the spleen was an expendable organ. Aristotle's conclusion was accepted and propagated by many surgeons beginning with the first recorded successful splenectomy in the 16th century. Aristotle was not seriously challenged for nearly 400 years. By the end of the 18th century reports of patients surviving splenectomy without apparent sequelae provided little evidence of value that the spleen served a useful function in man. Experimental studies conducted throughout the 18th and 19th centures were poorly

37

designed, uncontrolled, and added nothing useful to the knowledge of splenic function. Following the first successful splenectomy for blunt abdominal trauma, reported by Riegner in 1893, trauma surgeons were quick to adopt this procedure. Case reports of successful splenectomy for traumatic rupture multiplied, and the concept that the spleen served no useful function was apparently confirmed.

The second major misconception was that the spleen could not heal spontaneously. Berger, in his painstaking statistical review of the literature prior to 1900, added credence to this misconception by noting that nonoperative management of patients with ruptured spleens resulted in mortalities of 90%–100%.[2] Although the possibility that a ruptured spleen might heal without surgical intervention was considered unlikely, there was some controversy over the issue. Bilroth reported autopsy findings in the spleen of a patient dying 5 days after a severe head injury, as follows: "From the appearance of the rent, and the small quantity of blood effused, we concluded that the injury might have healed completely."[3] Conjecture concerning the ability of the spleen to repair itself, stimulated by occasional case reports of healed splenic injuries, began to appear in the literature.[4-6] Turnbull,[7] McCartney,[8] and other pathologists contended that they had never seen evidence at autopsy of a healed splenic injury.

Bailey resolved the controversy to his satisfaction by stating, "The whole question of the natural repair of a splenic injury is an unimportant one. Nature fails so frequently that we must assume that surgical aid is always needed."[9]

Belief that the spleen could not heal spontaneously contributed significantly to the development of the third major misconception: "delayed rupture" of the spleen. Evans, in 1866, reported the case of a patient who apparently stabilized following injury to the spleen, only to bleed again on the fourth postinjury day.[10] In the following years a number of other authors added to the literature many examples of so-called delayed rupture of the spleen. These instances of bleeding from a ruptured spleen at a time somewhat remote from the time of injury were interpreted as strong evidence that the injured spleen had to be removed if fatal hemorrhage was to be avoided.

Kocher, in 1911, embraced and authoritatively crystallized these three major misconceptions concerning the management of rupture of the spleen in his widely read *Textbook of Operative Surgery:* "Injuries of the spleen demand excision of the gland. No evil effects follow its removal, while the danger of hemorrhage is effectively stopped."[11]

Based on such apparent inviolable evidence, splenectomy became the most common operation for injuries to the spleen. Nevertheless, surgical management of many patients in the first few decades of the 20th century was accomplished successfully with lesser procedures. Conservative measures including tamponade, suture repair, partial splenectomy, and ligation of the splenic artery were reported by a number of surgeons.[3, 12, 13]

The evolution of surgical management of injuries to the spleen, with particular reference to conservative surgical procedures versus splenectomy, reflected a fourth major misconception held by many surgeons: the presumption that the number of complications following conservative procedures on the spleen was increasing at the same time that splenectomy was becoming increasingly safe. For these reasons, by the middle of the 20th century all reports of procedures less than total splenectomy had vanished from the literature.

Contemporary review of many early reports of conservative management of splenic injuries, however, fails to reveal an increasing number of complications following these procedures. The dictum that removal of the spleen was the procedure of choice, was clearly based on lack of evidence that the spleen could heal itself and on lack of evidence of harm to the spleen-deprived patient rather than on failure of more conservative measures.

THE SPLEEN AND INFECTION

Just when the first reference to the possible role of the spleen in resistance to infection appeared in the early literature is not clear. No doubt, enlargement of the spleen during acute specific fevers and in other conditions associated with serious infections was interpreted to indicate that the spleen might play an active part in defense against infection. Only a few experimental studies on the spleen and infection were reported during the 19th century, and those published in the early 20th century were poorly controlled and conflicting.

It was not until 1919 that the first scientifically sound exper-

imental study on the relationship of the spleen and infection
was published. The landmark report of Morris and Bullock, en-
titled "The Importance of the Spleen in Resistance to Infection," was the first clear indication that the spleen serves an
important role in host defense.[14] In a series of well-controlled
experiments in splenectomized rats infected with the rat
plague bacillus, they found significantly increased mortality in
splenectomized rats over controls.

The final conclusion of these authors was prophetic: "The
surgical bearing of these results is obvious. If, as we may reasonably infer, the physiological process of mammals are similar, it is not improbable that the human body deprived of its
spleen shows a similar increased susceptibility to infection.
Bearing this in mind, some of the fatalities following splenectomy, especially where death was attributed to infection, may
find a ready explanation and tend to increase our caution in
the removal of this organ." It is of interest, and certainly significant, that this paper was published not in a journal of bac-
teriology but in the *Annals of Surgery*.

Prominent surgeons of the time refuted the conclusions of
Morris and Bullock and agreed from their personal experience
that resistance to infection was not altered by splenectomy.[15–17] Attention to mortality, however, with little attention
to possible late results following splenectomy, is apparent in
the case reports that rapidly accumulated in the literature of
the first half of the 20th century. Mortality fell from a high of
60% reported by Connors in 1928[15] to 0% in some series[18, 19] by
the mid-1950s.

The first undisputed challenge to the long-held belief that
the spleen played no role in resistance to infection came in
1952, when King and Shumacker published a report on the increased susceptibility to infections in infants following splenectomy.[20] They reported a series of five patients who had episodes
of severe sepsis following splenectomy for congenital spherocy-
tosis. Two of the patients died. These cases prompted the authors to suggest a relationship between splenectomy and resistance to infection. They concluded their report with the
following suggestion: "It certainly makes it desirable to ana-
lyze other clinical material in order to establish or rule out the
causal relationship between the removal of the spleen in in-

fants and the serious infections we have observed to follow this procedure."

Others soon confirmed that severe infection and death in children due to fulminating sepsis did occur after splenectomy for hematologic disorders, particularly in younger children.[21-25] Several workers reported that fulminating sepsis following splenectomy for trauma had not been encountered.[21, 26-28] Because of the apparent lack of serious infections following splenectomy for trauma, Huntley proposed that patients splenectomized for disease have a lower resistance to infection not because of absence of the spleen but because of the primary disease for which the spleen was removed.[23]

The concept that serious sepsis was not associated with splenectomy for trauma was short-lived. Smith et al., just 5 years after the publication of King and Shumacker, reported the first severe infections in children following splenectomy for traumatic rupture.[25] Other reports followed, including the first report of deaths in children from overwhelming sepsis following splenectomy for trauma.[29]

Reports of adults dying from sepsis related to splenectomy for underlying disease began to appear in the literature.[30, 31] Soon thereafter, episodes of sepsis and death in adults following splenectomy for trauma were reported.[32, 33] By then it had become clear that splenectomy in otherwise healthy individuals, both children and adults, was associated with severe and often fatal sepsis.

Overwhelming Postsplenectomy Infection

The characteristic syndrome of severe sepsis seen in asplenic individuals has been termed "overwhelming postsplenectomy infection" by Diamond in a report in which, incidentally, he discounted the risk of infection after splenectomy for trauma.[34] The syndrome of overwhelming postsplenectomy infection is quite unlike fulminating bacteremias and septicemias in individuals with normal splenic function. It is a rare patient with bacteremia whose course from good health to death occurs in less than 24 hours, whereas the overwhelming postsplenectomy infection syndrome constitutes a distinct entity that often lasts only 12–18 hours.

The onset is sudden, with nausea, vomiting, headache, and confusion leading to coma. The infecting organism is *Pneumococcus* in just over one half of cases. *Meningococcus, Escherichia coli, Hemophilus influenzae, Staphylococcus,* and *Streptococcus* organisms are found with decreasing frequency. Disseminated intravascular coagulation is common. Severe hypoglycemia, electrolyte imbalance, and shock are often present. Of particular interest is the occasional presence of diplococci on peripheral blood smears. Blood culture reports in these patients indicate that there may be as many as 10^6 organisms/cu mm, which clearly separates this syndrome from the bacteremia accompanying pneumonia and other ordinary infections. At autopsy, multiorgan hemorrhage and Waterhouse-Fridericksen syndrome is seen in many cases. Rapidity of course from onset until death with failure of antibiotic therapy is characteristic. The overall mortality is 50% and is highest in pneumococcal infections, which have a mortality of 50%–80%. It is of interest that types 6, 22, and 23 pneumococci cause a much higher percentage of bacteremic sepsis in splenectomized patients than in the general population.

INCIDENCE

In 1973, Singer, in his often quoted survey of his and 23 other reported series of infection following splenectomy, attempted to establish the incidence of sepsis following splenectomy in nine categories of disease. There were 2,795 total patients in the combined series, of whom 119 (4.25%) developed sepsis and 71 (2.52%) died from it.[35] Singer asked, "Is the incidence of postsplenectomy sepsis greater than that of sepsis in the population at large?" In attempting to answer this question he reviewed a 5-year study of 1,000 families in Newcastle-upon-Tyne, in whom an incidence of meningitis and sepsis of 0.7% but no deaths were reported.

Using annual morbidity and mortality data and multiplying by 5 for 5 years and by 2 to "provide a safety factor," Singer obtained the following results:

- In infants less than 1 year old, mortality from infection occurs in 0.3% of the population born alive.
- In children aged 1–7 years, the mortality from infection is 0.07%.

- In children aged 5–14 years, the mortality from infection is 0.02%.
- In the general population, including all ages, the mortality from sepsis is 0.01%.

Singer's extrapolations from general nonmatched control groups are of course subject to error; however, in lieu of a larger prospective study that might establish the incidence of serious infection following splenectomy, his comparison has been used as a rough approximation of the hazard.

With specific reference to trauma, Singer reviewed the cases of 688 patients (388 children, 300 adults) who underwent splenectomy for injury to the spleen. Among these were 10 patients with sepsis, 4 of whom died, for a mortality of 0.58%; when combined with 4 deaths from sepsis following splenectomy for trauma in a series of 342 children reported by Eraklis and Filler, the incidence of mortality from sepsis is 0.78%, for a total of 78 times the expected rate as calculated by Singer in the general population.[36]

Francke and Neu, in a later review of the literature on postoperative infections occurring more than 8 weeks postsplenectomy, divided the case reports into those dealing with pediatric patients (less than 17 years old) and those dealing with adult patients. The data for the pediatric patients were categorized according to the reason for splenectomy. The incidence of sepsis ranged from 1.5% to 24%, with the highest incidence in patients with congenital and acquired anemias, portal hypertension, and lymphoreticular malignant tumors. The overall incidence of sepsis from all causes was 5% of 3,430 splenectomized patients. Mortality, too, was highest among patients with those underlying diseases. When both pediatric and adult data are combined, sepsis occurred in 3.9% of 4,846 patients, with a mortality of 2.4% for 5,485 patients.[37]

O'Neal and McDonald have reported on the risk of sepsis in the adult asplenic patient as determined from a review of all adults who underwent splenectomy in three hospitals of the Louisiana State University Medical Center during a 10-year period.[38] Two hundred fifty-six asplenic patients were followed for an average of 45 months. A group of 250 surgery patients who had either gastrectomy (100 patients) or choleceptectomy (150 patients) without splenectomy were followed for an average of 61 months as a control group. One hundred eighty-seven patients (74%) had splenectomy for trauma, including 59 patients that had splenectomy incidental to other surgery. Sixtynine patients (26%) had splenectomy in association with other disease. There were seven deaths. Splenectomy was performed in four patients for trauma incidental to other surgery. Two patients had direct extension of cancer from an adjacent organ, and one patient underwent splenectomy as a staging procedure for Hodgkin's disease. The interval between splenectomy and the onset of sepsis ranged between 1 and 72 months. The organisms isolated included *Pneumococcus* in two patients, *Pseudomonas* in two patients, *Staphylococcus* alone in one patient and *Staphylococcus* plus *Escherichia* in one patient. The overall incidence of lethal sepsis was 2.7%. In the control group there were no cases of septicemia.

O'Neal and McDonald quote the annual incidence of death due to sepsis in all ages of the general population of the south central United States as 12.8 per 100,000 people, or .001%. Although admittedly subject to error, a rough approximation of the risk of lethal sepsis in the group of asplenic patients was 540 times greater than for the population at large. The four patients who underwent splenectomy with no underlying disease and succumbed to lethal sepsis represent an incidence of 2.2% in this group.

Singer also included patients with splenectomy incidental to other surgical operations in his survey of the literature prior to 1973. His reports included 43 children and 190 adults. The indications for operations are not clearly stated but consisted of gastrectomy for ulcer and hiatal hernia repair in many cases. Five of the 233 patients (2.1%) had severe sepsis, and two patients (.86%) died. Using Singer's estimations of annual morbidity and mortality from sepsis in the general population (0.1%), these figures represent an 86-fold increase over that of the general population for patients in this category.

Standage and Goss included 107 patients with incidental splenectomy in their report on 277 adult patients who underwent splenectomy. The incidental group included patients that had gastrectomy (47.7%) and colon procedures, primarily left colectomy (16.8%). Pancreatectomy was the primary operation in 13.1%, hiatal hernia repair in 12.2%, left nephrectomy in 3.7%, and miscellaneous operations in 11.3%. One patient in this group died of pneumococcal sepsis 11 months after a left hemicolectomy and incidental splenectomy (0.96%).[39]

Gopal and Bisno reported fulminant pneumococcal infections in "normal" asplenic hosts. Twenty of a total of 25 patients had undergone splenectomy. Seventeen patients were splenectomized for trauma and three patients underwent splenectomy during operations for benign disease. The other five patients had "splenic atrophy," congenital asplenia, or remote splenic infection.[40] Of the 25 subjects, 13 (52%) were over 20 years old at the time of their infection (mean age, 27.7 years). The average interval between splenectomy and infection was 5.6 years. Six episodes of infection occurred 10 or more years following splenectomy. The case fatality rate among postsplenectomy patients was 71%. Serotyping of the infecting pneumococci was available in eight patients. Half of the isolates belonged to type 12. Since this type generally accounts for less than 10% of blood isolates of pneumococci, the possible significance of this finding is intriguing.

Since the study by Gopal and Bisno appeared, additional cases of overwhelming postsplenectomy pneumococcal septicemia in patients without underlying disease continue to be reported. Oakes described 14 additional patients with overwhelming well-documented postsplenectomy pneumococcal septicemia. Thirteen patients underwent splenectomy for trauma and one patient had splenectomy incidental to surgery for peptic ulcer disease.[41] Age at splenectomy ranged from 4 to 46 years (average, 16.4 years). Nine of the 14 patients were over 15 years of age at the time of splenic injury. The onset of sepsis occurred between 6 months and 31 years after splenectomy (average, 8.1 years). Nine patients developed sepsis 5 or more years after splenectomy. Mortality was 93%.

Other case reports continue to accumulate[42, 43]; undoubtedly some cases have gone unrecognized.

Schwartz et al., in a study of postsplenectomy sepsis and mortality in 193 adults who underwent splenectomy in Rochester, Minnesota from 1955 to 1979,[44] list a number of valid reasons why the reviews of Singer and Eraklis may not reflect the true incidence of fulminant sepsis after splenectomy in the general population. Their study is important since the data were derived by applying actuarial methods to a population free of selection bias and for which nearly complete follow-up data were available. The mean age of the patients in this series was 46 years. Only two patients had documented fulminant sepsis during the 1,090 person-years of follow-up (0.18 cases per 100 person-years) in this unselected population. One patient, a 24-year-old woman with recurrent Hodgkin's disease who was receiving radiation and cytotoxic therapy, died of a fulminant gram-negative bacillary bacteremia. The other patient, who survived, was a 20-year-old woman who had undergone splenectomy for trauma 17 months earlier, after which she had received pneumococcal vaccine. She recovered from a *Nisseria meningitidis* bacteremia. Mortality from fulminant sepsis following splenectomy was 0.9 per 1,000 person-years of follow-up. The incidence of any type of serious infection in these patients was estimated at 7.16 infections per 100 person-years of follow-up (78 cases). The incidence of infections was significantly increased among patients undergoing incidental splenectomy in conjunction with abdominal operations for malignant neoplasms or other conditions. Immunosupression, radiation, and chemotherapy also significantly increased the risk of subsequent infection. Based on this study, the authors conclude "that fulminant sepsis after splenectomy is indeed a potential problem, but that the risk in the general adult population is very low."

It is clear that the true incidence of overwhelming postsplenectomy infection cannot be calculated with any great accuracy.

There are many unanswered questions on the fascinating problem of overwhelming postsplenectomy sepsis. It is estimated that 35–40,000 patients undergo splenectomy each year in the United States, yet only a small number of people for variable periods after splenectomy are subject to the syndrome. Is there, as suggested by Baue, some unique abnormality in these people?[45]

Regardless of the controversy surrounding the entire subject of postsplenectomy infection, there is no doubt that a small number of patients who have undergone splenectomy for trauma are at indefinite risk of a characteristic, highly lethal septic syndrome. At present it is not possible to identify which postsplenectomy patients are possible candidates for this disaster.

Splenic Structure

The postsplenectomy sepsis syndrome has generated renewed interest in the structure and functions of the spleen. Phylogenetically, the thymus and the spleen are the earliest elements of the lymphoreticular system to appear. As specialization progresses in phylogeny, the spleen becomes more and more specialized as a tissue in its relationship to the circulation. Ontogenetically, the spleen begins in humans as a collection of mesenchymal cells in the dorsal mesogastrium at the beginning of the sixth week. It becomes evident as an organ by the beginning of the third month and assumes its final position in the left upper quadrant in relation to the stomach and other organs by the fourth month of fetal life. At birth it is larger in relationship to body weight than at any other time during life. It increases in weight during the first year of life by 300%–400%, exceeding the rate of growth of all other organs in this respect. At birth very few primitive lymphoid follicles, and no germinal centers, are present. By age 1, the white pulp is highly developed, with many lymphoid follicles and germinal centers. At this stage the maturation of the spleen, as expressed in its morphological elements, is apparently complete

The splenic artery, which delivers 4% of the circulating blood volume per minute, divides in the hilum into trabecular branches that enter the spleen surrounded by the white pulp, where they are known as central arteries. At this point the arteries are surrounded by collections of lymphocytes, plasma cells, and fixed macrophages. Leaving the white pulp, the blood passes through an ill-defined vascular space called the marginal zone prior to entering the venous sinuses of the red pulp. There is considerable controversy over the details of the microcirculation of this region, but under normal circumstances most of the perfusing blood flows into the sinusoid of the red pulp; from there, at a slow flow rate, it sloshes around a reticulum comprised of a variety of lymphoreticular cells, including a transient population of large and small lymphocytes, plasma cells in addition to fixed cells, and transient macrophages and histiocytes. It is here that phagocytes engulf effete elements of the blood, bacteria, and other particulate material. Blood from the sinusoids ultimately collects in the splenic vein, which returns the blood into the portal system.

The anatomical arrangement of the spleen provides for the interaction of immunologically competent tissue with elements introduced via the blood in addition to a slow sinusoidal circulation through a bed of macrophages capable of clearing elements recognized as foreign.

Early in the 19th century experimental studies dealing with the segmental nature of distribution of the central blood supply of the spleen began to be reported. In 1802, Assolant showed that in dogs, ligation of a branch of the terminal division of the splenic artery produced necrosis of the portion of the spleen supplied by the ligated branch.[46] Funaioli, in 1901, published a description of partial splenectomy and splenic hemostasis in dogs using segmental arterial ligation.[47] He proposed the application of these techniques to man.

The segmental distribution of the parenchymal branches of the splenic artery is responsible for the more commonly encountered types of splenic injuries following blunt adbominal trauma. Most injuries result in transverse ruptures of the spleen following the trabeculae and segmental blood supply. They include incomplete transverse rents of the spleen not involving the hilus (Fig 1), rents that may extend to the hilus without dividing it (Fig 2), and more extensive rents that involve not only the hilus but tear the hilar vessels as well (Fig 3). The friability of the spleen, despite the segmental trabecu-

Fig 1 (left).—Incomplete transverse rent in the direction of the segmental artery.

Fig 2 (right).—Incomplete transverse rent along a segmental artery extending to the hilus.

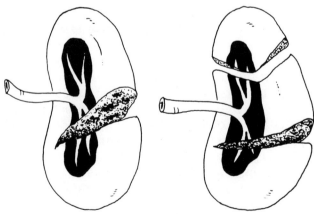

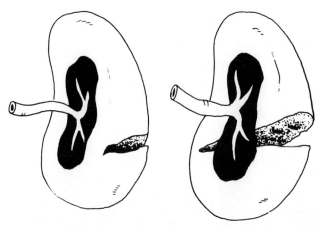

Fig 3 (left).—Transverse rent into the hilus dividing the vessels to the lower pole.
Fig 4 (right).—Complete fragmentation of the spleen not following segmental planes.

lar arrangement of the parenchymal arterial branches, is responsible for other types of injury, including complete fragmentation of the spleen (Fig 4).

Splenic Function

The functions of the spleen have captivated the imaginations of historians and physicians since ancient times. The Babylonian *Talmud* (second to sixth centuries) propagated the belief that the spleen produced laughter, a concept that continued to appear in ancient Jewish writings. Judah Halevi (1086–1145) prophetically related: "The spleen is called laughing because of its nature to cleanse the blood and spirit from unclean and obscuring matter." By the mid-12th century, Maimonides, in his *Aphorisms of Moses,* no longer attributed laughter to the spleen but reemphasized, correctly, its blood-purifying properties.[48]

More modern studies of splenic function have demonstrated that the spleen serves a distinct role in host defense mechanisms by removal of particulate matter by phagocytosis. The phagocytic functions of the spleen are dependent on both cellular and humoral mechanisms. In addition, the spleen is a site of antibody production. The optimal function of the splenic macrophage system in removing particulate matter (especially encapsulated bacteria) depends on the prior elaboration of specific antibodies to facilitate phagocytosis.[49]

PHAGOCYTOSIS

In the normal host the reticuloendothelial cells of the liver, as well as those of the spleen, share in the clearance from the bloodstream of such foreign elements as bacteria and old or imperfect cellular elements. The optimal function of the macrophage system is dependent on opsonizing antibody. When such opsonins are present, the liver becomes an important clearance site, yet it is still less active than the spleen on a weight for weight basis. When these opsonizing proteins are absent, pneumococci in the blood are cleared primarily through the spleen rather than the liver. Accordingly, in the nonimmune host, the spleen is of major importance in processing certain foreign materials.[50]

In addition to the cellular phagocytic function, the spleen is the site of production of a humoral substance that stimulates phagocytosis. Najjar et al., in 1970, reported identifying leukokinin, a specific cell-bound leukophilic γ-globulin fraction essential for maximal stimulation of phagocytic activity of the blood neutrophiles and macrophages in man.[51] The entire stimulatory effect of this substance is due to a single peptide fragment named tuftsin, after Tufts University, where it was discovered. Production of tuftsin occurs exclusively in the spleen. The mechanism by which tuftsin is delivered to the cell after manufacture in the spleen is intriguing. The tuftsin fragment is cleaved from the parent leukophilic γ-globulin (leukokinin) molecule by an enzyme (leukokinase) produced by neutrophil cell membrane. The remnant γ-globulin molecule is returned to the spleen where a replacement tuftsin molecule is added.

Tuftsin, in addition to augmenting the phagocytic activity of both blood neutrophiles and tissue macrophages, stimulates the bactericidal capability of polymorphonuclear leukocytes. These effects result in increased clearing of bacteria from the circulation and considerable diminution of the bacterial population of the host.[52]

Antibody Production

Although the spleen has been shown to have a special phagocytic function in the absence of antibody, it has also been shown to be a major source of early-appearing antibody when particulate antigen is presented by the intravenous route.

Rowley demonstrated that when a dose of particulate antigen is both small and presented by the intravenous route, splenectomized humans respond with insignificant amounts of antibody, compared to controls.[53] When splenectomized rats were given a dose of antigen by an other than intravenous route, antibody titers were the same as in control animals, establishing that the spleen appears necessary for a normal primary response to some intravenously administered antigens.

A number of other immunologic studies have been carried out in man in an attempt to corroborate findings in experimental animals. There have been studies on antibody levels, response to pneumococcal antigens, complement function, phagocyte function, and cellular immunity in splenectomized patients.

Immunoglobulin levels after splenectomy have been studied in different age groups and depend in part on the time after splenectomy when they are measured. Maturation of splenic follicles that produce antibody is not complete for a year or more after birth, although newborn infants produce IgM for months. Production of IgG starts sometime between age 16 days and after 1 year. Therefore, 15%–20% or more of children under 1 year of age have no measurable opsonic IgM against pneumococci, among other organisms. In older children and adults, IgM levels usually fall after splenectomy to levels significantly below preoperative levels. The decrease in IgM lasts more than 1 year. IgA levels increase continually postoperatively for about 3 years before leveling off. IgG levels remain constant or increase after splenectomy.[37]

Since IgM is the first species of immunoglobulin produced after primary exposure to an antigen, its reduction following splenectomy may be related to the failure of primary response to intravenous antigen that has been demonstrated.

Studies of the alternative complement pathway have revealed deficits after splenectomy. Since a high concentration of pneumococci ($> 10^6$ organisms/ml) may activate this pathway even in the absence of antibody, complement may contribute to mortality in overwhelming postsplenectomy infection.

The evidence of the immunologic role of the spleen discussed above provides an explanation of overwhelming postsplenectomy infection. When the spleen encounters relatively few blood-borne pneumococcal organisms, it effectively and rapidly mobilizes an immune response. The spleen initiates rapid specific antibody synthesis and releases the antibody in high local concentration into the slow-moving capillary bed, where efficient phagocytosis occurs. The way is thus prepared to deal effectively with the subsequent phases of the bacteremia that determine the outcome of infection.

Without a spleen the patient, deprived of an organ capable of recognizing both small doses of particulate antigen and of phagocytosis in the absence of antibody, would not react to the small antigenic challenge presented by the few organisms in the circulation in the early bacteremic episode. Since the liver is relatively inefficient in phagocytosis of pneumococci in the absence of antibody, increasing numbers of organisms would circulate freely. Rapidly fulminating pneumococcal sepsis would ensue. Oakes concludes his lucid discussion of the pathophysiology of overwhelming postsplenectomy infection: "Since 'natural antibody' appears only gradually during the first year or two of life, one would predict an increased incidence of overwhelming sepsis in asplenic infants and young children. A previously unencountered type of encapsulated bacteria could enter the circulation at any time, however, and thus account for the occurrence of fulminating postsplenectomy sepsis at any age."[41]

Splenic Salvage

Although the incidence of overwhelming sepsis following splenectomy for trauma is apparently low, the consequences are so devastating that a number of measures to reduce or eliminate this complication have been employed. In the past 10 years a large volume of evidence has accumulated supporting the fact that the spleen can heal itself both spontaneously and following surgical repair.

Nonoperative Management

Douglas and Simpson, in 1971, reported on a series of 16 children with strongly suspected splenic injury on clinical grounds who were managed without operative intervention.[54] Their interest in nonoperative management was sparked by an autopsy observation of a child with a completely healed total transection of the spleen from an injury in the past.

Successful nonoperative management was contingent on development of precise techniques for diagnosis and continued evaluation of the course of traumatic lesions of the spleen. Confirmation of the reliability of peritoneal lavage for establishing the presence of hemoperitoneum and utilization of radioisotope scanning for diagnosis and follow-up have permitted the successful nonoperative management of large numbers of carefully selected adult and pediatric patients.[55-57]

Collective experience with nonoperative management indicates that patients with isolated splenic injury who are hemodynamically stable and are in an appropriate hospital setting for close observation can be satisfactorily managed without laparotomy.

It has been our practice to admit adult candidates for nonoperative management of splenic injury to the surgical intensive care unit for 48–72 hours of bed rest and observation. Replacement of initial blood loss of up to 2 units over the first few hours after injury may be required. Vigorous respiratory therapy is avoided unless it is absolutely necessary. Continued evidence of blood loss is followed by surgical exploration. Patients who remain stable after initial resuscitation are kept in the hospital with limited activity for 7–10 days. After discharge, patients may not undertake vigorous physical activity but may return to nonstrenuous daily routines. Follow-up spleen scans at monthly intervals usually indicate either resorption of a subcapsular hematoma or healing of a splenic rent within 3 months after injury.

Children who remain stable following splenic injury are managed in the surgical intensive care unit similarly to adults. Total hospitalization, however, is usually 2–3 weeks since restriction of activity of younger children after discharge may be more difficult than for adults.[58]

As the number of patients treated without operative intervention continues to grow, we must ask ourselves what the possible complications are that may be produced by this method of management and whether such complications are more frequent than or as serious as the risk of postsplenectomy sepsis.

The risk of a missed intra-abdominal injury associated with an injured spleen is always possible when nonoperative management is elected. Close observation and utilization of arteriography, radioisotopic scans, computerized tomography, and other sophisticated diagnostic modalities, where indicated, make the possibility of a missed serious concomitant abdominal injury highly unlikely.

The possibility of delayed rupture of the spleen following nonoperative management of patients with splenic injury is a major objection of a number of surgeons who advocate laparotomy for all patients with splenic injury. It is most interesting that to date, no patients who have been managed without operative intervention, as outlined above, and who have been followed by splenic scans, have been reported to have delayed rupture of the spleen.

Since the first report in 1866 of a sudden splenic bleed some time after injury, the entity of delayed rupture of the spleen has been the subject of numerous reports.[55, 59] There is no question that delayed rupture of the spleen has been clearly identified in the older literature as a real risk, but it must be remembered that most of these patients were described before definitive diagnostic procedures for identification of splenic injury were available. Furthermore, these patients did not have the close observation and in-hospital management currently prescribed.

Development of posttraumatic cysts of the spleen is another possible complication of nonoperative management of splenic injury. Although a history of trauma was present in 23% of 137 nonparasitic cysts reviewed in the world's literature, that represents a very small number of reported cases.[60] It may be anticipated that nonoperative management will be responsible for an increased number of posttraumatic splenic cysts, but the consequences of an increased incidence of this entity remain to be seen.

Splenosis following splenectomy for trauma was found to be

present in half of the patients studied by Pearson et al.[61] It is possible that nonoperative management of patients with splenic injury might produce an even higher incidence of autotransplantation of splenic tissue than in patients with removal of a ruptured spleen; however, experimental observation documents that splenectomy is a powerful growth stimulus to autografted splenic tissue.[62] With the spleen in place, autotransplanted splenic tissue may not grow significantly in man.

Trimble and Eason reviewed 54 reported cases of splenosis and added one of their own in a review of the literature.[63] Forty-eight patients had splenosis after splenectomy for trauma, three had had splenectomy for medical reasons, and four had not had splenectomy, although splenic trauma may have previously occurred. Morbidity related directly to splenosis consisted largely of intestinal obstruction. Of the 17 patients operated on for this complication, at least six had obstruction directly attributed to adhesion or a bowel kink originating at an autotransplanted nodule. Of the 14 patients that had exploratory laparotomy, most were operated on for vague abdominal complaints possibly caused by splenosis. Of the six patients whose diagnosis of splenosis was made at emergency appendectomy, the pathology of acute appendicitis was not evident in most.

These few cases of complications from splenosis, in light of the fact that splenosis is clearly more common following splenectomy for trauma than was previously thought, do not contraindicate nonoperative management of splenic injury.

A high index of suspicion of splenosis followed by radioisotope scanning of patients presenting with intestinal obstruction and a history of splenectomy for trauma or of nonoperative management of splenic injury should quickly identify these patients and suggest the appropriate diagnosis.

Evidence that many patients already have accidental posttraumatic autotransplantation of splenic tissue without an apparent high incidence of complications would seem to make the risk of little consequence.

There may be other, as yet unrecognized complications in addition to those already discussed. Nevertheless, the risk of overwhelming postsplenectomy infection, with its high mortality, appears to outweigh the possible complications of nonoperative management presently identified.

Splenorrhaphy or Partial Resection

Reports of surgical procedures less than total splenectomy in the management of patients with splenic injury have appeared in the literature since the 16th century. Rosetti, in 1590, described a successful partial splenectomy in a patient presenting with evisceration of a portion of the spleen through a wound in the left side.[55] Reports of successful suture repair began to appear in the surgical literature in the late 19th century. Berger collected reports of 14 patients who were treated by suture of splenic wounds prior to 1900. There were only two deaths among these patients.[2] Sporadic reports of successful management of splenic injuries by suture continued to appear in the literature, but it was not until 1930 that modern surgeons rediscovered that lesser procedures than splenectomy could suffice. Dretzka reported a series of 27 patients with rupture of the spleen.[64] Three of them were treated by suture of the spleen; all survived. Included among these is the first reported instance of an extensive laceration of the spleen in a child successfully treated by mattress suture. In his concluding remarks, Dretzka established principles for successful splenorraphy, to which little has been added since then: "A suture of the organ cannot be done unless the incision is ample. A rent in the capsule may be conveniently treated by a mattress suture and this is also true of a puncture or stab wound. Catgut is preferable to the nonabsorbable material. The suture must be inserted with gentleness and tied with caution. No case of secondary hemorrhage was encountered in this series" (Fig 5).[64]

Dretzka's report and a similar one by Mazel in 1945 were largely ignored because the concept of low mortality and absent sequelae associated with splenectomy for trauma was the standard of the time.[65]

The first report of successful partial splenectomy in modern times was a publication in 1962 by Christo.[66] After treating experimental segmental splenectomy in animals, he applied his techniques to eight patients with splenic injuries. Six patients had penetrating injuries, four from gunshot wounds and two from knife wounds. Two patients had blunt injuries received in automobile accidents. The splenic pedicle was approached through the gastrosplenic ligament. The vessels in the hilus of the spleen supplying the injured portion of the spleen were li-

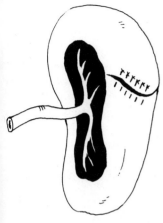

Fig 5.—Interrupted catgut vertical mattress sutures for repair of simple rents.

gated. Demarcation of the devascularized segment was apparent, allowing accurate segmental resection of the injured tissue. Bleeding from the cut surface was controlled by ligation of the individual bleeding points and by application of Gelfoam or omentum. One patient died 30 days postoperatively following drainage of a subphrenic abscess secondary to a gastric perforation sustained with the original wounds. No late complications were observed. Christo concluded his report: "partial systematized splenectomy can be adapted to every traumatic lesion of the spleen limited to one defined vascular segment."

Following the well-documented report of Christo, others began to revive the usefulness of splenic suture and splenorrhaphy for patients with splenic injury. Trauma surgeons, finally convinced that the spleen could heal itself spontaneously or after suture repair, developed operative approaches and additional operative techniques for managing injuries to the spleen.

LaMura et al., in 1974, reported treating an 18-month-old child with a longitudinal rupture of the spleen after a fall from a building. Repair with 3-0 catgut simple sutures led to successful splenic salvage.[67] Mishalany reported successful splenic salvage in 1974, utilizing through-and-through 3-0 chromic catgut sutures followed by simple fine catgut sutures in the capsule, some of which incorporated a pedicle of omentum over the injury site (Fig 6).

Morgenstern, in 1974, described the use of microfibrillar collagen (Avitene) as a hemostatic agent in a patient with a capsular alvusion injury of the lower pole of the spleen during gastric surgery (Fig 7).[68] Morgenstern continued to use microfibrillar collagen in patients with splenic injury and in 1977 described an additional 15 patients in whom successful hemostasis of splenic injuries had been achieved with that agent.[69] His report confirmed the usefulness of Avitene, which is particularly well suited for control of bleeding from the injured surface of the spleen because of its ability to adhere to wet surfaces.

Ratner et al., in 1977, reported successful surgical salvage of the spleen in 15 patients. They used large chromic catgut sutures placed as simple figure-of-eight sutures. No complications were observed secondary to splenic repair.[70]

In the same year Burrington described eight patients who were managed by splenic salvage techniques, including partial splenectomy. His technique entailed placing mattress sutures of 0-0 or 2-0 chromic catgut to compress the raw surface. An omental pedicle was added to reinforce the suture line (Fig 8).[71]

Following these reports, experience with increasing numbers of patients with splenic injury managed by suture repair and partial splenectomy provided the necessary essentials of tech-

Fig 6 (left).—Through-and-through 3-0 catgut in addition to fine catgut sutures to the capsule over an omental pedicle.

Fig 7 (center).—Hemostasis by microfibrillar collagen of a common iatrogenic lower pole capsular avulsion.

Fig 8 (right).—Catgut mattress sutures for compression of raw surfaces with an omental pedicle reinforcement. The pedicle is not essential.

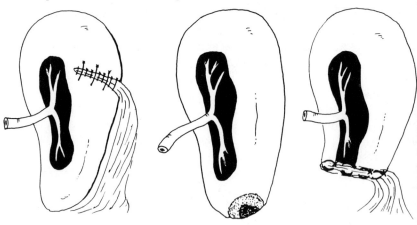

nique and methods for successful splenic surgery. Morgenstern
and Shapiro, in 1979, outlined techniques of splenic conservation, emphasizing the important points in management.[72] The
abdominal incision must permit easy access to the spleen for
adequate mobilization. Capsular avulsion injuries must be
avoided during mobilization of the spleen onto the anterior abdominal wall. Avoiding capsular injuries requires identifying
and ligating the peritoneal folds that may arise from the
greater omentum, parietal peritoneum, splenic flexure of the
colon, gastrosplenic omentum, or the diaphragm. The posterior
parietal peritoneum should be incised parallel to the entire
length of the spleen. Gentle blunt dissection of the spleen and
pancreas is satisfactory for mobilization. Control of the splenic
artery in its course above the pancreas should be achieved
when time permits under controlled conditions. Identification
of hilar divisions of the splenic artery should be carried out
when indicated. Control of parenchymatous bleeding during
splenic resection is afforded by temporary occlusion of the
splenic artery. Intraparenchymal splenic vessels should be in-
dividually ligated or clipped. Through-and-through 2-0 catgut
sutures are adequate for hemostasis. Raw surfaces should be
managed with microfibrillar collagen.

Following these principles of management, several hundred
reported patients have been managed by partial splenectomy or surgical repair of the spleen. Many more patients
whose cases have never been reported have been similarly managed.

Ligation of the splenic artery as a method for control of parenchymal hemorrhage was reported as early as 1903[55] but
generated little enthusiasm, although it was apparently a useful procedure. Modern surgeons have achieved control of hemorrhage from the splenic hilus that could otherwise have not
been successfully repaired.[73] Splenic artery ligation in combination with splenorraphy has also been reported.[74] Postoperative spleen scans show uptake in the spleen in both of these
reports.

Reoperation for continued or delayed bleeding following suture repair or splenorrhaphy is infrequent. Strauch cites one
patient who required splenectomy following partial splenectomy from among 277 patients reviewed.[75] Oakes described one
patient in a series of 20 patients that had splenic repair who

required reoperation on the sixth postoperative day for extensive areas of subcapsular and intraparenchymal hemorrhage.[41] The original injury to the spleen was thought to be only moderately severe, with no evidence of hilar involvement.

Traub and Perry,[76] in their report of 41 patients who underwent splenic preservation, noted that one patient had to return to the operating room for control of bleeding from a hilar laceration of the spleen missed at the time of original exploratory laparotomy. They cite the case of another patient, reported elsewhere, with failure of splenic repair. They conclude their report: "Early complications are, as in the present study, equal to or less than those found following splenectomy. The technique is safe and is as applicable to adults as to children. But most important, a policy of operation to access splenic injury offers the surgeon the opportunity to evaluate and treat associated intra-abdominal injuries. Convalescence is shortened, and therefore hospital costs are minimized. The spleens that undergo repair are not at increased risk to future injury, but undergo healing with preservation of viable tissue that appears, by present standards, to be adequate to perform the functions of the spleen."

Regardless of the clear evidence that splenic preservation procedures are safe and probably effective in preserving splenic function, there will always be patients who require total splenectomy. The primary indications for splenectomy after traumatic rupture are total avulsion or extensive fragmentation of the spleen, severe associated injuries requiring prompt attention, and continued bleeding after attempted splenic repair. In patients with multiple intra-abdominal injuries or extensive peritoneal contamination from visceral perforation, it is good surgical judgment to weigh the benefits of splenic salvage against the safer course of splenectomy.

Protection Against Overwhelming Postsplenectomy Infection

There are currently three possible avenues for protecting patients that have undergone splenectomy from overwhelming postsplenectomy infection. These are deliberate splenic autotransplantation, antibiotic prophylaxis, and immunization with polyvalent pneumococcal vaccine.

DELIBERATE AUTOTRANSPLANTATION

The deliberate autotransplantation of portions of the spleen as possible protection against overwhelming postsplenectomy sepsis has been the object of great interest since Pearson et al., in 1978, proposed that accidental autotransplantation (splenosis) following traumatic rupture of the spleen could provide normal splenic functions.[61] In an effort to explain the reduced incidence of postsplenectomy sepsis following splenectomy for trauma as compared to splenectomy for hematologic-oncologic diseases, they measured "pitted" red blood cells (RBCs) in the circulating blood as an index of splenic function. RBC membrane abnormalities ("pits") can be recognized in hyposplenic persons by means of interference phase microscopy. The percentage of pitted RBCs was significantly lower in children splenectomized for trauma than for other indications. [99m]Tc sulfer colloid scans confirmed the presence of aberrant splenic tissue in five patients with a lower percentage of pitted cells. Moncada has shown by ^{99m}Tc sulfer colloid scans that 11 of 21 patients studied after splenectomy for trauma had evidence of accidental autotransplantation of splenic tissue.[55]

Experimental evidence demonstrates that autotransplanted splenic tissue placed within the peritoneal cavity of rats will grow. Although these implants restore ability to form antibody, raise leukophilic γ-globulin levels, remove RBC imperfections, and take up injected radiocolloid, their ability to protect against pneumococcal challenge is in question.[77]

Clinical reports of overwhelming sepsis in splenectomized patients with remaining accessory spleens or splenosis discovered at autopsy raise questions about the ability of autotransplanted splenic tissue to deter overwhelming sepsis.[41, 55]

Experimental studies of the function of the replanted spleen in animals have been reported extensively by many investigators, but there are conflicting findings of the ability of autotransplanted splenic tissue to protect against or to ameliorate overwhelming sepsis in the experimental animal. Although there are conflicting findings on whether the replanted spleen functions adequately, most investigators in the past few years have identified a protective function of autotransplanted splenic tissue against bacterial challenge.[78–83] Others have reported that autotransplanted splenic tissue offers no protection against bacterial challenge.[84, 85] The difference in findings in experimental animals is related to various factors: the different types of animals used, the size and location of autotransplanted splenic segments, the vascular supply and venous drainage of the autotransplants, the bacteria used to challenge the experimental animals, and the dose and route of entry of the challenge.

A number of surgeons believe that deliberate splenic autotransplantation provides a logical and simple alternative for preserving some splenic function.[86, 87]

Suggested technical procedures for splenic reimplantation include use of thin splenic slices (3 mm thick) from the central portion of the spleen, implantation of two or three cross-section slices side by side into a pocket of omentum made by folding the omentum back upon itself, and careful search for and removal of splenic fragments from the peritoneal cavity.

Thin slices of spleen increase the ability of the transplant to vascularize. Placement of the transplant into omental pouches permits venous drainage of the splenic tissue into the portal system, which is apparently important and should prevent the complication of bowel obstruction seen in patients with peritoneal implants.

Antibiotic Prophylaxis

Antibiotic prophylaxis with 250 mg of oral penicillin, once or twice daily, or depot penicillin injections on a monthly basis, would seem to be an attractive option, and this regimen is recommended by many physicians. There are, however, a number of disadvantages. Chief among these are the problems of compliance and inadequate dosage. Patient compliance, especially with long-term antibiotic prophylaxis programs (rheumatic fever), has been disappointing. Case reports of postsplenectomy sepsis due to penicillin-sensitive organisms in patients purporting to be on prophylactic penicillin are disturbing.[88] The emergence of penicillin-resistant as well as erythromycin-resistant and clindamycin-resistant strains of not only pneumococci but also *H. influenzae* is an additional problem with antibiotic prophylaxis.[89, 90] The reliability of antibiotic prophylaxis is further compromised by the fact that a number of penicillin-resistant organisms may produce the syndrome of overwhelming postsplenectomy infection. Finally, the possibility of inducing penicillin-resistant strains of pneumococci in patients on long-term prophylactic regimens cannot be ruled out.

Because there are no controlled studies to validate the efficacy of prophylactic administration of penicillin in preventing postsplenectomy sepsis, and because patients may have a false sense of security while taking antibiotics, alternatives such as those recommended by Pearson are worthy of serious consideration.[91]

For children, Pearson recommends that parents bring the child to the hospital emergency room whenever an illness is associated with a temperature of 102 F or more. A loading dose of penicillin is given intravenously, followed by appropriate evaluation. A temperature of 102 F as an indication for a trip to the emergency room is admittedly arbitrary, but postsplenectomy sepsis is usually accompanied by elevations of temperature as high as 104 F.

Because, as far as can be determined, splenectomized patients are at risk for postsplenectomy sepsis for their lifetime, older children and adults must be impressed with the importance of immediate medical attention whenever an illness with significant fever or toxicity occurs.

Vaccine Prophylaxis

A safe, licensed vaccine for the prevention of infection caused by 14 of the serotypes most often responsible for bacteremic infection with *Streptococcus pneumoniae* is available. The vaccine has been shown to be well tolerated and offers great promise for effective control of illness caused by pneumococci in normal individuals. Sullivan et al. reported significant seroconversions in response to pneumococcal polysaccharide antigens in asplenic patients (excluding those with Hodgkin's disease) and concluded: "Since the majority of cases of overwhelming postsplenectomy infections are caused by *Streptococcus pneumoniae* all patients with either anatomical or functional asplenia should receive pneumococcal polysaccharide vaccine."[92]

Unfortunately, pneumococcal vaccine cannot be relied on for protection in a number of clinical situations. The antigens for the 14 serotypes contained in the vaccine account for about

85% of pneumococcal infections encountered in the United States. This, of course, leaves the patient unprotected from 15% of pneumococcal pathogens. Even if the vaccine were 100% effective, the pneumococcus accounts for just over one half of reported cases of overwhelming postsplenectomy infection, leaving the remaining patients at risk for the many other organisms incriminated in postsplenectomy sepsis.

Soon after introduction of the vaccine, reports of failure began to appear.[93] Especially important is the report by Applebaum et al. of a 6-year-old boy who developed fatal pneumococcal sepsis following splenectomy for trauma despite prophylactic vaccination.[94] All vaccines have failures, which is not surprising, considering that susceptibility to pneumococcal disease depends on the levels of antibody classes for specific serotypes, the particular serotypes involved, and the underlying illness of the host, among other factors.

Another limitation of the vaccine is that it is variably effective in children under 2 years of age, whose immune response to encapsulated bacteria is immature.

All patients with splenectomy for trauma should receive polyvalent pneumococcal vaccine. As suggested by Oakes, patients who have sustained major splenic injury, even if splenorraphy has been successfully performed, should be immunized as well, as the long-term ability of such spleens to protect against pneumococcal sepsis has not been established.[41] The duration of protection induced by vaccination is unknown, with currently available data showing elevation of titers 3–5 years after immunization. Because of marked increase in adverse reactions with reinjection of pneumococcal vaccine, second or "booster" doses should not be given, at least at this time.[95]

Since adequate antibody titers require 2–3 weeks to develop, prophylactic penicillin, or erythromycin in patients allergic to penicillin, should be administered for 2–4 weeks after vaccination. Because of the variable response to pneumococcal vaccine in children under the age of 2, antibiotic prophylaxis is indicated in addition to immunization in this age group.

Summary

1. Throughout history, until quite recently, surgeons based the management of trauma to the spleen on four major miscon-

ceptions concerning the function and structure of the spleen: A. The spleen served no useful function in man and could be sacrificed with impunity. B. The spleen cannot heal itself and therefore cannot be left in place. C. An injured spleen, if left in place, will be subject to "delayed rupture" and subsequent fatal hemorrhage. D. Attempts to suture or repair an injured spleen lead to many complications.

2. Beginning with the 1919 report that the spleen protected against infection in experimental animals, and later in the 1952 clinical report of deaths from infection in infants following splenectomy, the syndrome of postsplenectomy infection has been elucidated.

3. The overwhelming postsplenectomy infection syndrome is characterized by rapid onset, a fulminating course, massive bacteremia, and a frequently fatal outcome despite vigorous treatment. The syndrome is most often produced by the pneumococcus but *Meningococcus, E. coli, H. influenzae, Staphylococcus,* and *Streptococcus* organisms are also found, in order of decreasing frequency. At autopsy multiorgan hemorrhage and Waterhouse-Fridericksen syndrome is seen in many cases.

4. The exact incidence of overwhelming postsplenectomy infection is unknown, but it is in the neighborhood of 0.5%–0.78%, which is considerably higher than the incidence in the general population (0.01%). Children with splenectomy for hemato-oncologic indications are at highest risk. Postsplenectomy sepsis can occur many years after splenectomy. The small number of reported cases of overwhelming postsplenectomy infection in light of the large number of splenectomies performed each year (35,000–40,000) suggests the possibility of some unique abnormality among these individuals.

5. The anatomical arrangement of the spleen permits the interaction of immunologically competent tissue with elements introduced via the bloodstream in addition to a slow sinusoidal circulation through a bed of macrophages capable of clearing elements recognized as foreign. The segmental distribution of the parenchymal branches of the splenic artery is responsible for fractures of the spleen along segmental planes.

6. The role of the spleen in host defense mechanisms includes the removal of particulate matter by phagocytosis by both cellular and humoral mechanisms and the production of antibodies and of proteins that activate the alternative pathway of

complement. Overwhelming postsplenectomy infection occurs in patients who have been deprived of an organ capable both of recognizing particulate antigens and of phagocytosis in the absence of antibody. Since the liver is relatively inefficient in phagocytosis of pneumococci, in the absence of antibody, increasing numbers of organisms circulate freely, leading to fulminating pneumococcal sepsis.

6. Verification that the spleen can heal spontaneously as well as after suture repair and partial resection has allowed increasing numbers of patients with splenic injuries to be managed without surgical intervention—by splenorraphy or by partial resection of the spleen.

7. To date there is little evidence to suggest that nonoperative intervention for patients with injury to the spleen will result in significant complications. Complications of splenorraphy and of partial resection of the spleen, consisting of continued or delayed bleeding, have been reported in only three patients.

8. Regardless of clear evidence that splenic preservation procedures are safe, many patients will still require splenectomy following injury to the spleen. The primary indications for splenectomy are total avulsion or extensive fragmentation of the spleen, severe associated injuries requiring prompt attention, and continued bleeding after attempted splenic repair. In patients with multiple intra-abdominal injuries or extensive peritoneal contamination from visceral perforation, the benefits of splenic salvage should be weighed against the safer course of splenectomy.

9. The deliberate autotransplantation of splenic tissue as possible protection against overwhelming postsplenectomy in section patients requiring splenectomy for trauma has received much attention. Patients with demonstrable splenic remnants have reportedly developed fulminant sepsis despite accidental autotransplantation of variable amounts of splenic tissue. Animal experiments have yielded conflicting findings; however, most investigators in the past few years have identified a protective function of autotransplanted splenic tissue against bacterial challenge. Several surgeons have advocated implantation of thin splenic slices in omental pouches in man following splenectomy for trauma. The protective effect of deliberate autotransplantation of splenic tissue in man has not been demonstrated.

10. Patients who have undergone splenectomy must be fully informed of their possible vulnerability to severe sepsis. They should receive polyvalent pneumococcal vaccine and be instructed to seek early medical attention whenever an illness with significant fever or toxicity occurs.

11. All patients who have undergone nonoperative management or splenic salvage procedures should receive polyvalent pneumococcal vaccine. The duration of protection induced by vaccination is unknown. Because of the marked increase in adverse reactions with reinjection of pneumococcal vaccine, second or "booster" doses probably should not be given at this time.

REFERENCES

1. Aristotle: *Parts of Animals* 3.12, Peck A.L. (trans.). Cambridge, Mass., Harvard University Press, 1955.
2. Berger E.: Die Verletzungen der Milz und ihre Chirurgische Behandlung. *Arch. Klin. Chir.* 68:56, 1902.
3. Billroth T.: *Clinical Surgery* London, New Sydenham Society, 1881, p. 229.
4. Gerrard P.N.: Traumatic rupture of the spleen, followed by recovery. *Dublin J. Med. Sci.* 117:425–428, 1904.
5. Gunther C.E.M.: Spontaneous healing of an injured spleen, discovered at autopsy. *Med. J. Aust.* 1:655–656, 1939.
6. Hunter E.A.: Ruptured spleen with delayed hemorrhage and spontaneous cure. *Br. Med. J.* 2:256, 1935.
7. Turnbull H.M. cited in: Bailey H.: Traumatic rupture of the normal spleen. *Br. J. Surg.* 15:43, 1927.
8. McCartney J.S., cited by Webb R.C.: Traumatic rupture of the normal spleen with delayed hemorrhage. *Lancet* 59:545, 1939.
9. Bailey H.: Traumatic rupture of the normal spleen. *Br. J. Surg.* 15:40–46, 1927.
10. Evans C.: Ductless glands: Rupture of the spleen from external violence. *Trans. Pathol. Soc. London* 17:299–301, 1866.
11. Kocher E.T.: *Textbook of Operative Surgery,* ed. 3. London, A. & C. Black, 1911, pp. 565–566.
12. Senn H.: The surgical treatment of traumatic hemorrhage of the spleen. *JAMA* 41:1241–1245, 1903.
13. Quenu J.: Diagnostic et traitement des ruptures traumatiques de la rate avec hemorragie en peritone libre. *J. Chir.* 28:393–420, 1926.
14. Morris D.H., Bullock F.D.: The importance of the spleen in resistance to infection. *Ann. Surg.* 70:513–521, 1919.
15. Connors J.F.: Splenectomy for trauma. *Ann. Surg.* 88:388–403, 1928.
16. Wright L.T., Prigot A.: Traumatic subcutaneous rupture of the normal spleen. *Arch. Surg.* 39:551–576, 1939.
17. Rousselot L.M., Illyne C.A.: Traumatic rupture of the spleen with a con-

sideration of early features and late sequelae in seventeen cases. *Surg. Clin. North Am.* 21:455–467, 1941.

18. Mansfield R.D.: Traumatic rupture of the normal spleen. *Am. J. Surg.* 89:759–768, 1955.
19. Parsons L., Thompson J.E.: Traumatic rupture of the spleen from nonpenetrating injuries. *Ann. Surg.* 147:214–223, 1958.
20. King H., Shumacker H.B. Jr.: Splenic studies: I. Susceptibility to infection after splenectomy performed in infancy. *Ann. Surg.* 136:239–242, 1952.
21. Gofstein R., Gellis S.S.: Splenectomy in infancy and childhood. *Am. J. Dis. Child.* 91:566–569, 1956.
22. Hoefnagel R.: Susceptibility of infection after splenectomy performed in children. *Clin. Proc. Child. Hosp.* 12:48–55, 1956.
23. Huntley C.C.: Infection following splenectomy in infants and children. *Am. J. Dis. Child.* 95:477–480, 1958.
24. Laski B., MacMillan A.: Incidence of infection in children after splenectomy. *Pediatrics* 24:523–527, 1959.
25. Smith C.H., Erlandson M., Schulman I., et al.: Hazard of severe infections in splenectomized infants and children. *Am. J. Med.* 22:390–403, 1957.
26. Ek J.I., Rayner S.: An analytical study of splenectomized cases after traumatic rupture of healthy spleens. *Acta Med. Scand.* 137:417–435, 1950.
27. McKinnon W.M.P., Boley S.J., Manpel J.: Infection in children following splenectomy for traumatic rupture. *Am. J. Dis. Child.* 98:710–712, 1959.
28. Walter L.E., Chaffin L.: Splenectomy in infants and children. *Ann. Surg.* 142:798–803, 1955.
29. Coler R.S.: Postsplenectomy sepsis: A review of the literature and two new cases. *Northwest Med.* 62:865–870, 1963.
30. Doan C.A., Bouroncle B.A., Wiseman B.K.: Idiopathic and secondary thrombocytopenic purpura: Clinical study and evaluation of 381 cases over a period of 28 years. *Ann. Intern. Med.* 53:861–876, 1960.
31. Hitzrot J.M.: A discussion of G.C. Penberthy's "Results of splenectomy in childhood." *Ann. Surg.* 102:654, 1935.
32. Stossel T.P., Levy R.: Intravascular coagulation associated with pneumococcal bacteremia and symmetrical peripheral gangrene. *Arch. Intern. Med.* 125:876–878, 1970.
33. Hodam R.P.: The risk of splenectomy: A review of 310 cases. *Am. J. Surg.* 119:709–713, 1970.
34. Diamond L.K.: Splenectomy in childhood and the hazard of overwhelming infection. *Pediatrics* 43:886, 1969.
35. Singer D.B.: Postsplenectomy sepsis. *Perspect. Pediatr. Pathol.* 1:285–311, 1973.
36. Eraklis A.J., Filler R.M.: Splenectomy in childhood: A review of 1413 cases. *J. Pediatr. Surg.* 7:382, 1972.
37. Francke E.L., Neu H.C.: Postsplenectomy infection. *Surg. Clin. North Am.* 61:135, 1981.

38. O'Neal B.J., McDonald J.C.: The risk of sepsis in the asplenic adult. *Ann. Surg.* 194:775, 1981.
39. Standage B.A., Goss J.C.: Outcome and sepsis after splenectomy in adults. *Am. J. Surg.* 143:545, 1982.
40. Gopal V., Bisno A.L.: Fulminant pneumococcal infections in "normal" asplenic hosts. *Arch. Intern. Med.* 137:1526, 1977.
41. Oakes D.D.: Splenic trauma. *Curr. Probl. Surg.* 18:342, 1981.
42. Francioli P., Schaller M.D., Glauser M.P.: Overwhelming pneumococci septicemias in patients who underwent splenectomy. *Schweiz. Med. Wochenschr.* 111:2014, 1981.
43. Mufson M.A., Oley G., Hulhey D.: Pneumococcal disease in a medium sized community in the United States. *JAMA* 248:1486, 1982.
44. Schwartz P.E., Ste25rioff S., Mucha P., et al.: Postsplenectomy sepsis and mortality in adults. *JAMA* 248:2278, 1982.
45. Baue A.E.: Editorial comment. *Arch. Surg.* 116:363, 1981.
46. Pearce R.M., Krumbhaar E.B., Frazier C.H.: The history of extirpation of the spleen, in Pearce R.M. et al.: *The Spleen and Anemia: Experimental and Clinical Studies.* Philadelphia, J.B. Lippincott Co., 1918, pp. 3–10.
47. Funaioli G.: Splenectomia parzalie ed emostasi splenicia. *G. Med. Esercito* 49:1160–1166, 1901.
48. Rosner F.: The spleen in the Talmud and other early Jewish writings. *Bull. Hist. Med.* 46:82–85, 1972.
49. Dickerman J.D.: Bacterial infection and the asplenic host: A review. *J. Trauma* 16:662, 1976.
50. Schulkind M.L., Ellis E.F., Smith R.T.: Effect of antibody upon clearance of I^{125} labeled pneumococci by the spleen and liver. *Pediatr. Res.* 1:178, 1967.
51. Najjar V.A., Nishioka K.: 'Tuftsin': A natural phagocytosis stimulating peptide. *Nature* 228:672–673, 1970.
52. Najjar V.A., Schmidt J.J.: The chemistry and biology of Tuftsin. *Lymphokine Rep.* 1:157, 1980.
53. Rowley D.A.: The formation of circulating antibody in the splenectomized human being following intravenous injection of heterologous erythrocytes. *J. Immunol.* 65:515–521, 1950.
54. Douglas G.L., Simpson J.S.: The conservative management of splenic trauma. *J. Pediatr. Surg.* 6:565–570, 1971.
55. Sherman R.: Perspectives in management of trauma to the spleen: 1979 Presidential Address, American Association for the Surgery of Trauma. *J. Trauma* 20:1, 1980.
56. Hebler R.F., Ward R.E., Miller P.W., Ben-Menachem Y.: The management of splenic injury. *J. Trauma* 22:492, 1982.
57. Morgenstern L.: Personal communication, 1982.
58. Ein S.E., Shandling B., Simpson J.S., et al.: Nonoperative management of traumatized spleen in children: How and why. *J. Pediatr. Surg.* 13:117–119, 1978.
59. Zabinski E.J., Harkins H.N.: Delayed splenic rupture: A clinical syndrome following trauma. Report of four cases with analysis of 177 cases collected from the literature. *Arch. Surg.* 46:186–213, 1943.

60. Fowler R.H.: Cystic tumors of the spleen. *Int. Abst. Surg.* 70:213, 1940.
61. Pearson H.A., Johnston D., Smith K.A., et al.: The born-again spleen: Return of splenic function after splenectomy for trauma. *N. Engl. J. Med.* 298:1389–1392, 1978.
62. Metcalf D.: Spleen graft growth in splenectomized mice. *Aust. J. Exp. Biol. Med. Sci.* 41:51, 1963.
63. Trimble C., Eason F.J.: A complication of splenosis. *J. Trauma* 12:358, 1972.
64. Dretzka L.: Rupture of the spleen: A report of 27 cases. *Surg. Gynecol. Obstet.* 51:258–261, 1930.
65. Mazel M.S.: Traumatic rupture of the spleen; with special reference to its characteristics in young children. *J. Pediatr.* 26:82–88, 1945.
66. Christo M.C.: Segmental resections of the spleen: Report on the first eight cases operated on. *O. Hospital (RIO),* 62:575, 1962.
67. LaMura J., Chung-Fat S.P., San Filippo J.A.: Splenorraphy for the treatment of splenic rupture in infants and children. *Surgery* 81:497–501, 1977.
68. Morgenstern L.: Microcrystalline collagen used in experimental splenic injury. *Arch. Surg.* 109:44, 1974.
69. Morgenstern L.: The avoidable complications of splenectomy. *Surg. Gynecol. Obstet.* 145:525–528, 1977.
70. Ratner M.H., Garrow E., Valda V., et al.: Surgical repair of the injured spleen. *J. Pediatr. Surg.* 12:1019–1025, 1977.
71. Burrington J.D.: Surgical repair of a ruptured spleen in children. *Arch. Surg.* 112:417–419, 1977.
72. Morgenstern L., Shapiro S.J.: Techniques of splenic conservation. *Arch. Surg.* 114:449, 1979.
73. Conti S.: Splenic artery ligation for trauma: An alternative to splenectomy. *Am. J. Surg.* 140:445, 1980.
74. Keramidas D.C.: The ligation of the splenic artery in the treatment of traumatic rupture of the spleen. *Surgery* 85:530, 1979.
75. Strauch G.O.: Preservation of splenic function in adults and children with injured spleens. *Am. J. Surg.* 137:478–483, 1979.
76. Traub A.C., Perry J.F. Jr.: Splenic preservation following splenic trauma. *J. Trauma* 22:496, 1982.
77. Schwartz A.D., Goldthorn J.F., Winkelstein J.A., et al.: Lack of protective effect of autotransplanted splenic tissue to pneumococcal challenge. *Blood* 51:475–478, 1978.
78. Cooney D.R., Dearth J.C., Swanson S.E., et al.: Relative merits of partial splenectomy, splenic reimplantation, and immunization in preventing postsplenectomy infection. *Surgery* 86:561, 1979.
79. Cooney D.R., Michalar S.A., Michalak, D.M., et al.: Comparative methods of splenic preservation. *J. Pediatr. Surg.* 16:327, 1981.
80. Cooney D.R., Swanson S.E., Dearth J.C., et al.: Heterotopic splenic autotransplantation in prevention of overwhelming post-splenectomy infection. *J. Pediatr. Surg.* 14:336, 1979.
81. Dickerman J.D., Horner S.R., Coil J.A., et al.: The protective effect of intraperitoneal splenic autotransplants in mice exposed to an aerosolized suspension of type III *Streptococcus pneumoniae. Blood* 54:354, 1979.

82. Fasching M.C., Cooney D.R.: Reimmunization and splenic autotransplantation: A long-term study of immunologic response and survival following pneumococcal challenge. *J. Surg. Res.* 28:449, 1980.
83. Likhite V.V.: Protection against fulminant sepsis in splenectomized mice by implantation of autochthonous splenic tissue. *Exp. Hematol.* 6:433, 1978.
84. Pringle K.C., Rowley D., Burrington J.D.: Immunologic response in splenectomized and partially splenectomized rats. *J. Pediatr. Surg.* 15:531, 1980.
85. Weiss S.M., Rosato F.E., Stewart E., et al.: Splenic autotransplant function in experimental bacteremia. *Surg. Forum* 30:30, 1979.
86. Patel J., Williams J.C., Naim J.O., et al.: Protection against pneumococcal sepsis in splenectomized rats by implantation of splenic tissue into an omental pouch. *Surgery* 91:638, 1982.
87. Kusminsky R.E., Chang H., Hossino H., et al.: An omental implant technique for salvage of the spleen. *Surg. Gynecol. Obstet.* 155:407, 1982.
88. Ertel I.J., Boles E.T., Newton W.A.: Infection after splenectomy. *N. Engl. J. Med.* 296:1174, 1977.
89. Applebaum P.C., Bhamjee A., Scragg J.N., et al.: *Streptococcus pneumoniae* resistant to penicillin and chloramphenicol. *Lancet* 2:995–997, 1977.
90. Champion L.A.A., Wald E.R., Luddy R.E., et al.: *Streptococcus pneumoniae* resistant to erythromycin and clindamycin. *J. Pediatr.* 92:505–506, 1978.
91. Pearson H.H.: Splenectomy: Its risks and its roles. *Hosp. Pract.,* pp. 85–94, August 1980.
92. Sullivan J.L., Ochs H.D., Schiffman G., et al.: Immune response after splenectomy. *Lancet* 1:178–181, 1978.
93. Ahonkhai V.I., Landesman S.H., Fikrig S.M., et al.: Failure of pneumococcal vaccine in children with sickle-cell disease. *N. Engl. J. Med.* 301:26–27, 1979.
94. Applebaum P.C., Shaikh B.S., Widome M.D., et al.: Fatal pneumococcal bacteremia in a vaccinated, splenectomized child. *N. Engl. J. Med.* 300:203–204, 1979.
95. Pneumococcal polysaccharide vaccine: Recommendation of the Immunization Practices Advisory Committee. *Ann. Intern. Med.* 96:203–205, 1982.

Microsurgery: Replantation, and Free Flaps

FOAD NAHAI, M.D. AND M. J. JURKIEWICZ, M.D.

Division of Plastic and Reconstructive Surgery, Department of Surgery
Emory University Medical School, Atlanta, Georgia

THE TERM "microsurgery" was introduced in the *Surgical Forum* in 1960 by Jacobson and Suarez, who described miniaturized instruments and new techniques to repair small vessels under the dissecting microscope.[1] They concluded, "it is our belief that the techniques presented will extend vascular surgery to many previously inaccessible areas." Since then the development of precision needles, finer suture material, and the microvascular approximating clamp[2] has led to the successful anastomosis of blood vessels with lumen diameters as small as 0.5 mm and even smaller. After a variable period of practice time in the laboratory an individual may acquire the necessary technical skill to construct consistently successful microvascular anatomoses. Concurrent with technical advances, interest in the blood supply to skin and muscle was rekindled. An exact and detailed description of the blood supply to the skin and muscle was made available to the scientific world, and numerous flaps of skin, muscle, or muscle and skin based on a single artery and vein have been tested for clinical utility. These two factors, technical capability and anatomical description of new flaps, opened up the young, exciting, and rapidly advancing field of microvascular surgery. The prediction of Jacobson and Suarez has been realized—vascular surgery has been extended into many previously inaccessible areas.

0065-3411/84/0017-0073-0098-$04.00

Our colleagues in otolaryngology were among the first surgical specialists to use the microscope to facilitate operations, particularly on the inner ear. Most neurosurgical and ophthalmic procedures are now performed under microscopic magnification. Gynecologists and urologists reverse tubal ligations and vasectomies with microscope magnification. Microsurgery is so relevant to today's medicine that soon each surgical resident may need access to a laboratory where microsurgical techniques can be learned and perfected.

Because the uses of the microscope in surgery are many and varied, this review will be limited to the application of microsurgery in the field of plastic and reconstructive surgery. Two major aspects that will be described are replantation of acral parts and composite tissue transplantation, or free flap transfer. The former is always an emergency procedure, whereas the latter is usually a well-planned elective surgical procedure.

Replantation

Limbs, digits, scalp, ears, the penis, and composite facial tissue have all been successfully replanted, but by far the most common procedure is digital replantation.

Malt and McKhann[3] reported the first replantation of an arm, and in 1963 Chen in China performed the first hand replant.[4] Kleinert and Kasdan[5] reported the first successful anastomosis of digital vessels in a devascularized thumb in 1965, and in 1968 Komatsu and Tamai[6] from Japan reported the first successful replantation of an amputated thumb. In the early 1970s there were numerous reports of successful digital replants. In those early days it appeared that digit survival was the end point, with little emphasis on the final result, particularly eventual function, sensibility, cold intolerance, recovery time, and, most important, time lost from work. In 1977 Weiland et al.[7] reported a series of 86 replantations in 71 patients, emphasizing not survival only but functional results and patient selection as well. Success in digit replantation is measured not in terms of digit survival but function, sensory return, and the patient's return to gainful employment. The question no longer is can it be replanted, but should it be replanted.

DIGITAL REPLANTATION

Certain factors influence not only immediate survival but also long-term function; obviously these factors play a great part in the decision to replant or not. They include characteristics of the patient, the nature of injury, and the digit or digits involved (Table 1).

In patient selection, age, sex, occupation, and general health are considered. Age as such is not a contraindication to replantation, but in general younger patients, especially children, have better functional results. In terms of return to employment, patient motivation is far more important.[8] The patient's job must be taken into account when considering a single digit replant. A musician may be totally disabled by the loss of an index finger, whereas a laborer may be as effective without it and in fact may return to work far more rapidly if the digit is not replanted. The patient's general health must be good enough to permit several hours of general anesthesia. Any associated life-threatening injuries take priority over replanta-

TABLE 1.—FACTORS INFLUENCING DIGITAL REPLANTATION:
RELATIVE INDICATIONS AND CONTRAINDICATIONS

FACTORS	RELATIVE INDICATION	RELATIVE CONTRAINDICATION
Patient factors		
Associated injuries		X
Preexisting conditions		X
Occupation	X	X
Age	X	X
Sex	X	
Injury factors		
Type:		
Cut	X	
Crush		X
Avulsion		X
Severity		X
Contamination		X
Level	Beyond proximal interphalangeal joint	
Digit factors		
Thumb	X	
Multiple digit	X	
Single digit		X

tion. Aesthetics are taken into account when considering replantation in women.

The injury itself is the key to immediate success and eventual function. The type, severity, and level of the injury must be considered. Sharp, clean injuries are obviously preferred to avulsion or crush injuries. In our experience over the last 5 years there has been no loss of a replanted digit that was cleanly and sharply amputated. Crush or avulsion injury often results in tissue damage far beyond the actual amputation. This damage affects not only efforts to reestablish vascular flow, but also the final functional result. Replant survival following crush or avulsion injuries is reduced significantly. Interpositional vein grafts have proved most useful in replacing the damaged portions of crushed and avulsed vessels (Fig 1).[9] Bone shortening is avoided with vein grafts. An amputated digit that is damaged or lacerated beyond the point of amputation is less likely to be useful after replantation. The level of injury affects the functional result. If the digit is amputated beyond the insertion of the sublimus tendon, proximal interphalangeal joint

Fig 1.—Partial thumb replantation. **A** and **B**, diagonal partial amputation of the left thumb in a 42-year-old butcher. **C**, venous drainage re-established with 4-cm vein graft. **D**, postoperative result.

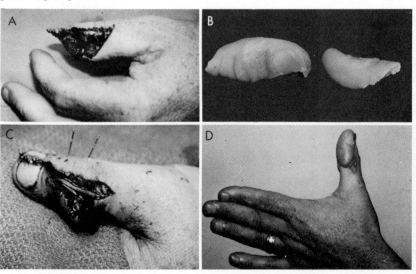

motion is preserved, rendering the finger more useful. In this situation we feel that single digit replants are indicated.

The digit or digits involved are also taken into account. Every attempt is made to replant a thumb, regardless of the type of injury (Fig 2). Similarly, if a number of digits are amputated, every attempt is made to replant at least one or two. Whether to replant a single digit remains a matter for debate, and a number of factors are weighed in such a decision.

While the foregoing are guidelines to selecting patients and digits for replantation, the patient's wishes, together with the judgment of the surgeon, play a key part in the decision to replant. Digital replantation is time-consuming and expensive. It places a burden on limited health care resources. Lost time from work and compensation add to this cost. Good clinical judgment is essential. A stiff, insensitive finger may be a tribute to technical skill, but it is also a monument to poor judgment.

Are there any clear, absolute contraindications to replantation? No. There are, however, a number of relative contraindications, which include the following:

1. Elderly patients or patients with serious preexisting disease.

2. Severe avulsion or crush injuries with significant damage to the part.

3. Other life-threatening injuries.

4. Single digit amputation of the index or little finger.

Are there any clear and absolute indications for replantation? Provided the patient's well-being is not threatened, yes! Every attempt should be made to replant a thumb and at least some digits in multiple digit amputations.

Because not all hospitals and emergency centers are equipped for replantation, most patients with amputated acral parts are referred to replant centers. The initial evaluation, care, and transport of the patient may influence the final result. The patient is first examined to rule out other urgent or life-threatening conditions. The amputated parts and the amputation stump are also examined. If there is any doubt whether the patient is a candidate for replantation or not, the patient should be referred to the replant center and the final decision made there. The amputation stump should be dressed with sterile dressings and elevated. If there is any active bleed-

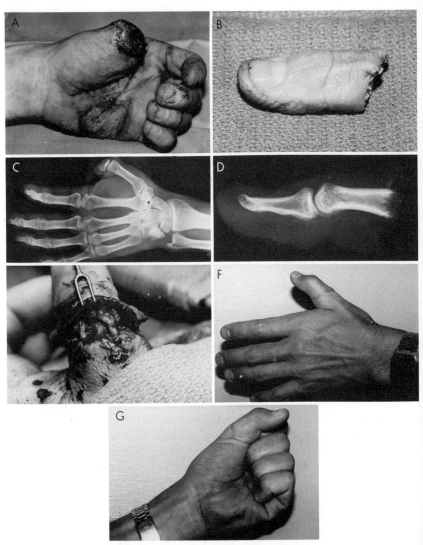

Fig 2.—Total thumb replantation. **A** and **B,** complete power saw amputation of left thumb in a right-handed 28-year-old man. **C** and **D,** radiographs of hand and amputated specimen demonstrate clean, sharp, saw cut. **E,** two dorsal veins repaired. **F** and **G,** postoperative results at 1 year.

ing, clamping of the vessels should be avoided. Dressings, elevation, and appropriate medication for pain will usually control the bleeding. Clamping will inflict further damage on the vessels. The amputated part is cleansed with saline, wrapped in moist gauze (moistened with saline or Ringer's solution), placed in a plastic bag, and then placed over ice for transportation. The amputated part should not be placed directly in the ice, as this may lead to tissue damage from freezing. Similarly, dry ice is to be avoided for transportation as it may lead to freezing. If the amputation is incomplete and a devascularized part is hanging by a tendon, nerve, or skin bridge, these connections are preserved. They should never be cut. Under these circumstances, the part is untwisted, and whenever possible, under local anesthesia, the bone stabilized with a K-wire in the emergency room prior to transfer to a replant center. Transfer of the part and patient should be swift. Cold ischemia time should be kept to a minimum. Digits will tolerate cold ischemia up to 24 hours, but in cases of major extremity amputations this time is reduced to approximately 6–8 hours. Digits have no muscle and therefore are able to withstand longer ischemia time.

On arrival at the replant center, the patient and the part or parts are examined; roentgenograms of the amputation stump and the amputated parts are also examined. If a decision is made to replant, the amputated parts are taken to the operating room by one team of surgeons while a second team prepares the patient. Blood is crossmatched for the patient and intravenous broad-spectrum antibiotics are begun. In the meantime the amputated part is cleaned in the operating room. Additional incisions are made to expose and label digital arteries, nerves, and dorsal veins. The vessels in the amputated part are not irrigated or flushed. When the patient arrives in the operating room, the amputation stump is cleaned under general anesthesia. Additional incisions are made and the digital vessels, veins, and nerves are identified and labeled. A general anesthetic is preferred because of the length of the procedure. At this stage it will be obvious if interpositional vein grafts will be necessary. If so, the vein grafts are harvested at this stage. We prefer to use the small vein on the volar aspect of the wrist. The vein grafts are labeled and stored in moist gauze sponges.

OPERATIVE TECHNIQUE

Replantation then commences. The bone is stabilized first, if possible. We prefer interosseous wiring of the bony fragments.[10] Next the flexor and extensor tendons are repaired. The microscope is then brought back into the field and the nerves and artery or arteries are repaired, in that order. The patient is not heparinized, but a heparin solution is used to irrigate the vessel ends. If possible, we repair both digital arteries, even though the digit will survive with only one artery.

Fig 3.—Replantation of right arm. **A,** saw amputation of right arm just beyond the elbow. **B,** late result following replantation. **C,** multiple vein grafts were used.

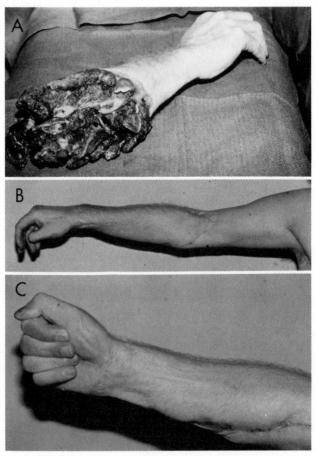

Urbaniak et al. have shown that when both vessels are repaired there is better return of sensibility.[11] The veins are repaired next. Again, we make every attempt to repair at least two or more veins. Finally, the soft tissues are closed, very loosely, and if necessary skin grafts are used to cover the wound. Skin grafts may be placed directly over the vein grafts. The hand is then dressed. Our average time for an uncomplicated replant is approximately 4 hours per digit. The patient is started on intravenous low molecular weight dextran, which is continued for 5 days. Aspirin, 2 tablets daily, is also administered for its effect on platelets. Smoking by the patient or visitors in the room is prohibited for 3 weeks. The patients are usually discharged from the hospital on day 6. Early postoperative hand therapy is initiated after discharge.

MAJOR LIMB REPLANTATIONS

Major limb replantations are technically less difficult than digit replantation. The success of replantation is judged by return of muscle function and sensibility. Nerve regeneration is therefore the key. A major extremity replant is successful only if it surpasses a prosthetic device in function and is acceptable in appearance (Fig 3). This is usually true of upper extremity replants. However, lower extremity replants are successful only if the patient can bear weight on the replanted extremity without heel ulceration. While lower extremity replants are still a matter of debate, a very good case has been made by Jupiter et al.[12] for replantation of parts of lower extremity amputation to preserve the knee joint.

REPLANTATION OF OTHER ACRAL PARTS

While function is an essential consideration to replantation of limbs and digits, the replantation of other acral parts, such as scalp,[13] ear[14], penis,[15] and composite facial tissue,[16] should always be attempted. Our efforts at reconstruction of these tissues often fall short in terms of appearance and function.

We have successfully replanted an entire scalp,[17] a partial scalp, and two penises.[18] Both patients with scalp replants have full hair growth. There is no available method of scalp reconstruction to match a successful replant. Both patients with penile replants also have had full return of sexual function and voiding with near normal sensory return. Again, no other method of penile reconstruction can match these results.

Composite Tissue Transplantation or Free Tissue Transfer

In parallel with the technical advances and the development of digital replantation, experience was gained in the laboratory with experimental composite tissue transplantation.[19-21] Krizek et al. in 1965 reported the successful transfer of free skin flaps in dogs.[20] In 1966 Buncke and co-workers reported experimental replantation of rabbit ears[22] and toe-to-thumb transfers in the Rhesus monkey.[23] McClean and Buncke in 1972 reported the successful transfer of the omentum by microvascular technique to cover a scalp defect.[24] The groin flap described by McGregor and Jackson[25] in 1973 was then successfully transferred by microsurgical techniques by Daniel and Taylor[26] and O'Brien et al.[27] These early reports of successful skin flap transfer were followed by reports of successful microsurgical transplantation of bone,[28] muscle,[29] muscle skin units,[30-32] nerve,[33] skin and bone units,[34] and rib.[35]

The description of the anatomical basis of the groin flap and its successful transfer by microsurgical technique provided an impetus for the search for other skin areas suitable for heterotopic transfer.[36-38]

Concurrently, interest in muscle flaps was rekindled by the work of Ger.[39] Orticochea had shown that skin overlying the gracilis muscle would survive when elevated as an island based only on the underlying muscle.[40] McCraw and co-workers then described a number of musculocutaneous flaps, some of which proved suitable for transfer as free flaps.[41, 42] A detailed description and classification of the blood supply of muscle then followed.[43]

Initially skin flaps, particularly the groin flap, were the most widely utilized tissue for microvacular transfer, but with the evolution of the musculocutaneous flap and the recognition of its many advantages over skin flaps, muscle-based flaps have become universally accepted and transferred as the tissue of choice. The reasons for this are twofold: the anatomy of muscle and the physiology of muscle. Anatomically, the vessels that provide the dominant blood supply to the muscles most useful for tissue transfer are larger in size, longer, and more constant in location than those on which skin flaps are based. This predictable anatomy, longer length, and wider lumen size make muscle flaps easier to transfer and more reliable. Physiologically, the greater vascularity of and oxygen tension within muscle render it more suitable for transfer into contaminated or infected wounds.[44]

Over the past decade, free tissue transfer has evolved from the early phase of amazement to the current period of refinement. Flap survival is not the end point; it is only a step (often taken for granted) in the entire reconstructive process. Our attention is focused more on flap selection and restoration of form and function in the defect, with preservation of form and function in the donor area.[45] Free tissue transfer is firmly established as a method for distant tissue transfer.[46] As such, it has essentially replaced the more traditionally multistaged methods of tissue transfer. This has resulted in a reduction in the number of operations, length of hospital stay, and, importantly, cost.[47]

The essence of reconstructive surgery is to reconstruct the defective body part with tissue similar to that destroyed by trauma, resected for neoplastic disease, or congenitally deformed or absent. The goal of the plastic surgeon is to select suitable tissue or tissues, to transfer the tissue or combination of tissues in one stage, and to restore a defect to its original form while preserving the form and function of the donor area. Microvascular free tissue transfer has been a great step toward the realization of this goal.

Microsurgical free tissue transfer is safe and reliable. Our results over the past 6 years with various tissue transfers are tabulated in Table 2. Success with free tissue transfer depends on appropriate selection of the patient, of the flap or tissues for transfer, and of recipient vessels. While technical skill in constructing the actual microsurgical anastomosis is essential, we consider selection of suitable vessels the single most important factor. Although vascular complications have been few, in each patient the cause of vascular failure has been related to poor selection of the recipient vessels. Ideally, the recipient vessels are normal vessels of adequate size, have excellent flow, and are free of intimal disease or posttraumatic perivascular scarring. Vein grafts are used if suitable recipient vessels are not

TABLE 2.—EMORY UNIVERSITY AFFILIATED
HOSPITALS: FREE TRANSPLANTATION, 1976–1982

TISSUE	NO.	SUCCESS RATE (%)
Muscle & musculocutaneous	64	92
Skin	14	92
Jejunum	38	95
Colon	5	80
Omentum	24	96
Digits (toe to hand)	8	100
Osteocutaneous	4	100

available close to the defect. Although ideally one would like to avoid irradiated vessels, successful microvascular anastomosis of vessels in an irradiated field can be achieved in vessels that have excellent flow.

Although microsurgical free tissue transfer has been undertaken for transplantation of tissue to all parts of the body, we shall concentrate on tissue transfer to the head and neck and lower extremities.

HEAD AND NECK RECONSTRUCTION

Microvascular free tissue transfer is our method of choice for esophageal reconstruction, coverge of large scalp defects, and correction of soft tissue deformities of the face.

ESOPHAGEAL RECONSTRUCTION.—The early experimental work and clinical applications of Seidenberg and colleagues[48] and others[49, 50] suggested the feasibility of esophageal reconstruction with a segment of jejunum. Use of the microscope and microsurgical technique have made this an excellent, safe, and predictable one-stage method for reconstruction of the pharynx and cervical esophagus following tumor resection.[51, 52]

In the last 6 years we have used the jejunum as a free vascularized graft for the immediate reconstruction of the esophagus, pharynx, and oral cavity in 38 patients following resection for tumor or strictures. The operation is performed by two teams. One team resects the tumor while the second team harvests the jejunum. A suitable loop of jejunum is selected and isolated on a single artery and vein (branches of the superior mesenteric artery) usually 1½–2 mm in lumen diameter. Each end of the loop is then divided and the proximal end is labeled with suture so that it can be sutured in an isoperistaltic fashion in the neck. This loop of bowel, now totally isolated on its blood supply, is wrapped in moist gauze. Continuity of the rest of the bowel is then reestablished through a bowel anastomosis and the mesentery is repaired. Meanwhile, the resection in the neck is completed and suitable recipient vessels, usually a branch of the external carotid artery and a tributary of the internal jugular vein, are isolated and prepared for the microvascular anastomosis. This part of the dissection is performed under loupe magnification. The choice of vessels is made on an individual basis and varies from patient to patient. On occasion, the bowel vessels have been sutured end to side into the external or common carotid arteries and into the internal jugular vein. Once the recipient vessels in the neck are prepared, the loop of bowel is transferred from the abdomen to the neck. Usually the proximal anastomosis of the bowel into the floor of the mouth or pharynx is made first, then microvascular anastomosis of the vessels under microscope magnification, and finally the distal anastomosis to the esophagus. In the meantime the second team closes the abdominal wall. The skin flaps in the neck are then closed. If the jejunum has been sutured into the oropharynx, bowel viability can be easily followed by intra-oral examination. If not, a small window is left in the incision over the bowel, a small piece of Silastic is placed in the window to prevent dessication, and the bowel is monitored through the window. The Silastic is removed on day 5 and the skin edges are closed at the bedside. Most patients are able to take fluid by mouth 6 or 7 days after the operation and are usually discharged after 10 days.

There have been no intra-abdominal complications, and other complications have been few. There have been only 2 losses out of 38 replantations, a success rate of 95%. Vessels in irradiated necks have been used without difficulty, and many patients have undergone postoperative radiation with no complications to the transferred loop of bowel.

On occasion, soft tissue coverage in the neck is not adequate to cover the bowel loop. In these cases, a meshed, split-thickness skin graft is placed directly over the bowel and mesentery (Fig 4).

LARGE SCALP DEFECTS.—Most defects of the scalp, whether the result of trauma or tumor resection, can be closed with lo-

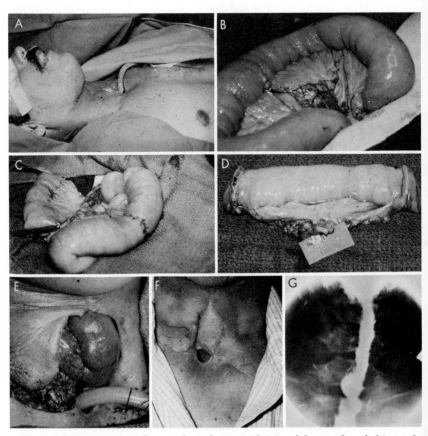

Fig 4.—Reconstruction of cervical esophagus with jejunal free graft and skin graft. **A,** 45-year-old man with breakdown of flap reconstruction of esophagus following tumor resection in an irradiated field. **B,** loop of jejunum is selected and mesentry is divided. **C,** loop of jejunum is isolated and continuity of bowel is restored. **D,** isolated loop of bowel. Note vessels. **E,** jejunum revascularized and sutured in neck. **F,** 6-month follow-up showing healed skin graft. Patient swallows with no difficulty. **G,** contrast study demonstrates loop of bowel.

cal scalp flaps.[53, 54] Up to one third of the scalp can be covered by this method. Larger defects or defects in irradiated tissue require distant tissue transfer. We prefer to transfer the distant tissue by microvascular technique as a free flap.[55] Our flap of choice is the latissimus dorsi. It is a large flap of muscle which will cover a large area and has a long vascular pedicle, 11–12 cm. Thus the vascular anastomoses are constructed in the upper neck, out of the area of trauma or previous irradiation.

The facial and superior thyroid arteries make suitable recipient arteries, and the posterior facial vein is usually our recipient vein of choice. We avoid the temporal artery because it is usually too small to receive the thoracodorsal, or right gastroepigastric vessels.

We have covered the scalp with the latissimus dorsi (10) and with omentum (2) in 12 patients with uniform success. If the latissimus dorsi is not available, then the omentum is transferred because it has a long vascular pedicle and can cover a large area of scalp (Fig 5).

OMENTUM IN HEAD AND NECK RECONSTRUCTION.—The omentum is admirably suited for free vascularized transfer to the head and neck for control of infection,[56] restoration of contour,[56, 57] or revascularization of free grafts of rib and skin.[58] The omentum is suitable and reliable for transplantation as a vascularized free graft because it has a predictable anatomy, long vascular pedicle, and vessels of relatively large lumen diameter, 1½–2 mm. Although it can be based on either the right or left gastroepigastric vessels, we prefer to base it on the right vessels, as these vessels are larger and dissection around the spleen is avoided. The omentum has a disadvantage in that

Fig 5.—Omental flap. Reconstruction of scalp defect. **A,** radionecrotic, infected, exposed skull following tumor resection and radiation. Wounds are debrided and covered with omental free flap and skin graft. Latissimus dorsi was not available following right radical mastectomy with ligating thoracodorsal vessel and left pneumonectomy. **B,** wound is stable with omentum and skin graft, several months postoperatively.

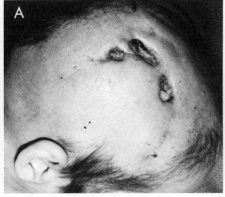
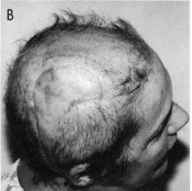

a laparotomy is necessary to harvest the omentum. In our experience, however, with 29 patients over the last 7 years, we have not had a single intra-abdominal complication.

The omentum has been successfully transferred for control of posttraumatic chronic, recalcitrant frontal sinus infection following trauma in three patients. In another three patients the omentum has been used to revascularize a skeleton of split rib grafts, constructed to replace the facial skeleton destroyed by trauma. The omentum was then skin grafted. In the remainder of our patients, the omentum has been transferred to cover contour deformities of differing etiology, including tumor resection, congenital deformities, radiation growth arrest, or Romberg's disease (hemifacial atrophy). The vascular anatomy and reliability of the omentum enables the surgeon to fashion a small finger of omentum to insert in each part where tissue is required, a great advantage when correcting the deformity of Romberg's disease.

MANDIBULAR RECONSTRUCTION.—Reconstruction of the mandible following tumor resection, especially in the irradiated field, remains an obdurate problem for the surgeon and his patient. Microvascular free composite tissue transfer may prove to be an acceptable solution. Initial experimental work with free vascularized rib transfers[59, 60] was followed by clinical applications.[61–63] Rib transfers were followed by compound osteocutaneous flaps of iliac crest bone with overlying skin initially based on the superficial circumflex iliac artery and later on the deep circumflex iliac artery. Taylor et al.[64] have performed good mandibular reconstructions using this osteocutaneous flap based on the deep circumflex iliac artery. The deep circumflex iliac vessels are larger in lumen diameter and length than the superficial, making them more reliable for tissue transfer. Our experience with flap for mandibular reconstruction is limited to three patients. The initial results have been satisfactory.

LOWER EXTREMITY RECONSTRUCTION

Over the last decade, muscle flaps and microvascular free tissue transfer have revolutionized soft tissue coverage of the lower extremity. Simple solutions are now available for complex problems. Hitherto unsalvageable extremities that would have been amputated are now being saved. The indications for local muscle flaps or free tissue transfer depend on the level of the defect. Defects of the knee and upper third of the tibia are covered by transposition of the lateral or medial head of the gastrocnemius muscle, defects of the middle third are covered by the soleus muscle, and defects of the lower third and ankle are best covered by distant flap transfer using microsurgical techniques. Small defects in the lower third may occationally be covered by local muscle flaps.

Muscle, muscle skin units, skin flaps, the omentum, and composite bone-containing flaps have all been transferred as free flaps for coverage and reconstruction of the lower extremity. The choice of tissue is based on the requirement posed by the defect. By far the most useful are muscle and musculocutaneous flap. In 1946 Stark demonstrated the value of pedicled muscle flaps for control of chronic osteomyelitis.[65] Mathes et al. have confirmed the work of Stark with muscle flaps transferred by microsurgical techniques.[44] In addition to the capability of muscle to control infection, muscle may also promote more rapid healing of fractures.[66] The predictable anatomy and large vascular pedicle make muscle the flap of choice for transfer to the lower extremity for coverage of posttraumatic defects or control of osteomyelitis. We have had experience with the gracilis,[32] tensor fasciae latae,[31, 67] latissimus dorsi,[68] and more recently rectus abdominis as free muscle flaps for transfer to the lower extremity. If the defect is large, the latissimus is the flap of choice. For smaller defects, hitherto, the gracilis had been our flap of choice, but because the rectus abdominis based on its lower pedicle (the inferior epigastric artery) has a large pedicle, with larger lumen diameter than the gracilis, it may well replace the gracilis as the flap of choice for smaller defects. If the defect is deep, the flap is transferred with the overlying skin as a musculocutaneous flap. If the defect is shallow, muscle alone is transferred and skin grafted, thus avoiding the excessive bulk of subcutaneous tissue included in a musculocutaneous unit. We choose skin flaps when dealing with stable noncontaminated wounds where aesthetic considerations are of importance. The groin flap, the original standard flap, has been superceded in our practice by a flap of lower abdominal skin based on the superficial inferior epigstric artery. This flap has a larger pedicle than the groin flap and a very acceptable donor deformity, an "abdominoplasty" scar.

The omentum is an excellent alternative to the muscle flaps but is only indicated under special circumstances.

PREOPERATIVE EVALUATION

Although there are no definite contraindications to free tissue transplantation to the lower extremity, certain factors will influence the final result. These are taken into account before a final decision to proceed is made.

Again, age as such is not a contraindication. We have successfully operated on children 3 years old and on adults in their 60s. However, the patient's general health must be good enough to tolerate a 4- to 12-hour procedure. Our average time for an uncomplicated free tissue transfer to the lower extremity is 5–6 hours. Patients with significant peripheral vascular disease or severe diabetes are not candidates.

Patients who have had significant trauma to an extremity and patients with absent or poor pulse at the level of the ankle are evaluated by arteriography. Arteriography is helpful in selecting recipient vessels. Arteriographic evaluation of the donor area is not necessary.

If osteomyelitis is present or if bone viability is in question, oral tetracycline, 250 mg four times a day, is administered to the patient 48 hours before operation. This tetracycline labeling has proved useful in evaluating the necessary bone debridement at the time of operation.

OPERATING TECHNIQUES

The extremity wound is first debrided, then all devitalized soft tissue and bone is removed. A Wood's light is used to evaluate the tetracycline-labeled bone. Any bone that does not fluoresce is debrided. The wound is then irrigated and the exposure and isolation of the recipient vessels are begun. The posterior tibial or anterior tibial vessels are exposed. The choice is guided by the location of the wound and findings on preoperative arteriography. Under loupe magnification the vessels are exposed, isolated, and evaluated. Only normal vessels out of the field of injury are selected.

Once the wound has been debrided and recipient vessels exposed, the final selection of the suitable flap is made and the flap is elevated. The flap is then transferred to the leg and temporarily sutured in place, and microsurgical anastomosis is constructed under microscopic magnification. In the lower extremity we routinely construct on end-to-side arterial anastomosis. This not only preserves all the blood supply to the foot, but also eliminates the technical problems involved in end-to-end anastomosis of vessels of different lumen size.[69] In a single vessel, leg (Fig 6) end to side is the only choice. The venous anastomosis is next constructed, either end to end or end to side, depending on the size of the recipient vessels. After the anastomoses are completed, the flap is trimmed and inset. The donor area is usually closed by the second team while the flap is sutured in place.

As with replants, the patient receives Dextran 40, 30 cc every hour for 5 days, and refrains from smoking for 3 weeks after the operation.

RESULTS AND COMPLICATIONS

Our overall survival rate over the last 6 years with muscle and musculocutaneous free flaps has been approximately 92% (see Table 2). Most of the flap losses came early in our experience and were related to poor selection of recipient vessels and delay in recognizing vascular complications. There has not been a loss of a flap in the last 2 years.

Complications have been few. Early recognition of vascular complications, usually venous, has led to early exploration and salvage of three flaps in the last 2 years. The only other complications have been related to the donor site, specifically seroma of the back when the latissimus dorsi muscle has been harvested.

Successful flap transfer does not necessarily mean that the patient's problem has been corrected, nor does it mean the limb has been salvaged. We have operated on 26 patients with chronic osteomyelitis and unstable lower extremity wounds in the last 6 years. All but two of the patients now have healed wounds and control of the infection. One patient subsequently had a below-knee amputation, and another patient has recurrent infection. We believe that the wound in this second patient is factitious. Mathes et al.[44] and May et al.[70] have reported uniform success in their series.

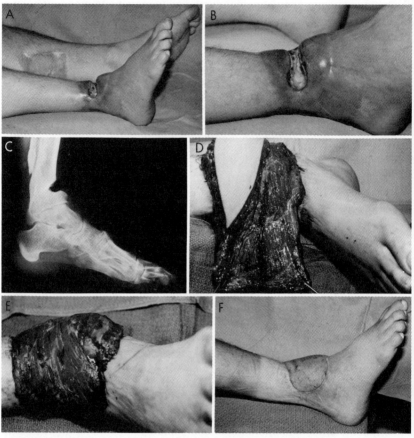

Fig 6.—Reconstruction of ankle defect and chronic osteomylitis of tibia with latissimus dorsi free muscle flap and skin graft. A, 40-year-old man with posttraumatic
ankle defect. B, chronic osteomyelitis of right lower tibia. Note failed previous cross-
leg flap. C, radiograph demonstrating bony deformity. On arteriography, only the posterior tibial artery was patent below the knee. D, revascularized latissimus dorsi musculocutaneous free flap. Muscle will be divided so that a portion is placed into bony
defect. E, skin island is reserved, and muscle is sutured into defect. The skin from the
island was harvested and placed directly on the muscle as a skin graft. F, postoperative result demonstrates stable coverage and control of infection.

Although in this discussion we have emphasized the role of
free muscle flaps in coverage of wounds and control of infection,
muscle may be transferred and reanimated for functional purposes. Harrii et al.[71] and O'Brien et al.[72] have used the gracilis
muscle for correction of facial paralysis, and Manktelow and

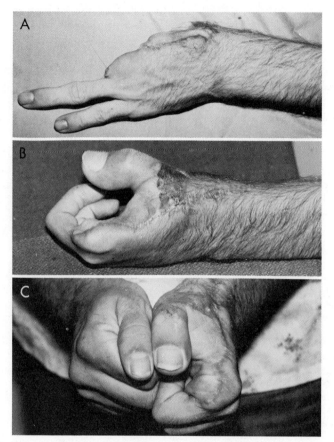

Fig 7.—Great toe to thumb transfer. **A,** dominant left hand of a 21-year-old saw-mill worker. He had lost the thumb, index, and long finger in an accident. **B,** with transfer of great toe, some thumb function is restored, as evidenced by pinch to left hand. **C,** comparision of right thumb with left great toe thumb.

McKee[73] have refined free muscle transplantation with micro-neurovascular anastomosis to replace destroyed forearm flexor muscle following Volkman's ischemic contracture.

TOE-TO-HAND TRANSFERS

The initial laboratory work of Buncke et al.[23] on toe-to-hand transfers in primates led to the first clinical application of toe-to-hand transfers by Cobbett,[74] who transferred the great toe to replace a thumb based on the plantar digital arteries and dorsal veins. Buncke et al.[75] then transferred the great toe based on the first dorsal metatarsal artery and dorsal vein, and O'Brien et al.[76] advocated basing the great toe on the dorsalis pedis artery and saphenous vein, which provide a larger pedicle with vessels of large lumen diameter, thereby making the procedure simpler and more reliable. The transfer of the great toe has proved to be an excellent one-stage reconstruction for the thumb, with excellent return of sensibility and function. (Fig 7). The donor deformity in the foot, though, is rather obvious. The second toe may also be transferred, based on the dorsalis pedis artery and the saphenous vein.[77] The donor deformity in the foot is more acceptable and the functional result in the hand is comparable to the function of the great toe. The resemblance of the second toe to the thumb is less good than the resemblance of the great toe to the thumb.

REFERENCES

1. Jacobson J.H., Suarez E.L.: Microsurgery in anastomosis of small vessels. *Surg. Forum* 11:243, 1960.
2. Acland R.D.: Microvascular anastomosis: A device for holding stay sutures and a new vascular clamp. *Surgery* 75:185, 1974.
3. Malt R.A., McKhann C.F.: Replantation of severed arms. *JAMA* 198:716, 1964.
4. Gonzalez E.R.: China, rest of technical world share replantation data. *JAMA* 242:1593, 1979.
5. Kleinert H.E., Kasdan M.L.: Anastomosis of digital vessels. *J. Ky. Med. Assoc.* 63:106, 1965.
6. Komatsu S., Tamai S.: Successful replantation of a completely cut off thumb. *Plast. Reconstr. Surg.* 42:347, 1968.
7. Weiland A.J., Villareal-Rios A., Kleinert H.E., et al.: Replantation of digits and hands: Analysis of surgical techniques and functional results in 71 patients with 86 replantations. *J. Hand Surg.* 21:1, 1977.
8. Kleinert H.E., Jablon M., Tsai T.-M.: An overview of replantation and results of 347 replants in 245 patients. *J. Trauma* 20:390, 1980.
9. Alpert B.S., Buncke H.J., Brownstein M.: Replacement of damaged arteries and veins with vein grafts when replacing crushed, amputated fingers. *Plast. Reconstr. Surg.* 61:17, 1978.
10. Lister G.: Interosseus wiring of the digital skeleton. *J. Hand Surg.* 3:427, 1978.
11. Urbaniak J.R., Evans J.P., Bright D.S.: Microvascular management of ring avulsion injuries. *J. Hand Surg.* 6:25, 1981.
12. Jupiter J.B., Tsai T.-M., Kleinert H.E.: Salvage replantation of lower limb amputations. *Plast. Reconstr. Surg.* 69:1, 1982.
13. Alpert B.S., Buncke H.J., Mathes S.J.: Surgical treatment of the totally avulsed scalp. *Clin. Plast. Surg.* 9:145, 1982.

14. Nahai F., Hayhurst J.W., Salibian A.H. Microvascular surgery in avulsive trauma of the ear. *Clin. Plast. Surg.* 5:423, 1978.
15. Cohen B.E., May J.W., Daly J.S.F., et al.: Successful clinical replantation of an amputated penis by microneurovascular repair: Case report. *Plast. Reconstr. Surg.* 59:276, 1977.
16. James N.J., Survival of large replanted segment of lower lip and nose. *Plast. Reconstr. Surg.* 58:623, 1976.
17. Nahai F., Hurteau J., Vasconez L.O.: Successful microsurgical replantation of an entire scalp and ear by microvascular anastomosis of only one artery and one vein. *Br. J. Plast. Surg.* 31:339, 1978.
18. O'Brien D.: Penile replantation following traumatic amputation, in *Proceedings of the International Urological Society,* to be published.
19. Goldwyn R.M., Lamb D.L., White W.L.: An experimental study of large island flaps in dogs. *Plast. Reconstr. Surg.* 31:438, 1963.
20. Krizek T.J., Taimi T., DesPrez J.D., et al.: Experimental transplantation of composite grafts by microsurgical vascular anastomosis. *Plast. Reconstr. Surg.* 36:538, 1965.
21. Strauch B., Murray D.E.: Transfer of composite graft with immediate suture anastomosis of its vascular pedicle measuring less than one millimeter in external diameter using microsurgical techniques. *Plast. Reconstr. Surg.* 40:325, 1967.
22. Buncke H.J., Schulz W.P.: Total ear reimplantation in the rabbit utilizing microminiature vascular anastomosis. *Br. J. Plast. Surg.* 19:15, 1966.
23. Buncke H.J., Buncke C.M., Schulz W.P.: Immediate nicoladone procedure in the rhesus monkey or hallux-to-hand transplantation using microminiature vascular anastomosis. *Br. J. Plast. Surg.* 19:332, 1966.
24. McLean D.H., Buncke H.J.: Autotransplant of the omentum to a large scalp defect with microsurgical revascularization. *Plast. Reconstr. Surg.* 49:268, 1972.
25. McGregor I.A., Jackson I.T.: The groin flap. *Br. J. Plast. Surg.* 23:173, 1973.
26. Daniel R.K., Taylor G.I.: Distant transfer of an island flap by microvascular anastomosis. *Plast. Reconstr. Surg.* 52:111, 1973.
27. O'Brien B.McC., MacCleod A.M., Hayhurst J.W., et al.: Successful transfer of a large island flap from the groin to the foot by microvascular anastomosis. *Plast. Reconstr. Surg.* 52:291, 1972.
28. Taylor G.I., Miller G.D.H., Ham F.J.: The free vascularized bone graft. *Plast. Reconstr. Surg.* 55:553, 1975.
29. Harii K., Ohmori K., Torii S.: Free gracilis muscle transplantation with microvascular anastomosis for the treatment of facial paralysis. *Plast. Reconstr. Surg.* 57:133, 1976.
30. Harii K., Ohmori K., Sekeguchi J.: The free musculocutaneous flap. *Plast. Reconstr. Surg.* 57:294, 1976.
31. Hill H.L., Nahai F., Vasconez L.O.: The tensor fascia lata myocutaneous free flap. *Plast. Reconstr. Surg.* 61:517, 1978.
32. Mathes S.J., Nahai F., Vasconez L.O.: Myocutaneous free flap transfer: Anatomical and experimental considerations. *Plast. Reconstr. Surg.* 62:162, 1978.
33. Taylor G.I., Ham F.J., The free vascularized nerve graft: A further ex-

perimental and clinical application of microvascular techniques. *Plast. Reconstr. Surg.* 57:413, 1976.

34. Taylor G.I., Watson H.: One stage repair of compound leg defects with revascularized flaps of groin skin and iliac bone. *Plast. Reconstr. Surg.* 61:494, 1978.
35. Buncke H.J., Furnas D.V., Gordon L., et al.: Free osteocutaneous flap from a rib to tibia. *Plast. Reconstr. Surg.* 59;799, 1977.
36. McCraw J.B., Furlow L.T.: The dorsalis pedis arteriolized flap: A clinical study. *Plast. Reconstr. Surg.* 55:177, 1975.
37. Taylor G.I., Daniel R.K., The anatomy of severed free flap donor sites. *Plast. Reconstr. Surg.* 56:243, 1975.
38. Baudet J., Guimberteau J.C., Nascimento E.: Successful clinical transfer of two free thoracodorsal axillary flaps. *Plast. Reconstr. Surg.* 58:680, 1976.
39. Ger R.: The management of pre-tibial skin loss. *Surgery* 63:757, 1968.
40. Orticochea M.: The musculo-cutaneous flap method: An immediate and heroic substitute for the method of delay. *Br. J. Plast. Surg.* 25:106, 1972.
41. McCraw J.B., Dibbell D.G.: Experimental definition of independent myocutaneous vascular territories. *Plast. Reconstr. Surg.* 60:212, 1977.
42. McCraw J.B., Dibbell D.G., Carraway J.H.: Clinical definition of independent myocutaneous vascular territories. *Plast. Reconstr. Surg.* 60:341, 1977.
43. Mathes S.J., Nahai F.: Classification of the vascular anatomy of muscles: Experimental and clinical correlation. *Plast. Reconstr. Surg.* 67:177, 1981.
44. Mathes S.J., Alpert B., Chang N.: Use of the muscle flap in chronic osteomyelitis: Experimental and clinical correlation. *Plast. Reconstr. Surg.* 69:815, 1982.
45. Nahai F., Mathes S.J.: Esthetic aspects of reconstructive surgery of the lower extremity. *Clin. Plast. Surg.* 8:369, 1981.
46. Mathes S.J., Nahai F.: *Clinical Application for Muscle and Musculocutaneous Flaps.* St. Louis, C.V. Mosby Co., 1982, chap. 1.
47. Serafin D., Georgiade N., Smith D.N.: Comparison of free flaps with pedicled flaps for coverage of defects of the leg or foot. *Plast. Reconstr. Surg.* 59:492, 1977.
48. Seidenberg B., Rosenak S.S., Hurwitt E.S., et al.: Immediate reconstruction of the cervical esophagus by a revascularized isolated jejunal segment. *Ann. Surg.* 149:162, 1959.
49. Jurkiewicz M.J.: Vascularized intestinal graft for reconstruction of the cervical oesophagus and pharynx. *Plast. Reconstr. Surg.* 36:509, 1965.
50. Peters C.R., McKee D.M., Berry B.E.: Pharyngoesophageal reconstruction with revascularized jejunal transplant. *Am. J. Surg.* 121:675, 1971.
51. Hester T.R., McConnell F.M.S., Nahai F., et al.: Reconstruction of the cervical oesophagus, hypopharynx, and oral cavity using free jejunal transfer. *Am. J. Surg.* 140:487, 1980.
52. McConnell F.M.S., Hester T.R., Nahai F., et al.: Free jejunal graft for reconstruction of pharynx and oesophagus. *Arch. Otolaryngol.* 107:476, 1981.

53. Orticochea M.: Four-flap scalp reconstruction technique. *Br. J. Plast. Surg.* 41:323, 1968.
54. Jurkiewicz M.J.: Open wounds of the scalp: An account of methods of repair. *J. Trauma Scalp* 21:769, 1981.
55. Barrow D.L., Nahai F., Fleischer A.S.: Utilization of free latissimus dorsi musculocutaneous flaps in various neurosurgical disorders. *J. Neurosurg.* 58:252, 1983.
56. Jurkiewicz M.J., Nahai F.: The omentum: Its use as a free vascularized graft for reconstruction of the head and neck. *Ann. Surg.* 195:756, 1982.
57. Wallace J.C., Schneider W.J., Brown R.G., et al.: Reconstruction of hemifacial atrophy with a free flap of omentum. *Br. J. Plast. Surg.* 32:15, 1979.
58. Brown R.G., Nahai F., Silverton J.S.: The omentum in facial reconstruction. *Br. J. Plast. Surg.* 31:58, 1978.
59. Strauch B., Bloomberg A.E., Lewin M.L.: An experimental approach to mandibular replacement: Island vascular composite rib grafts. *Br. J. Plast. Surg.* 24:334, 1971.
60. Ostrup L.T., Fredrickson J.M.: Distant transfer of a free living bone graft by microvascular anastomosis: An experimental study. *Plast. Reconstr. Surg.* 54:274, 1974.
61. Ostrup L.T., Fredrickson J.M.: Reconstruction of mandibular defects after radiation using a free living bone graft transferred by microvascular anastomosis. *Plast. Reconstr. Surg.* 55:563, 1975.
62. Serafin D., Villareal-Rios A., Georgiade N.G.: A rib containing free flap to reconstruct mandibular defects. *Br. J. Plast. Surg.* 30:263, 1977.
63. Daniel R.K.: Mandibular reconstruction with free tissue transfers. *Ann. Plast. Surg.* 1:346, 1978.
64. Taylor G.I., Acland R.D., Schusterman M., et al.: The saphenous neurovascular free flap. *Plast. Reconstr. Surg.* 67:763, 1981.
65. Stark W.J.: The use of pedicled muscle flaps in the surgical treatment of chronic osteomyelitis resulting from compound fractures. *J. Bone Joint Surg.* 28:343, 1946.
66. Byrd H.S., Cierny G. III, Tebbetts J.B.: The management of open tibial fractures with associated soft tissue loss: External pin fixation with early flap coverage. *Plast. Reconstr. Surg.* 68:73, 1981.
67. Nahai F., Hill H.L., Hester T.R.: Experiences with the tensor fascia lata flap. *Plast. Reconstr. Surg.* 63:788, 1979.
68. Bostwick J. III, Nahai F., Wallace J.G., et al.: Sixty latissimus dorsi flaps. *Plast. Reconstr. Surg.* 63:31, 1979.
69. Godina T.M.: Preferential use of end to side arterial anastomosis in free flap transfers. *Plast. Reconstr. Surg.* 64:673, 1979.
70. May J.W., Gallico G.G. III, Lukash F.N.: Microvascular transfer of free tissue for closure of bone wounds of the distal lower extremity. *N. Engl. J. Med.* 306:253, 1982.
71. Harrii K., Ohmor K., Thorii S.: Free gracilis muscle transplantation with microvascular anastomosis for treatment of facial paralysis. *Plast. Reconstr. Surg.* 57:133, 1976.
72. O'Brien B.M., Franklin J.D., Morrilon W.A.: Cross-facial nerve grafts and microvascular free muscle transfer for early established facial palsy. *Br. J. Plast. Surg.* 33:202, 1980.

73. Manktelow R.T., McKee N.M.: Free muscle transplantation to provide active finger flexion. *J. Hand Surg.* 3:416, 1978.
74. Cobbett J.R.: Free digital transfer: Report of a case of transfer of a great toe to replace an amputated thumb. *J. Bone Joint Surg.* 51B:677, 1969.
75. Buncke H.J., McLean M.C., George P.T., et al.: Thumb replacement: Great toe transplantation by microvascular anastomosis. *Br. J. Plast. Surg.* 26:194, 1973.
76. O'Brien B.McC., MacLeod A.M., Sykes P.J., et al.: Hallux to hand transfer. *Hand* 7:128, 1975.
77. O'Brien B.McC., Brennen M.D., Macleod A.M.: Microvascular second toe transfer for digital reconstruction. *Clin. Plast. Surg.* 5:223, 1978.

The Impact of Cyclosporin A on Transplantation

PETER J. MORRIS, M.D.

Nuffield Department of Surgery, University of Oxford, John Radcliffe Hospital, Oxford, England

CYCLOSPORIN A (CyA) is an exciting new immunosuppressive agent that has proved to be potent in a wide variety of experimental models of tissue transplantation and promises to be a valuable addition to our immunosuppressive armamentarium in clinical organ transplantation.[1] First isolated from two strains of fungi imperfecti at Sandoz in Basel (*Cylindrocarpon lucidum* Booth and *Trichoderma polysporum* [Link ex Pers.]. Rifai, more correctly known as *Tolypocladium inflatum* Gams) as an antifungal agent of limited activity, it was shown by Jean Borel to have potent immunosuppressive activity in a variety of in vitro and in vivo experiments.[2-4] The drug has a molecular weight of 1,200 daltons and comprises 11 amino acids, one of which is unique and most of which are hydrophobic. Thus, CyA is only soluble in lipids or organic solvents. Recently the drug has been synthesized,[5] which should allow many questions concerning mechanism of action and toxicity to be explored precisely and also allow other molecules with similar immunosuppressive properties but less toxicity to be synthesized.

Following the initial description of the immunosuppressive properties of this drug by Borel, CyA was shown to suppress rejection of vascularized organ allografts in the rat, rabbit, and dog,[6-8] followed soon after by similar observations in various

99

models of vascularized organ allografts in other species.[1] Clinical trials of CyA began in Cambridge in 1978,[9] and over the last 3 years, numerous centers have been accumulating experience with its use.

This chapter briefly outlines the effects of CyA in experimental tissue transplantation, including current knowledge of the drug's mechanism of action and a detailed summary of the initial clinical experience with CyA. It will be evident that the impact of CyA on transplantation has already been considerable, and promises to be even greater when one remembers that CyA is but the first of a new generation of immunosuppressive agents possessing such uniquely valuable properties.

Experimental Transplantation

KIDNEY

Much of the experimental work with CyA in vascularized organ allografts has been performed with a kidney allograft model in the rat. Rejection of a kidney allograft in the rat is readily suppressed by a short course of CyA given orally in olive oil.[10] However it is striking how dose- and time-dependent this effect is, as shown in Tables 1 and 2. Thus, a short course of CyA given during the first few critical days of exposure to the allograft results in prolonged and even indefinite survival time of renal allografts. In the rat the humoral response to the allograft is suppressed by the drug, but not the cell-mediated immune response,[10] while the drug appears relatively ineffec-

TABLE 1.—DOSE-DEPENDENT EFFECTS
OF CYCLOSPORIN A ON REJECTION OF DA
RENAL ALLOGRAFTS IN LEWIS RATS*

DOSE OF CyA	NUMBER	SURVIVAL IN DAYS
Nil	9	10 × 3, 11 × 6
2 mg/kg	5	10 × 2, 11 × 3
5 mg/day	7	24, 66, 100 × 5
10 mg/kg	5	77,† 100 × 5

*CyA was given for 14 days after transplantation or for as long as the animal survived. An orthotopic renal transplant was performed with removal of the remaining kidney on day 7.
†Death not due to rejection.

TABLE 2.—EFFECT OF CYCLOSPORIN A ON REJECTION OF DA
RENAL ALLOGRAFTS IN LEWIS RATS DEPENDING ON TIME OF
ADMINISTRATION*

PERIOD OF TREATMENT (DAYS)	NUMBER	SURVIVAL (DAYS)
−2 to 0	6	12, 12, 12, 12, 14, 14
0 to 2	5	16, 21, 22, 28, >60
−1 to 2	6	12, 17, 18, 19, 20, >100
0 to 3	5	17, 19, 24, 91, 105
0 to 4	5	20, 23, 28, 34, >140
0 to 14	2	>140, >140
2 to 14	6	13, 13,† 77, >140, >140, >140
4 to 14	5	11, 12, 13, 13, 14

*CyA was given orally at a dose of 10 mg/kg. An orthotopic renal
transplant was performed on day 0 with removal of the remaining kidney on day 7.
†Died from infection.

tive in a specifically presensitized animal.[11] The specificity of
the tolerance to a renal allograft induced by CyA is partial in
that a third-party allograft will be rejected when implanted
100 days after the induction of the tolerant state, but the cytotoxic antibody response to the third-party allograft is suppressed.[12] Of particular interest is the marked synergism seen
in the rat with heterologous antilymphocyte serum, a finding
that may be particularly relevant to clinical practice.[13]

Just as in the rat, a short course of CyA in the rabbit will
produce prolonged survival time of renal allografts,[8, 14] where
the tolerance so induced has appeared to be specific in some
experiments but not in others.[15–16] These differing results can
probably be attributed to the timing of the tests for specificity
and to the particular assays used.[12, 17]

In contrast to the rodent, renal allografts in the dog are rejected after cessation of CyA administration even after 3
months. But provided an initial therapeutic dosage of 20 mg/
kg/day of CyA is used, rejection is completely suppressed.[18, 19]
Of relevance to clinical practice is the observation that the use
of prednisolone with CyA does not appear to increase the incidence of infectious complications, and that conversion from
CyA to Azathioprine and prednisolone at 3 months in dogs can
be accomplished without loss of the allograft.[20, 21] Delay in the
administration of CyA until day 4, at which time rejection of a
renal allograft should have been initiated, still resulted in pro-

longed survival time in some animals,[22] in contrast to the rat. This finding suggests that it might be possible to use CyA to treat a rejection reaction, although theoretically this would not be expected as will become evident in the later discussion on the mechanism of action of CyA. Further work is needed to clarify this important point, for anecdotal data is now available in the human suggesting that CyA may indeed be effective in steroid-resistant acute rejection.[23]

In the primate, early studies in the rhesus monkey showed that a CyA dosage of 25 mg/kg/day suppressed rejection of renal allografts, although rejection occurred some 10 days after cessation of the drug.[24] Borleffs and his colleagues[25] confirmed these findings with a lower dose of CyA but, more importantly, proved that continued administration of CyA at a dosage of 10 mg/kg/day led to a prolonged period of survival of all renal allografts with continuing survival of three of five animals at 6 months. The transfusion effect was still evident in these experiments, and there were no instances of nephrotoxicity, lymphomas, or infections even when CyA was combined with Azathioprine and prednisolone. In contrast to the impressive results obtained in the rhesus monkey, which are very similar to those obtained in the dog, CyA has proved less effective in prolonging the renal allograft survival rate in the chacma baboon. A dosage of 20 mg/kg/daily given indefinitely only increased survival time from a median of 11 days to 22.5 days. A modest improvement in this survival time was obtained by pretreatment with a dosage of 30 mg/day and indefinite administration of this dose afterwards, although what might be considered therapeutic levels of CyA in the blood were obtained.[26]

HEART

Heterotopic heart allografts in the rat show an indefinite survival time with CyA treatment, and reported results are very similar to those seen with renal allografts.[6, 26-29] In the pig, a striking prolongation of orthotopic heart allografts was obtained with CyA, and in some instances hearts did not reject when CyA was discontinued at some months after transplantation.[30] Extensive studies of orthotopic heart allografts in the primate have been performed by the Stanford group using CyA alone and in combination with other immunosuppressive agents. There was a marked prolongation in the survival time of heart allografts in cynomologous monkeys after a 14-day course of CyA (25 mg/kg/day), while continued administration of CyA led to marked prolongation of survival time.[31, 32] The same researchers also found prolonged survival times of combined heart-lung transplants.[33] A striking finding in the Stanford studies was the very high incidence of malignant lymphomas.[34]

PANCREAS

CyA has proved less effective in pancreatic transplantation than in transplantation of other organs. In the rat, suppression of rejection of isolated pancreatic islets, or of fetal pancreas transplanted across a major histocompatibility barrier, is only modest despite the use of quite large doses of CyA.[35, 36] However, transplantation of isolated islets as a vascularized composite graft of kidney and islets beneath the renal capsule, seems to reduce the apparent immunogenicity of islets, such that CyA can produce prolonged survival time of the diabetic rat.[37] CyA does produce prolonged survival time of the vascularized pancreas in the rat, but the effect is not as striking as that seen with the heart or the kidney.[36, 38]

In the dog, CyA does prolong the survival time of vascularized segmental pancreatic allografts in total pancreatectomized recipients,[19, 39, 40] but only in a dosage considerably larger than required for renal allografts, namely 40 mg/kg/day (Table 3).[39] This may have been due to poor absorption of CyA as a result of the loss of the pancreatic exocrine secretions in these pancreatectomized dogs. Although a number of dogs survived over 6 months, their response to an IV glucose challenge was abnormal as measured by both glucose and insulin levels. However, the onset of rejection in two dogs at 6–7 months, as the dose of CyA was reduced, was reversed with methylprednisolone.[19] Gingival hypertrophy and widespread development of warts were common in dogs receiving high doses of CyA for a long time. The transplantation of a crude pancreatic islet preparation into the spleen of totally pancreatectomized dogs did restore normoglycemia as an autologous graft, but not as an allograft at CyA doses of 25 mg/kg, although these dogs did survive longer than control animals.[19, 41]

TABLE 3.—DURATION OF NORMOGLYCEMIA IN TOTALLY PANCREATECTOMIZED DOGS GIVEN A VASCULARIZED SEGMENTAL PANCREATIC AUTOGRAFT OR ALLOGRAFT, WITH/WITHOUT ORAL CyA*

TREATMENT	VASCULARIZED PANCREATIC GRAFT	NUMBER	DURATION OF NORMOGLYCEMIA (DAYS)
Nil	—	10	<1 × 10
Nil	Autograft	10	>180 × 10
Nil	Allograft	5	8, 9, 9, 9, 10
CyA 25 mg/kg/day	Allograft	10	7,† 8,† 13, 15, 17, 17, 18, 18, 22, 40
CyA 40 mg/kg/day—reducing after 120 days	Allograft	8	6,† 8, 9, 120, 195, 205, 220, >250

*The pancreatic duct was blocked with Ethibloc.
†Died of intussusception.

LIVER

There is not a great deal of information about CyA in experimental liver transplantation. Orthotopic liver allografts in the rat are not rejected in many strain combinations,[42] but in combinations where rejection does occur, a short course of CyA will prevent rejection.[43] However, auxillary heterotopic liver allografts in the rat are rejected in strain combinations where orthotopic livers are not rejected, and here a short course of CyA will prevent rejection.[44]

LUNG

Single-lung allografts in the dog showed prolonged survival in the dog with CyA treatment, either alone or with other agents, with 7 of 16 dogs surviving longer than 100 days.[45] Of the protocols tested by Veith and colleagues, the addition of a 2-week course of Azathioprine immediately after transplantation perhaps produced the best results. These results are quite striking when one considers how difficult it is to obtain a significant number of long-surviving lung allografts with other immunosuppressive agents.[46] The initial success of combined heart-lung transplants in the primate, referred to in an earlier section, further reaffirms the potency of CyA in this experimental model.

SKIN

Skin allografts in the mouse, rat, rabbit, and dog have a survival time lasting as long as CyA continues to be administered but are rejected soon after cessation of the drug.[2, 17, 47–50] In the dog, the onset of rejection of a skin allograft after cessation of CyA can be reversed by restarting the drug.[50]

ORGAN XENOGRAFTS

Heterotopic cardiac xenografts from hamsters to rats (concordant species) survived for around 21 days compared to 2 days in controls, but nearly toxic dosages of CyA in the rat (35 mg/kg/day) were required.[51] Similarly, in another example of a xenograft between concordant species, namely hare kidney to rabbit, CyA administered in a dosage of 15 mg/kg/day produced prolonged graft survival time although hyperacute rejection occurred in untreated animals.[52] However, the survival time of renal xenografts between more disparate species, such as rabbit to cat, was not influenced by CyA.[53]

BONE MARROW

CyA has proved less effective in preventing acute graft versus host disease (GVHD) in a radiation-induced marrow chimera in the mouse,[54] in comparison to the rat where acute GVHD after allogeneic marrow transplantation in rats prepared by total irradiation or cyclophosphamide is prevented and tends not to recur on cessation of the drug.[2, 55] However, an established GVHD does not respond to CyA treatment. Successfully transplanted recipients have been shown to be chimeras with specific tolerance to donor and recipient but not third-party grafts.[56, 57] However, in the dog, Deeg and his colleagues[35] found CyA relatively ineffective in preventing acute GVHD in unrelated irradiated recipients of allogeneic marrow and less effective than methotrexate in DLA-identical littermate recipients. And so too in the rabbit the effect of CyA in preventing acute GVHD was not striking.[59] However, a combination of CyA and methotrexate after transplantation in unrelated recipients was most effective, producing survival times of greater than 100 days in 7 of 13 animals.[60]

Mechanism of Action

It is apparent from a number of in vivo experiments that CyA exerts its effect at a very early stage after exposure of the recipient to a tissue allograft. This was clearly illustrated in a rat renal allograft model cited earlier,[10, 61] (see Table 2), which showed that CyA is relatively ineffective after the immune response has been induced or before the recipient animal has been exposed to the allogeneic histocompatibility antigens.

In vitro experiments correlate well with these in vivo observations. In several species, including man, CyA has been shown to inhibit the proliferative response of lymphocytes to concanaval in A, phytohemagglutinin and pokeweek mitogen in vitro.[62–68] If CyA is added 48 hours after the addition of mitogen to a culture then there is no inhibition of proliferation, and the effect is reversed by washing the lymphocytes and reexposing them to the mitogen.[62, 67] Complete inhibition of the mixed lymphocyte reaction (MLR) by CyA has been demonstrated in several species including man.[66, 69–72] The generation of cytotoxic lymphocytes in the MLR is prevented by CyA, but once generated CyA has no effect on their cytotoxic activity.[70–74] Thus, in vivo CyA does not prevent allograft rejection in sensitized animals,[11, 49] and as might be expected, it does not inhibit the secondary MLR response nor the generation of cytotoxic T lymphocytes in such a secondary reaction.[66, 71] Lymphocytes extracted from a rejecting renal allograft in the rat can be shown to exhibit both specific cytotoxic activity and nonspecific natural killer cell activity in vitro, but in animals treated with CyA the lymphocytes are not cytotoxic to specific target cells, although still displaying normal natural killer cell activity (Mason and Morris, in preparation).

There is a growing amount of evidence that the action of CyA is directed predominantly against T helper lymphocytes,[2, 64, 65, 75–78] either preventing production of IL-2 (T cell growth factor) or inhibiting the response to IL-2.[63, 74, 79] In this way the generation of the cytotoxic T cells from the cytotoxic T cell precursor is prevented, and this may then also allow the uninhibited generation of suppressor T lymphocytes both nonspecific and specific as suggested by the work of Leapman and colleagues[66] and Hess and colleagues.[73, 80]

Although in general CyA has not been thought to inhibit the function of B lymphocytes,[3, 65, 75] there is now some evidence to the contrary, both in man[81] and in the mouse,[76, 129] the latter workers having demonstrated a CyA-sensitive subpopulation of T-independent B lymphocytes. There is also some evidence that CyA may have some inhibiting effect on the production of IL1 by macrophages,[74] although their response to lymphokines is not inhibited.[82] CyA does not appear to influence the inflammatory granulation response in vivo[83]; this finding is consistent with the normal wound healing seen in clinical practice in patients receiving CyA.

Thus, although the action of CyA remains to be completely elucidated, it is becoming more clear that its predominant effect is directed at T lymphocytes at an early stage of the induction of the immune response to an antigen and that a major part of this activity is related to the inhibition of IL2-induced proliferation of cytotoxic T cell precursors.

Clinical Experience

KIDNEY

Considerable experience is being gained with the use of CyA in renal transplantation, for somewhere around 1,000 patients had been treated with the drug by the end of 1982. CyA was first used in renal transplantation by Calne and colleagues in Cambridge.[9, 84] Initially it was used with other drugs, such as prednisolone or cytimum (a cyclophosphamide derivative), but this proved a dangerous combination, with a number of patients dying of infection. It also became apparent that CyA was nephrotoxic in humans, although the extensive use of this agent in studies on animals had given no indication of a nephrotoxic effect. In addition, three lymphomas were seen in these early patients, which did cause considerable alarm.

It was then that a new policy was adopted at Cambridge in which CyA was used only in patients whose grafts were diuresing; CyA was used alone, with methylprednisolone given only to treat rejection. If a dose of more than 6 gm of methylprednisolone was required, the patients were converted to Azathioprine and prednisolone. Following this policy, 60 cadaveric grafts have since been performed in 59 patients, all but one of whom had previously been transfused. The actuarial allograft survival rate at 1 year is 82%. Six deaths have occurred, five from infection. Ten patients were converted to Azathioprine and prednisolone because rejection of the allograft was not controlled with CyA.[85] Of considerable note is the fact that many of these patients were not receiving steroids, and indeed, had never received any steroids.

This early experience in Cambridge prompted a number of controlled trials of CyA, namely single-center trials at Minneapolis, Oxford, and Sydney, as well as multicenter trials in Europe and Canada, together with uncontrolled studies of its use at Denver, Pittsburgh, Stockholm, and Boston. In the European multicenter trial, only patients who were given grafts that were diuresing 6 hours after surgery were randomized to receive CyA alone or conventional treatment with Azathioprine and prednisolone, according to the custom of unit. The trial was closed at the end of 1981 after 1 year when just over 200 patients had been entered. Follow-up is obviously short but the actuarial survival rate at 6 months was 73% in the CyA group and 52% in the control group,[86] even though a considerable number of patients were converted to Azathioprine and steroids because of apparent rejection on CyA. However, undoubtedly many of the grafts considered to be rejecting were suffering from nephrotoxicity, an ever-present problem which shall be discussed later.

An excellent multicenter trial has been conducted in Canada where CyA with prednisone was compared with standard therapy based on Azathioprine and prednisone in 209 cadaveric renal allograft recipients.[128] The allograft survival rate at 1 year is predicted to be 84% in the CyA group compared to 67% in those receiving standard therapy, with patient allograft survival rates of 97% and 90% in the two groups respectively. No transfusion effect was seen in the CyA group, although this was evident in the control group. Of considerable interest is their observation that a detrimental effect on graft survival time was seen in CyA-treated patients if they received kidneys that had been machine perfused for longer than 24 hours or if the surgical anastomosis time took longer than 45 minutes, suggesting that CyA nephrotoxicity is more likely to occur in kidneys that have some ischemic damage.

In Minneapolis all HLA mismatched living or cadaveric donor transplants were eligible for their trial in which CyA plus prednisolone was compared with their conventional therapy of Azathioprine, steroids, and ALG.[87, 88] All patients had had a splenectomy and at least 5 units of blood. As of July 1982, 137 patients had been entered into the trial, 70 received CyA and 67 conventional therapy. Approximately 50% of the patients in each group were diabetic and 60% received cadaver kidneys. The trial is still in progress, but so far there is no difference in either the patient or graft survival rate. The patient survival rate is over 90% in each group and the graft survival rate is over 80%. However, there have been less acute rejection episodes in the CyA patients (17% vs. 54%), despite the use of one-half the total corticosteroid dose over the first 6 months in patients treated with CyA compared to conventional therapy.

There were fewer infection episodes in the CyA patients, and the incidence of overt CMV disease was a strikingly low—3% in the CyA patients compared to 33% in the conventional treatment patients. Acute tubular necrosis following transplant was no more of a problem in patients receiving CyA than conventional treatment, but delayed nephrotoxicity was a significant problem.

Similarly Starzl and his colleagues,[89, 90] first at Denver (where treatment was not standardized) and then at Pittsburgh, have reported most impressive results with CyA plus prednisone (at a maintenance dosage of 20 mg/day after a burst of high-dose prednisone) both in primary as well as secondary cadaveric transplants. The graft survival rate is about 90% at 6 months in primary cadaveric transplants, and of 26 patients receiving a cadaver retransplant, 20 are functioning 1–21 months after transplantation, although follow-up is still short in most of these patients. Early anuria was not considered a contraindication to CyA, being attributed to either rejection or sometimes to nephrotoxicity, although it did provide diagnostic problems.

The Stockholm group has used CyA with prednisolone in 20 high-risk patients, namely diabetics or patients over the age of 55, most of whom received a cadaver kidney. Twelve patients are alive and well with acceptable renal function at 6–30 months after transplantation.[132]

The Oxford study of CyA is rather different from the above studies in that the strategy is based on treatment of recipients of cadaveric kidneys with CyA alone for 3 months followed by conversion to Azathioprine and low-dose prednisolone. In the first trial, patients were not eligible for the trial if they were to receive an HLA-DR compatible kidney (because of the excellent results obtained with DR compatible kidneys in the Oxford unit) or if the allograft was not diuresing 6 hours after surgery. Thus, only patients receiving a DR-mismatched and diuresing kidney were entered into the trial. Furthermore, if more than two rejection episodes required treatment with IV methylprednisolone, then this was regarded as a treatment failure of CyA and either the patient converted to Azathioprine plus prednisolone or prednisolone was added to the CyA. After 35 patients had been entered into the first trial, there was no apparent difference between the two groups,[91] and so a second trial was begun in which all patients entered into the trial regardless of matching or initial function. Thus randomization is performed before transplantation, and in those patients who are to receive CyA the first dose can be given IV before transplantation, which theoretically might be important.

The strategy of conversion from CyA to Azathioprine and prednisolone at 3 months was suggested by the results of this protocol in dog experiments, and the concern about the apparent increased lymphoma risk and the nephrotoxicity of CyA at that time reinforced the rationale of this present-day approach.

Over 50 patients have now been entered into the second trial, and there appears to be a better graft survival rate in the CyA patients, the patient allograft survival rate being 95% at 1 year in both groups (Table 4). Obviously further evaluation of this strategy will be needed both in the short- and long-term period, although the first 3 years of experience are encouraging. Yet, as the concern about lymphomas recedes, this approach may seldom be used unless long-term side effects of CyA appear as in the case of chronic renal damage, which is still a cause of concern.

The Oxford group is also currently conducting a trial in which patients with long-surviving renal allografts in Azathioprine plus prednisolone, but with severe steroid side effects, are converted from Azathioprine to CyA with a subsequent gradual reduction in prednisolone doses until steroids can be discontinued altogether.[133] The conversion has been accomplished without problems in ten patients so far selected for the trial, apart

TABLE 4.—EXPERIENCE WITH CyA IN OXFORD IN TWO RANDOMIZED PROSPECTIVE CONTROLLED TRIALS OF CyA GIVEN FOR 3 MONTHS WITH CONVERSION TO AZATHIOPRINE AND LOW DOSE PREDNISOLONE VERSUS STANDARD THERAPY WITH AZATHIOPRINE AND LOW DOSE PREDNISOLONE*

	TREATMENT	NUMBER OF PATIENTS	PATIENT SURVIVAL % 3	12	GRAFT SURVIVAL % 3	12
Trial I:	Aza + pred	14	93	93	85	58
	CyA	21	95	95	75	73
Trial II:	Aza + pred	25	95	95	73	73
	CyA	29	98	98	80	80

*In the first trial patients receiving HLA-DR compatible kidneys or non-diuresing kidneys were excluded from randomization, while in the second trial all patients are randomized to 1 or another treatment (none of these differences are significant).

from the expected CyA associated deterioration in renal function. However some other rather serious problems have arisen in a few patients, such as recurrent skin cancers and continued deterioration of renal function. For the moment this strategy must continue to be reevaluated.

In living-related transplantation Kahan's group[92] has shown an impressive 100% patient survival rate and a 95% graft survival rate in 20 one-haplotype disparate and MLR-reactive living-donor transplants with a mean follow-up of 10 months. Fourteen of the 20 patients did not have a single rejection episode.

Thus, it can be seen that CyA either with or without steroids has made a most impressive debut in renal transplantation in terms of patient and graft survival rates, the major side effect of the drug being nephrotoxocity.

LIVER TRANSPLANTATION

It does appear that the results of liver transplantation are significantly improved in patients treated with CyA. Experience is relatively limited at this time, and is confined, in the main, to the units of Starzl in Denver and Pittsburgh and Calne in Cambridge.[9, 85, 89, 93] Starzl had previously used a triple-drug therapy for most patients given a liver transplant (azathioprine, prednisolone and horse ALG) with a 1-year allograft survival rate after 170 liver grafts of around 30%. However, during the last 2 years Starzl has used CyA with prednisone, following a similar protocol to that used for kidney transplantation, and this has resulted in a 1-year allograft survival rate in 67 patients of over 70%, a dramatic improvement.[93]

Nephrotoxicity has been a problem in many patients but generally has resolved with reduction of the dose of CyA. In some patients the renal impairment was so severe that CyA was discontinued and azathioprine used in its place temporarily before restarting CyA at a much lower dose level. Calne has been more concerned by the potential and actual renal impairment in his patients and has now adopted a protocol where the patient is immunosuppressed initially with azathioprine and prednisolone, and when liver and renal function are stable the immunosuppression is changed to CyA. Calne's overall graft survival rate at 1 year in 98 patients is just over 20% (a comparable experience to that of Starzl remembering that there are no pediatric patients in the Cambridge experience; children have done better than adults in Starzl's experience), but since using CyA the 1-year allograft survival rate in 20 patients is over 50%.[85] Thus, despite the lack of controlled trials of CyA versus conventional immunosuppression in liver transplantation, there seems little doubt that it has improved the outcome very significantly, the controversy lying with determining the most satisfactory protocol for its use.

CARDIAC TRANSPLANTATION

Trials with CyA in cardiac transplantation were begun at Stanford at the end of 1980, with patients receiving prednisone plus rabbit antithymocyte globulin. Early reports were encouraging, with not only an improvement in the patient survival rate, but also a marked reduction in the incidence of rejection and the length of initial hospital stay. Infectious complications were certainly no greater than in patients treated with the previous conventional therapy, namely azathioprine instead of CyA.[94] Similar good early results have been reported from Pittsburgh,[95] where CyA has been used with prednisone. Both groups have commented on the lack of any clinical or electrocardiographic evidence of rejection in patients treated with CyA, the only reliable method of diagnosis being endomyocardial biopsy. Several lymphomas occurring in the Stanford patients have caused considerable concern, but are probably attributable to excess immunosuppression. As a result they have excluded routine treatment with ATG from their current protocol. Altogether, over 70 heart transplants had been performed at nine centers by June 1982, with a 75% patient survival rate, the longest follow-up being at 15 months.[96] There seems little doubt that CyA will improve the results of cardiac transplantation quite markedly in the short-term period, and it appears to be associated with a decrease in morbidity.

Six combined heart-lung transplants have also been performed at Stanford in patients with primary cardiac or pulmonary disease with secondary involvement of the other organ.[96, 97] Four of six patients are alive 6–15 months after surgery.

PANCREAS

There is growing experience of the use of CyA in pancreatic transplantation, usually combined with renal transplantation, in the diabetic patient with renal failure. Most of the experience has been gathered at Minneapolis, Lyon, Cambridge, Stockholm, and Birmingham.[98] The overall success rate of segmental pancreatic transplantation has been poor with only 25% of allografts functioning at 1 year. Not only has allograft rejection been a cause of failure but also there have been numerous incidences of technical complications, either due to vascular thromboses or complications associated with the exocrine secretions. The majority of patients receiving CyA have had the pancreatic duct blocked with one of a number of polymers to prevent the exocrine secretions while still leaving the endocrine gland intact. However, this causes intense fibrosis of the gland, which no doubt contributes to a significant number of the late allograft failures (between 6 and 12 months) in association with rejection. The use of CyA is particularly appealing in pancreatic transplantation, because it offers the possibility of not using steroids or using relatively low doses of steroids,[99, 100] a major advantage in the diabetic. However, it is not really possible to evaluate the role of CyA in pancreatic transplantation at this time because so many other problems plague the procedure in patients who are generally poor risks for transplantation. Nevertheless, one has the impression that here, too, immunosuppression has been improved with the use of CyA.

BONE MARROW

There appears to have been a significant impact of CyA on the outcome of allogeneic bone marrow transplantation for acute leukemia and severe aplastic anemia, both in terms of graft takes and GVHD. There is much experience now with CyA in bone marrow transplantation, second only to that in renal transplantation. CyA was used initially by the Marsden group to treat acute GVHD but was found to be ineffective.[130] The same group then began to use it prophylactically from the time of transplantation in patients with acute leukemia given

HLA-identical sibling marrow. There was a dramatic reduction not only in the incidence of acute GVHD but also in its severity compared to a historical control group given methotrexate.[131] Patients were given CyA for approximately 6 months, but on discontinuance of CyA, approximately 60% of patients developed acute or chronic GVHD, that was generally responsive to reinitiation of CyA or Azathioprine plus prednisolone.[101] The Marsden group also noted that their major problem following bone marrow transplantation for acute leukemia has been recurrence of the leukemia, which probably has been due to the superior suppression of the GVHD by CyA.[101] The comparatively smaller experience of Speck's group has been, on the whole, similar to that of the Marsden group,[102] but Gluckman's group has experienced comparatively poor results, mainly due to CyA toxicity.[103] Similarly, the early results of marrow allografting in patients with severe aplastic anemia are most encouraging,[96, 102, 104] with a 1-year patient survival rate of around 70%.

Nevertheless the experiences cited compare the prophylactic use of CyA with the historical use of methotrexate, and thus there is considerable interest in the controlled trial of CyA versus methotrexate being conducted by the Seattle group in patients with acute nonlymphoblastic leukemia. The early results suggest first that neither the overall patient survival rate, nor the incidences of acute GVHD are altered by CyA treatment, and second, that the severity of acute GVHD is very much reduced by CyA.[105]

A small number of HLA nonidentical marrow allografts have also been performed using CyA prophylaxis either alone or with methotrexate, and although acute GVHD has inevitably occurred, with several patients dying as a result, a new problem of acute respiratory distress syndrome has appeared, the etiology of which is unclear but is thought to be related to high CyA levels and/or high doses of irradiation in mismatched marrow graft recipients.[106] The mortality has been high in this early experience of mismatched family marrow allografts, and it does not seem that CyA used alone will allow the extension of marrow allografting beyond the HLA-identical sibling combination. In all units, toxicity (mostly nephrotoxicity) has been a persistent major problem.

Cyclosporin A Toxicity and Monitoring of Blood Levels

A number of side effects have been observed in patients receiving CyA, the most worrisome of which has been nephrotoxicity (Table 5). Nephrotoxicity was noted quite quickly in patients given CyA after renal transplantation by Calne,[9] and for that reason Calne advocated the use of CyA only in patients whose kidneys were diuresing after transplantation.[85] The nephrotoxicity of CyA in humans came as a surprise, for in extensive animal experiments no evidence of nephrotoxicity had been observed, even in ischemic kidneys.[107] More recently however, large, almost toxic, doses of CyA (50–100 mg/kg) in the rat have been shown to cause proximal tubular damage especially of the straight segment or thick descending limb of Henle's loop.[108, 109] Nevertheless there is not the slightest doubt that in man CyA is nephrotoxic, nephrotoxicity not only having been observed in renal allografts, where differentiation from rejection may be difficult, but also after liver and bone marrow transplantation.[69, 110–113] There has been virtually no histologic or intrastructural evidence of tubular damage in humans, with

TABLE 5.—SIDE EFFECTS
OF CyA THERAPY

Nephrotoxicity
Hepatotoxicity
Tumors
   Lymphomas
   Fibroadenoma of breast
Skin
   Hirsutism
   Thickening
   Rashes
Gastrointestinal
   Anorexia
   Nausea
   Failure to gain weight
Central nervous system
   Tremor
   Burning sensation in limbs
   Malaise, depression
Cardiovascular
   Fluid retention
   Hypertension
Gingival hypertrophy

the exception of the description of three patients with severe renal failure and histological evidence of glomerular thromboses and severe tubular damage following bone marrow transplantation.[114] But the increase in urinary N-acetyl-β-D-glucosaminidase (NAG) in patients receiving CyA suggests that tubular damage is produced by CyA.

This nephrotoxicity appears to be dose-related and is reversible if CyA is discontinued. This was a striking observation made in the Oxford trial of CyA in renal transplantation where patients are converted to azathioprine and prednisolone 3 months after transplantation, which inevitably resulted in a rapid and significant improvement in renal function.[91, 115] Similarly after cessation of the drug in marrow grafted patients there was a return of renal function to normal, a situation not complicated by the possibility of renal allograft rejection.[112]

The concurrent use of aminoglycosides with CyA has been shown to enhance the likelihood of nephrotoxicity both in rat[116] and man,[104] as has ketoconazole,[103] amphotericin B,[69] trimethoprim and co-trimoxazole.[117] Perhaps of greater concern is the possibility of long-term nephrotoxicity in renal allograft patients receiving CyA, since biopsies at 3 months often show a marked degree of interstitial fibrosis.[91] Medium-term follow-up of 14 patients for 2 years at Cambridge does not suggest that there is a gradual deterioration in renal function, but obviously a much longer follow-up will be necessary to answer this question.[118]

Hepatotoxicity has been observed in patients on CyA after renal, cardiac and bone marrow transplantation.[94, 111–112] Generally, this has not been more than a temporary elevation in results of liver function tests, and has disappeared on reduction of the dosage. Very high doses of CyA in the rat produce ultrastructural changes in hepatocytes as well as deterioration of liver function.[109]

An apparent, increased incidence of lymphomas in the early patients having renal allografts treated with CyA caused considerable alarm.[119] But as time has passed this increased incidence of lymphoma, both in renal and cardiac allograft recipients may not be greater than that expected in recipients treated with conventional immunosuppressive therapy. Indeed most of the patients who have developed lymphomas have received other drugs as well, such as prednisone and ATG, suggesting that the occurrence of lymphoma is due to excessive immunosuppression rather than specifically to CyA. There appears to be an association between Epstein-Barr virus (EBV) reactivation or primary infection and the occurrence of lymphomas, with EBV nuclear antigen identified in two patients.[120] Theoretically lymphomas might be expected to occur more commonly in patients receiving CyA. Bird et al.[121] have demonstrated that EBV-infected B lymphocytes will proliferate unchecked in vitro in the presence of CyA, due to inhibition of the T cell-dependent control of this proliferation.

Most of the other side effects cause minimal problems in most patients and appear to be dose dependent. Hirsutism may be particularly troublesome in females and occurs in all patients to some extent, as does hypertrophy of the gums.

A good deal of effort has been expended in the measurement of blood and serum levels of CyA both by a radioimmune assay (RIA) and high performance liquid chromatography (HPLC). It appears that the drug is quite rapidly absorbed, reaching peak levels between 2 and 6 hours after oral ingestion and trough levels by 12 hours.[122–124] However there is considerable disagreement as to whether serum or blood levels correlate with either CyA toxicity or immunosuppression. In general, although some units have been able to show a correlation between high blood or serum trough levels and nephrotoxicity,[125] most have not.[126] As regards immunosuppression, on the other hand, most units find some crude correlation between blood or serum levels and suppression of rejection of renal allografts,[91] although this correlation is not strong enough to be of value in the individual patient.

Immunologic monitoring of T lymphocyte subpopulations in the peripheral blood of patients with a renal allograft using monoclonal antibodies has suggested that there is a reduction in the ratio of helper-inducer T cells to cytotoxic-suppressor T cells.[125, 127] Using monoclonal antibodies, the cellular infiltrate seen so commonly in renal allografts in patients receiving CyA, has been examined by the Oxford group, and the bulk of the cells in the kidney appear to belong to the cytotoxic-suppressor population, regardless of whether the patient shows clinical evidence of rejection or not (unpublished observations).

Conclusions

Cyclosporin A is an exciting new immunosuppressive agent, with a relatively specific action directed at T lymphocytes in all species. In experimental transplantation Cyclosporin A has produced impressive prolongation of the actuarial survival rate of most tissue allografts in many species. In clinical tissue, transplantation CyA has proved already to be a potent immunosuppressive drug. The allograft survival in renal transplantation appears to be improved significantly, and adequate immunosuppression has been achieved in many patients without or with minimal use of steroids. This is probably true also of liver and cardiac transplantation. The impact of CyA on pancreatic and bone marrow transplantation is less clear at this time but may represent an advance in immunosuppression. Although many side effects of the drug have been seen, nephrotoxicity is by far the major problem associated with the use of this drug in the human. Nevertheless, the impact of CyA on transplantation promises to be enormous, for in addition to a most impressive debut in the clinical arena, CyA will no doubt be the forerunner of a whole new family of immunosuppressive agents encompassing these unique properties.

REFERENCES

1. Morris P.J.: Cyclosporin A: Overview. *Transplantation* 32:349, 1981.
2. Borel, J.F., Feurer C., Gubler H.U., et al.: Biological effects of cyclosporin A: A new antilymphocytic agent. *Agents Actions* 6:468, 1976.
3. Borel J.F., Feurer C., Magnee C., et al.: Effects of the new anti-lymphocyte peptide cyclosporin A in animals. *Immunology* 32:1017, 1977.
4. Borel J.: The history of cyclosporin A and its significance, in White D.J. (ed.): *Cyclosporin A*. Elsevier Biomedical, p. 5.
5. Wenger R.: Chemistry of cyclosporin, in White D.J. (ed.): *Cyclosporin A*. Elsevier Biomedical, p. 19.
6. Kostakis A.J., White D.J.G., Calne R.Y.: Prolongation of rat heart allograft survival by cyclosporin A. *Ir. J. Med. Sci.* 5:280, 1977.
7. Calne R.Y., White D.J.G.: Cyclosporin A—A powerful immunosuppressant in dogs with renal allografts. *Ir. J. Med. Sci.* 5:595, 1977.
8. Green C.J., Allison A.C.: Extensive prolongation of rabbit kidney allograft survival after short term cyclosporin A treatment. *Lancet* 1:1182, 1978.
9. Calne R.Y., Rolles K., White D.J.G., et al.: Cyclosporin A initially as the only immunosuppressant in 34 recipients of cadaveric organs: 32 kidneys, 2 pancreases and 2 livers. *Lancet* 2:1033, 1979.
10. Homan W.P., Fabre J.W., Williams K.A., et al.: Studies on the immu-

nosuppressive properties of cyclosporin A in rats receiving renal allografts. *Transplantation* 29:361, 1980.

11. Homan W.P., Fabre J.W., Millard P.R., et al.: Effect of cyclosporin A upon second-set rejection of rat renal allografts. *Transplantation* 30:354, 1980.

12. Homan W.P., Fabre J.W., Morris P.J.: Nature of the unresponsiveness induced by cyclosporin A in rats bearing renal allografts. *Transplantation* 28:439, 1979.

13. Homan W.P., Fabre J.W., Millard P.R., et al.: Interaction of cyclosporin A with antilymphocyte serum and with enhancing serum for the suppression of renal allograft rejection in the rat. *Transplantation* 29:219, 1980.

14. Dunn D.C., White D.J.F., Herbertson B.M., et al.: Prolongation of kidney survival during and after cyclosporin A therapy. *Transplantation* 27:359, 1979.

15. Green C.J., Allison A.C., Precious S.: Induction of specific tolerance in rabbits by kidney allografting and short periods of cyclosporin A treatment. *Lancet* 2:123, 1979.

16. Dunn D.C.: The specificity of post-cyclosporin "tolerance." *Transplant. Proc.* 13:383, 1981.

17. White D.J.G., Rolles K., Ottawa T.: Cyclosporin-A-induced long-term survival of fully incompatible skin and heart grafts in rats. *Transplant. Proc.* 12:261, 1980.

18. Homan W.P., French M.E., Millard P.R., et al.: Studies on the effects of cyclosporin A upon renal allograft rejection in the dog. *Surgery* 88:168, 1980.

19. DuToit D.F., Homan W.P., Morris P.J.: The effect of cyclosporin A on experimental renal and pancreatic allografts in the dog, in D. White (ed.): *Cyclosporin A.* Elsevier, Biomedical, p. 101.

20. Homan W.P., French M.E., Fabre J.W., et al.: The interaction of cyclosporin A with other immunosuppressive agents in dog recipients of renal allografts. *Transplant. Proc.* 12:287, June 1980.

21. Homan W.P., French M.E., Millard P.J., et al.: A study of eleven drug regimens using cyclosporin A to suppress renal allograft rejection in the dog. *Transplant. Proc.* 13:397, 1981.

22. Homan W.P., Fabre J.W., French M.E., et al.: Reversal of acute rejection episodes by cyclosporin A in dogs receiving renal allografts. *Transplantation* 29:262, 1980.

23. Margreiter R., Huber C., Spielberger M., et al.: Cyclosporin (Cy) in the treatment of acute cadaveric kidney graft rejection refractory to high dose methylprednisolone (MP). *Transplantation* 36:203, 1983.

24. Cosimi A.B., Shield C.F., Peters C., et al.: Prolongation of allograft survival by cyclosporin A. *Surg. Forum* 30:287, 1978.

25. Borleffs J.C., Neuhaus P., Marquet R.L., et al.: Cyclosporin A and kidney transplantation in rhesus monkeys, in White D.J. (ed.): *Cyclosporin A.* Elsevier, Biomedical, p. 329, 1982.

26. Smit J.A., Drielsma R.F., Myburgh J.A., et al.: Renal allograft survival in the baboon using a pretreatment protocol with Cyclosporin A. *Transplantation.* 36:121, 1983.

27. Nagao T., White D.J.G., Calne R.Y.: Kinetics of unresponsiveness induced by a short course of cyclosporin A. *Transplantation* 33:31, 1982.
28. White D.J.G., Timmerman W., Davies Hff., et al.: Properties of cyclosporin-A-induced graft acceptance. *Transplant. Proc.* 13:379, 1981.
29. White D.J., Nagao T., Davies Hff.: Experimental transplantation in small animals, in White D. (ed.): *Cyclosporin A.* Elsevier Medical, p. 89, 1982.
30. Calne R.Y., White D.J.G., Rolles K., et al.: Prolonged survival of pig orthotopic heart grafts with cyclosporin A. *Lancet* 1:1183, 1978.
31. Jamieson S.W., Burton N.A., Beiber C.P. et al.: Cardiac allograft survival in primates treated with cyclosporin A. *Lancet* 1:545, 1979.
32. Pennock J., Reitz B.A., Bieber C.P., et al.: Cardiac allograft survival in cynomolgus monkeys treated with cyclosporin A in combination with conventional immune suppression. *Transplant. Proc.* 13:390, 1981.
33. Reitz B., Bieber C.P., Raney A.A., et al.: Orthotopic heart and combined heart and lung transplantation with cyclosporin A immune suppression. *Transplant. Proc.* 13:393, 1981.
34. Reitz B.A., Bieber C.B., Pennock J.L.: Cyclosporin A and lymphoma in non-human primates, in White D.J. (ed.): *Cyclosporin A.* Elsevier Biomedical, p. 317, 1982.
35. Garvey J.F.W., McShane P., Poole M.D., et al.: The effect of cyclosporin A on experimental pancreas allografts in the rat. *Transplant. Proc.* 12:266, 1980.
36. Rynasiewicz J.J., Sutherland D.E.R., Kawahara K., et al.: Cyclosporin A prolongation of segmental pancreatic and islet allograft function in rats. *Transplant. Proc.* 12:270, 1980.
37. Reece–Smith H., Homan W.P., DuToit D.F., et al.: A technique for transplanting pancreatic islets as a vascularized graft and prevention of rejection with cyclosporin A. *Transplantation* 31:442, 1981.
38. Morris P.J., Finch D.R., Garvey J.F., et al.: Suppression of rejection of allogeneic islet tissue in the rat. *Diabetes* 29:107, 1980.
39. DuToit D.F., Reece–Smith H., McShane P., et al.: Prolongation of segmental pancreatic allografts in dogs receiving cyclosporin A. *Transplantation* 33:432, 1982.
40. Calne R.Y., White D.J.G., Pentlow B.D., et al.: Cyclosporin A: Preliminary observations irt dogs with pancreatic duodenal allografts and patients with cadaveric renal transplants. *Transplant. Proc.* 11:860, 1979.
41. DuToit D.F., Reece–Smith H., McShane P., et al.: Effect of cyclosporin A on allotransplanted pancreatic fragments to the spleen of totally pancreatectomized dogs. *Transplantation* 33:302, 1982.
42. Zimmerman F.A., Butcher G.W., Davies H.S., et al.: Techniques for orthotopic liver transplantation in the rat and some studies of the immunologic responses to fully allogeneic liver grafts. *Transplant. Proc.* 11:571, 1979.
43. Kamada N.: Personal communication.
44. Müller G., Morris P.J.: Unresponsiveness induced by a short course of Cyclosporin A in liver grafted rats to subsequent kidney and heart grafts. (In preparation.)
45. Veith F.J., Norin A.J., Emeson E.E., et al.: Experimental lung trans-

plantation with cyclosporin A, in White D.J. (ed.): *Cyclosporin A*. Elsevier Biomedical, p. 143, 1982.

46. Veith F.J., Sinha S.B., Dougherty J.C.: Nature and evolution of lung allograft rejection with and without immunosuppression. *J. Thorac. Cardiovasc. Surg.* 63:509, 1972.

47. Lems S.P.M., Capel P.J.A., Koene R.A.P.: Prolongation of mouse skin allograft survival by cyclosporin A. Graft rejection after withdrawal of therapy. *Transplant. Proc.* 12:283, 1980.

48. Borel J.F., Meszaros J.: Skin transplantation in mice and dogs: Effect of cyclosporin A and dihydrocyclosporin C. *Transplantation* 29:161, 1980.

49. Gratwohl A., Forster I., Speck B.: Skin grafts in rabbits with cyclosporin A. Absence of induction of tolerance and untoward side effects. *Transplantation* 31:136, 1981.

50. Deeg H.J., Storb R., Gerhard–Miller L., et al.: Cyclosporin A, a powerful immunosuppressant in vivo and in vitro in the dog, fails to induce tolerance. *Transplantation* 29:230, 1980.

51. Homan W.P., Williams K.A., Fabre J.W., et al.: Prolongation of cardiac xenograft survival in rats receiving cyclosporin A. *Transplantation* 31:164, 1980.

52. Green C.J., Kemp E., Kemp G., et al.: Prolongation of concordant renal xenografts in rabbit recipients by a short course of cyclosporin A treatment, in White D.J. (ed.): *Cyclosporin A*. Elsevier Biomedical, pp. 156–163, 1982.

53. Green C.J., Kemp E., Kemp C.: The effects of cyclosporin A, ticlopidine hydrochloride and cobra venom factor in the hyperacute rejection of discordant renal xenografts. *J. Invest. Cell. Pathol.* 3:415, 1980.

54. van Bekkum D.W., Knaan S., Zurcher C.: Effects of cyclosporin A on experimental graft-versus-host disease (GvHD) in rodents. *Transplant. Proc.* 12:278, 1980.

55. Tutschka P.J., Beschorner W.E., Allison A.C., et al.: Use of cyclosporin A in allogeneic bone marrow transplantation in the rat. *Nature* 20:148, 1979.

56. Tutschka P.J., Hess A.D., Beschorner W.E., et al.: Suppressor cells in transplantation tolerance. I. Suppressor cells in the mechanism of tolerance in radiation chimera. *Transplantation* 32:203, 1981.

57. Tutschka P.J., King P.F., Beschorner W.E., et al.: Suppressor cells in transplantation tolerance. II. Maturation of suppressor cells in the bone marrow chimera. *Transplantation* 32:321, 1981.

58. Deeg H.J., Storb R., Weiden P.L., et al.: Cyclosporin-A effect on marrow engraftment and graft-versus-host disease in dogs. *Transplant. Proc.* 13:402, 1981.

59. Gratwohl A., Cornu P., Casanova S., et al.: Transplantation with cryopreserved allogeneic histocompatible rabbit bone marrow and cyclosporin A. *Exp. Hematol.* 8(suppl):13, 1980.

60. Deeg H.J., Storb R. Experimental marrow transplantation, in White D.J. (ed.): *Cyclosporin A*. Elsevier Biomedical, pp. 121–134, 1982.

61. Homan W.P., Williams K.A., Millard P.R., et al.: Prolongation of renal allograft survival in the rat by pretreatment with donor antigen and cyclosporin A. *Transplantation* 31:423, 1981.

62. Wiesinger D., Borel J.F.: Studies on mechanism of action of cyclosporin A. Immunobiology 156:454, 1979.
63. Larsson E.L.: Cyclosporin A and dexamethasone suppress T cell responses by selectively acting at distinct sites of the triggering process. J. Immunol. 124:2828, 1980.
64. Borel J.F.: Cyclosporin A—present experimental status. Transplant. Proc. 13:344, 1981.
65. Burckhardt J.J., Guggenheim B.: Cyclosporin A: In vivo and in vitro suppression of rat T-lymphocyte function. Immunology 36:753, 1979.
66. Leapman S.B., Filo R.S., Smith E.J., et al.: Differential effects of cyclosporin A on lymphocyte subpopulations. Transplant. Proc. 13:405, 1981.
67. Leoni P., Garcia R.C., Allison A.C.: Effects of cyclosporin A on human lymphocytes in culture. J. Clin. Lab. Immunol. 1:67, 1978.
68. White D.J.G., Plumb A.M., Pawelec G., et al.: Cyclosporin A: An immunosuppressive agent preferentially active against proliferating T cells. Transplantation 27:55, 1979.
69. Tutschka P.J., Hess A.D., Beschorner W.E., et al.: Cyclosporin A in allogeneic bone marrow transplantation: Preclinical and clinical studies, in White D.J. (ed.): Cyclosporin A. Elsevier Biomedical, pp. 519–538, 1982.
70. Horsburgh T., Wood P., Brent L.: Suppression of in vivo lymphocyte reactivity by cyclosporin A: Existence of a population of drug-resistant cytotoxic lymphocytes. Nature 286:609, 1980.
71. Hess A.D., Tutschka P.J.: Effect of cyclosporin A on human lymphocyte responses in vitro. I. CS-A allows for the expression of alloantigen-activated suppressor cells while preferentially inhibiting the induction of cytolytic effector lymphocytes in MLR. J. Immunol. 124:2601, 1980.
72. Keown P.A., Essery G.L., Stiller C.R., et al.: Mechanisms of immunosuppression by cyclosporin. Transplant. Proc. 13:386, 1981.
73. Hess A.D., Tutschka P.J., Santos G.W.: The effect of cyclosporin A on T-lymphocyte subpopulations, in White D.J. (ed.): Cyclosporin A. Elsevier Biomedical, pp. 209–231, 1982.
74. Bunjes D., Hardt C., Solbach W., et al.: Studies on the mechanism of action of cyclosporin A in the murine and human T-cell response in vitro, in White D.J. (ed.): Cyclosporin A. Elsevier Biomedical, pp. 261–280, 1982.
75. Gordon M.Y., Singer J.W.: Selective effects of cyclosporin A on colony-forming lymphoid and myeloid cells in man. Nature 279:433, 1979.
76. Kunkl A., Klaus G.G.B.: Selective effects of cyclosporin A on functional B cell subsets in the mouse. J. Immunol. 125:2526, 1980.
77. Cammisuli S.: The effect of cyclosporin A on cell interactions within the immune system, in White D.J. (ed.): Cyclosporin A. Elsevier Biomedical, pp. 243–259, 1982.
78. Kahan B.D., Kerman R.H., Agostino G., et al.: The action of cyclosporin A on human lymphocytes, in White D.J. (ed.): Cyclosporin A. Elsevier Biomedical, pp. 281–293, 1982.
79. Palacios R., Möller G.: Cyclosporin A blocks receptors for HLA-DR antigens on T cells. Nature 290:792, 1981.
80. Hess A.D., Tutschka P.J., Santos G.W.: Effect of cyclosporin A on hu-

man lymphocyte responses in vitro. II. Induction of specific alloantigen unresponsiveness mediated by a nylon wool adherent suppressor cell. *J. Immunol.* 126:961, 1981.

81. Paavonent T., Häyny P.: Effect of cyclosporin A on T-dependent and T-independent immunoglobulin synthesis in vitro. *Nature* 287:542, 1980.

82. Thomson A.W., Moon D.K., Geczy C.L., et al.: Cyclosporin A inhibits lymphokine production but not the responses of macrophages to lymphokines. *Immunology.* (In press.)

83. Nemlander A., Ahonen J., Wiktorowicz K., et al.: Effect of cyclosporin A on wound healing. An analysis with viscous cellulose sponges. *Transplantation* 36:1–6, 1983.

84. Calne R.Y., Rolles K., White D.J.G., et al.: Cyclosporin A in clinical organ grafting. *Transplant. Proc.* 13:349, 1981.

85. Calne R.Y., White D.J. The use of cyclosporin A in clinical organ grafting. *Ann. Surg.* 196:330–336, 1982.

86. European Multicentre Trial. Cyclosporin A as sole immunosuppressive agent in recipients of kidney allografts from cadaver donors. *Lancet* 2:57, 1982.

87. Ferguson R.M., Rynasiewicz J.J., Sutherland D.E., et al.: Cyclosporin A in renal transplantation: a prospective randomized trial. *Surgery* 92:175–181, 1982.

88. Najarian J.S., Ferguson R.M., Sutherland D.E., et al.: A prospective trial of the efficacy of cyclosporin in renal transplantation at the University of Minnesota. *Transplant. Proc.* 15:438, 1983.

89. Starzl T.E., Iwatsuki S., Klintmalm G., et al.: Liver transplantation 1980, with particular reference to cyclosporin A. *Transplant. Proc.* 13:281, 1981.

90. Starzl T.E., Hakula T.R., Iwatsuki S., et al.: Cyclosporin A and steroid treatment in 104 cadaveric renal transplantations, in White D.J. (ed.): *Cyclosporin A.* Elsevier Biomedical, pp. 364–377, 1982.

91. Morris P.J., French M.E., Ting A., et al.: A controlled trial of cyclosporin A in renal transplantation, in White D.J. (ed.): *Cyclosporin A.* Elsevier Biomedical, p. 355, 1982.

92. Fletchner S.M., Kerman R.H., van Bueen C., et al.: The use of cyclosporin and prednisone for high MLC haploidentical living related renal transplants. *Transplant. Proc.* 15:442, 1983.

93. Starzl T.E., Iwatsuki S., van Thiel D.H., et al.: Evolution of liver transplantation. *Hepatology.* 2:614, 1982.

94. Oyer P.E., Stinson E.B., Reitz B.A., et al.: Preliminary results with cyclosporin A in clinical cardiac transplantation, in White D.J. (ed.): *Cyclosporin A.* Elsevier Biomedical, p. 461, 1982.

95. Griffith B.P., Hardesty R.L., Deeb G.M., et al.: Cardiac transplantation with cyclosporin A and prednisone. *Ann. Surg.* 196:324, 1982.

96. Beveridge T.: Cyclosporin A: An evaluation of clinical results. *Transplant. Proc.* (In press.)

97. Reitz B.A., Wallwork J.L., Hunt S.A., et al.: Cyclosporin A for combined heart-lung transplantation, in White D.J. (ed.): *Cyclosporin A.* Elsevier Biomedical, pp. 473–478, 1982.

98. Sutherland D.E.: Current status of pancreas transplantation: Registry statistics and an overview. *Transplant. Proc.* 15:1303, 1983.
99. Rynasiewicz J.J., Sutherland D.E. Goetz F.C., et al.: Clinical pancreas transplantation with cyclosporin A at the University of Minnesota, in White D.J. (ed.): *Cyclosporin A.* Elsevier Biomedical, pp. 437–452, 1982.
100. McMaster P., Buckels J., Gibby D., et al.: Combined renal and pancreratic transplantation with cyclosporin A, in White D.J. (ed.): *Cyclosporin A.* Elsevier Biomedical, pp. 453–460, 1982.
101. Powles R.L., Morgenstern G.R.: Cyclosporin A to prevent graft-versus-host disease in man following HLA/MLC matched allogeneic bone marrow transplantation, in White D.J. (ed.): *Cyclosporin A.* Elsevier Biomedical, pp. 485–489, 1982.
102. Speck B., Gratwohl A., Nissen C., et al.: Bone marrow grafting for leukaemia and aplastic anaemia, in White D.J. (ed.): *Cyclosporin A.* Elsevier Biomedical, pp. 491–496, 1982.
103. Lokiec F., Porrier D., Gluckman E., et al.: A pharmacokinetic study of cyclosporin A: Preliminary results, in Touraine J., Gluckman E., Griscelli E. (eds.): *Bone Marrow Transplantation in Europe.* Excerpta Medica, Amsterdam, 1981, pp. 160–164.
104. Hows J.M., Palmer S., Gordon–Smith E.C.: Cyclosporin A in compatible grafting for severe aplastic anaemia, in D.J. White, (ed.): Cyclosporin A. Elsevier Biomedical, pp. 511–518, 1982.
105. Storb R., Thomas, E.D.: Current state of marrow transplantation, in *Contemporary Hematology and Oncology.* (In press.)
106. Powles R.L., Morgenstern G.R.: Allogeneic bone marrow transplantation using mismatched family donors, in White D.J. (ed.): *Cyclosporin A.* Elsevier Biomedical, pp. 539–543, 1982.
107. Homan W.P., French M.E., Morris P.J.: Effect of cyclosporin A upon the function of ischemically damaged renal autografts in the dog. *Transplantation* 30:228, 1980.
108. Whiting P.H., Thomson A.W., Blair J.T., et al.: Experimental cyclosporin A nephrotoxicity. *Br. J. Exp. Path.* 63:88, 1982.
109. Thompson A.W., Whiting P.H., Simpson J.G.: Pathobiology of cyclosporin A in experimental animals, in White D.J. (ed.): *Cyclosporin A.* Elsevier Biomedical, pp. 177–190, 1982.
110. Powell–Jackson P.R., Young B., Calne R.Y., Williams R.: Nephrotoxicity of parenterally administered cyclosporin A after orthotopic liver transplantation. *Transplantation.* (In press.)
111. Klintman G.B., Iwatsuki S., Starzl T.E.: Cyclosporin A hepatoxicity in 66 renal allograft recipients. *Transplantation* 32:488–489, 1981.
112. Hedley D., Powles R.L., Morgenstern G.R.: Toxicity of cyclosporin A in patients following bone marrow transplantation, in White D.J. (ed.): *Cyclosporin A.* Elsevier Biomedical, pp. 545–551, 1982.
113. Lokiec F., Poirier O., Gluckman E., et al.: Cyclosporin A: Pharmacokinetic monitoring during treatment of graft-versus-host disease following bone marrow transplantation, in White D.J. (ed.): *Cyclosporin A.* Elsevier, Biomedical, pp. 497–500, 1982.
114. Shulman H., Striker G., Deeg H.J., et al.: Nephrotoxicity of cyclosporin

A after allogeneic marrow transplantation—glomerular thromboses and tubular injury. *N. Engl. J. Med.* 305:1392–1395, 1981.

115. French M.E., Thompson J.F., Hunnisett A.G., et al.: Impaired function of renal allografts during treatment with cyclosporin A: Nephrotoxicity or rejection? *Transplant. Proc.* 15:485, 1983.

116. Whiting P.H., Simpson J.G., Davidson R.J., et al.: The toxic effects of combined administration of cyclosporin A and gentamycin. *Brit. J. Exp. Path.* 63:554, 1982.

117. Thompson J.F., Chalmers D.H., Hunnisett A.G., et al.: Nephrotoxicity of Trimethoprim and co-trimoxazole in renal allograft recipients treated with cyclosporin A. *Transplantation.* 36:204, 1983.

118. Hamilton D.V., Evans D.B., Henderson S., et al.: Long-term nephrotoxicity of cyclosporin A in transplantation. *Dialysis and Trans.* 11:146, 1982.

119. Thiru S., Calne R.Y., Nagington J.: Lymphoma in renal allograft patients treated with cyclosporin A as one of the immunosuppressive agents. *Transplant. Proc.* 13:359, 1981.

120. Bird A.G.: Cyclosporin A, lymphomata and Epstein–Barr virus, in White D.J. (ed.): *Cyclosporin A.* Elsevier Biomedical, pp. 307–315, 1982.

121. Bird A.G., McGlachlan S.M., Britton S.: Cyclosporin A promotes spontaneous outgrowth in vitro of Epstein–Barr virus induced B cell lines. *Nature (Lond.)* 289:300–301, 1981.

122. Beveridge T., Gratwohl A., Michot F., et al.: Cyclosporin A: Pharmacokinetics after a single dose in man and serum levels after multiple dosing in recipients of allogeneic bone marrow grafts. *Curr. Ther. Res.* 30:5, 1981.

123. Kahan B.D., Ried M., Newburger J.: Pharmacokinetics of cyclosporin in human renal transplantation. *Transplant. Proc.* 15:446, 1983.

124. Keown P.A., Stiller C.R., Ulan R.A., et al.: Immunological and pharmacological monitoring in the clinical use of cyclosporin A. *Lancet* 1:686, 1981.

125. Kahan B.D., van Buren C.T., Lin S.N., et al.: Immunopharmacological monitoring of cyclosporin A-treated recipients of cadaveric kidney allografts. *Transplantation* 34:36–45, 1982.

126. Attridge S.R., Powles R.L., Hedley D., et al.: Serum cyclosporin A levels in bone marrow transplant patients, in White D.J. (ed.): *Cyclosporin A.* Elsevier Biomedical, pp. 553–558, 1982.

127. Carter N.P., Cullen P.R., Thompson J.F., et al.: Monitoring lymphocyte subpopulations in renal allograft recipients. *Transplant. Proc.* 15:1157, 1983.

128. Canadian Multicentre Transplant Study Group. A randomized clinical trial of cyclosporin in cadaveric renal transplantation. *N. Eng. J. Med.* (In press.)

129. Klaus C.G., Dongworth D.W.: Effects of Cyclosporin A and B cell functioning in the mouse, in White D.J. (ed.): Cyclosporin A. Elsevier Biomedical, p. 233.

130. Powles R.L., Barrett A.J., Clink H., et al.: Cyclosporin A for the treatment of graft-versus-host disease in man. *Lancet* ii: 1327, 1978.

131. Powles R.L., Clink H.M., Spence D., et al.: Cyclosporin A to prevent

graft-versus-host disease in man after allogeneic bone-marrow transplantation. *Lancet* i: 327, 1980.
132. Ringden O., Collste H., Klintmalm G., et al.: Cyclosporin A in high-risk renal transplant recipients and in recipients with azathioprine intolerance. *Transplant. Proc.* 14:100, 1982.
133. Thompson J.F., Chalmers D.H., Carter N.P., et al.: Clinical and immunological effects of conversion to Cyclosporin A therapy in long-term renal allograft recipients. *Transplant. Proc.* (In press.)

Hepatic Resection in Trauma

DATÓ M. BALASEGARAM, M.B.

*Department of Surgery, National University of Malaysia Medical College,
and General Hospital, Kuala Lumpur, Malaysia*

IN RECENT YEARS the mortality and morbidity from hepatic trauma have steadily decreased, although the incidence of hepatic trauma is on the increase.[1] Mild injuries with only capsular splits and lacerations, without serious hemorrhage, and moderate injuries with deeper lacerations, tearing branches of the intrahepatic vessels and bile ducts, currently account for about 80%–85% of liver trauma. They can usually be successfully treated by suture ligation, hepatic artery ligation, hepatostomy and drainage and/or "resectional debridement" with drainage.

However, controversy persists about the management of the remaining 15%–20% of cases of severe hepatic trauma, in which there is major disruption of the hepatic parenchyma with tearing of the hepatic veins and inferior vena cava. Since the leading cause of death in liver trauma is hemorrhage and since the main complication is subsequent sepsis, hepatic resection offers the quickest, safest, and most definitive method of treatment, both for control of hemorrhage and for removal of devitalized liver tissue.[2] Survival rates are good. The formula for successful treatment of major hepatic trauma is the same as for successful hepatic resection: control of hemostasis (Fig 1).

Nevertheless, recently there has been a movement away from hepatic resection, mainly because of its reported high mortality, and toward more conservative management of severe injuries by nonresectional methods. However, careful analysis of the published series shows that the high mortalities

129

0065-3411/84/0017-0129-0170-$04.00

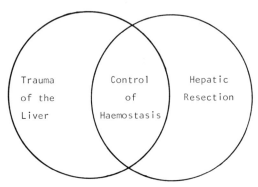

Fig 1.—Diagrammatic representation of management of extensive injury to the liver.

reported for hepatic resection could be misleading. Since many authors fail to indicate, first, whether the mortality is related to associated injuries or to the liver per se, and second, the type and extent of the resections performed; all patients are described as having "lobectomy."

This chapter discusses some precise indications for hepatic resection, correlating mortality rates with each type of resection. It also reviews an anatomical classification of the liver, based on cadaveric study of 100 normal human livers with rubber casts, and describes in simple terms the operative technique of hepatic resection using specially designed instruments and suture materials. The surgical unit at the General Hospital in Kuala Lumpur is the only referral center in Malaysia (population 14 million) for the more complicated problems of hepatic trauma and thus affords wide experience in diagnostic and therapeutic problems.

Historical Background

The historical background of hepatic injuries is of great interest and importance to an understanding of their incidence, diagnosis, and treatment. The serious consequences of liver injuries were observed more than 2,000 years ago by Hippocrates (ca. 460–360 BC), who noted that "a severe wound of the liver is deadly." Until the latter part of the 19th century, wounds of the liver were considered fatal and were treated nonoperatively, although isolated instances of successful management of civilian wounds were reported. In 1870, Bruns[3] resected a lacerated portion of the liver following a gunshot wound, and Burckhardt[4] in 1887 arrested hemorrhage from an injured liver by packing. By 1896, Kousnetzoff and Penski[5] were able to describe several methods of repair of liver wounds.

The vast majority of civilian surgeons continued to treat liver injuries conservatively, well into the 20th century. Since liver wounds were seen in large numbers during wartime, it was left to military surgeons to deal with the problem of penetrating wounds, but far less progress was made with blunt trauma. Understanding and progress in the treatment of penetrating wounds gradually improved during the two world wars. Hemorrhage came to be recognized as an immediate threat to life in liver injuries, and early operation was advocated for its control. Pringle's classic description of temporarily arresting hemorrhage from liver wounds was an outstanding contribution.[6]

Operative intervention for liver trauma was then followed by packing, suturing, and the use of free muscle grafts in an attempt to achieve permanent hemostasis and healing of repaired hepatic wounds. However, as no emphasis was placed on the importance of abdominal drainage, sepsis became a serious complication. In World War II, the experience of the Second Auxiliary Surgical Group of the United States Army[7] brought to light the importance of early surgical intervention, the disadvantage of packing as a definitive treatment, and the value of drainage. In a comparison of operations done in 1944 and 1945 by this surgical group for 695 liver injuries, nonoperative treatment decreased from 9.8% to 1.2% and packing of liver wounds from 65% to 9.6%, while drainage increased from 48.5% to 87.4% of cases.[7] Mortality was reduced from 34% in 1944 to 15% in 1945.

With the end of World War II, the treatment of liver wounds began to assume greater importance, owing to the tremendous increase in the incidence of hepatic trauma, both blunt and penetrating. High-speed road accidents and civil violence, including the use of high-velocity missiles, accounted for bursting or shattering wounds of the liver parenchyma. Since sepsis was the major late complication in such injuries, surgeons were forced to undertake more drastic forms of treatment such as debridement of devitalized tissue and hepatic resection.

As is usual in a complex field of surgery, there are widely differing views on the best methods of managing such major hepatic trauma, and particularly on the role of hepatic resection. Against this background, I will discuss my experience in managing 443 patients with hepatic trauma, with particular reference to hepatic resection.

Essentials for a Successful Hepatic Resection

The essentials for a successful hepatic resection are as follows:

1. Knowledge of hepatic anatomy and anomalies in relation to trauma and line of resections.
2. Knowledge of types of resections and bases for choosing.
3. Surgical instruments specifically designed for achieving hemostasis of the liver and aiding in resection.
4. Diagnostic accuracy and assessment of extent of injury.
5. Immediate laparotomy and readiness for resection. Mortality decreases in inverse proportion to the time spent on careful preoperative diagnostic studies.
6. Knowledge of diverse functions of liver and physiologic consequences of resections (jaundice, hypoproteinemia, coagulation factor deficiencies, liver failure pathways).
7. Aids to liver regeneration following resection (hyperalimentation with amino acids and vitamins).

Each of these factors is described in detail below.

KNOWLEDGE OF HEPATIC ANATOMY

An understanding of both the normal and anomalous features of the hepatic vasculature and biliary ductal system, and particularly knowledge of the divisions of the liver with respect to types of hepatic resection, are of vital importance in the surgical approach to the liver. A simplified and universal terminology is also important, as the classification of hepatic resection in the literature is quite confusing. Much of the confusion stems from incorrect usage of terms such as "surgical lobe," "clinical lobe," "lobar resection," or "lobectomy." Recent addition of the term "trisegmentectomy" has only compounded the already existing confusion. There is no technical basis for the term "trisegmentectomy" because the procedure concerns only two segments of the liver—the medial and lateral segments of the left lobe. Similarly, the term "middle lobectomy" should be avoided as there is no middle lobe to the liver. Moreover, the right lobe is divided into posterolateral and anteromedial segments.[8]

The liver is divided into right and left lobes by the principal plane, which extends vertically upward in a straight line from the apex of the gallbladder fossa just to the right of the inferior vena cava at the foramen, dividing the gallbladder bed inferiorly, bisecting the caudate lobe posteriorly, and separating the arteries, veins, and bile ducts. The quadrate lobe forms part of the left lobe. The middle hepatic vein lies along the principal plane in the depths of the liver.

The plane of the falciform ligament divides the left lobe of the liver into medial and lateral segments. The left hepatic vein drains the lateral segment of the left lobe, the so-called classical left lobe described previously, and enters the left anterior aspect of the inferior vena cava. Left lateral segmental resection is performed in this plane, with the hepatic vein tied at the plane or to its left. The middle hepatic vein drains parts of both lobes of the liver: the medial segment of the left lobe and the anteromedial segment of the right lobe. The actual line of resection must therefore be a little to one side or the other of the principal plane, to the right in right hemihepatectomy, and to the left in left hemihepatectomy.

The right hepatic vein drains the posterolateral segment of the right lobe and enters the right anterolateral aspect of the inferior vena cava. Although attempts have been made to demarcate the right lobe into two segments by external signs, the surgical importance of such a subdivision is limited. The surface of separation between the segments is a complicated curve and there is no anatomical landmark that might act as a guide to the position of the boundary. Therefore the term "right lobectomy" in surgery refers to removal of the lateral aspect of the right lobe.[9, 10]

By studying 100 normal human cadaveric livers by dissection, perfusion, and liver casts, using prevulcanized liquid rubber latex, I came to a thorough knowledge of the variations of the arterial, venous, and ductal system, as described in earlier reports.[8, 11] This information is of vital importance when major hepatic resection is performed.

KNOWLEDGE OF TYPES OF HEPATIC RESECTION

A thorough knowledge of the various types of hepatic resection is mandatory to the surgeon.[12] The following anatomical terms have therefore been clearly defined:

Right hemihepatectomy—resection of the right lobe of the liver along an axis corresponding to the right of the middle hepatic vein.

Extended right hemihepatectomy—removal of the liver to the right of the falciform ligament. The medial segment of the liver that is drained by the middle hepatic vein is also removed.

Extended hemihepatectomy—resection of the entire left lobe of the liver to the left of the middle hepatic vein.

Left hemihepatectomy—resection of the entire lobe of the liver to the left of the principal plane.

Right hepatic lobectomy—theoretically, removal of the anteromedial or the posterolateral segment of the right lobe, but there is no definite surgical demarcation. Surgically this is not important, and right hepatic lobectomy is defined as removal of the lateral aspect of the right lobe.

Middle wedge resection—removal of the medial segments of the right and left lobes of the liver drained by the middle hepatic vein. The types of resection and the parts of the liver resected are listed in Table 1.

Combined right hemihepatectomy and left lateral segmental resection—resection of the entire right lobe and the lateral segment of the left lobe, leaving intact the medial segment of the left lobe. This radical procedure is rarely performed.

SPECIFICALLY DESIGNED SURGICAL INSTRUMENTS

In the course of resecting a large number of nontraumatic hepatic lesions, particularly massive liver tumors, I have designed special liver instruments (Fig 2). These have been a deciding factor in the early arrest of hemorrhage and in simplifying and reducing operation time, an important factor in the

TABLE 1.—TYPES OF HEPATIC RESECTIONS FOR TRAUMA

LOCATION AND EXTENT OF INJURY IN THE LIVER	TYPE OF HEPATIC RESECTION	
	Our Terminology (see text)	Parts of Liver Resected
Right lobe, extensive	Right hemihepatectomy	Entire right lobe of liver, including its medial part drained by middle hepatic vein
Right lobe, beyond principal plane	Extended right hemihepatectomy	Entire right lobe and medial segment of left lobe
Right lobe, limited	Right lobectomy	Lateral aspect of the right lobe, not extending to the principal plane
Left lobe, beyond falciform ligament	Left hemihepatectomy	Entire left lobe of the liver
Left lobe, beyond medial segment	Extended left hemihepatectomy	Entire left lobe and medial portion of the right lobe
Left lobe, lateral segment only	Left lateral segmental resection	Lateral segment of the left lobe
Both right and left lobe, but sufficient healthy liver in middle portion	Combined right hemihepatectomy and left lateral segmental resection	Entire right lobe and lateral segment of left lobe
Hilar region	Middle wedge resection	Medial segments of the right and left lobe drained by middle hepatic vein

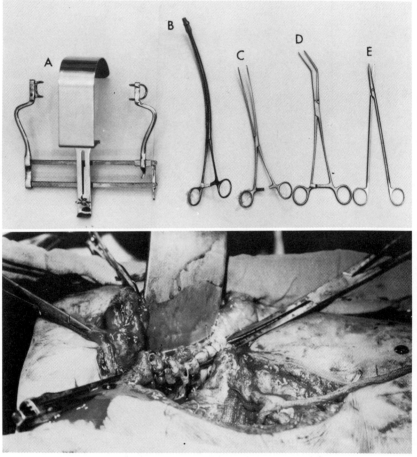

Fig 2 (top).—Instruments for hepatic resection. **A,** a self-retaining abdominohepatic retractor, which provides maximum exposure for right subcostal incisions. The additional adjustable blade permits the mobilized right lobe to be kept in position following rotation to the left side. This facilitates access to the hepatic veins, inferior vena cava, and portal hilum. **B,** large hemostatic liver clamp with 8½-inch (216-mm) curved atraugrip jaws with locking device. The clamp is 14½ inches (368 mm) long overall. **C,** a small liver clamp with 5½-inch (140 mm) curved atraugrip jaws. Clamp is 11 inches (279 mm) long overall. **D,** atraugrip vascular clamp. **E,** long dissecting scissors, 11 inches long, with curved diamond-edged blades and slender tips.

Fig 3 (bottom).—The liver clamp in position for an extended right hemihepatectomy following massive injury to the right lobe of the liver. The edges of the liver have been brought together and sutured prior to release of the clamp.

survival of exsanguinating, critically ill patients. The specially designed instruments are the following.

Self-retaining liver retractor—designed to provide maximum exposure, it contains a specially designed, curved adjustable blade that enables the surgeon to retract the mobilized and exteriorized lobe of the liver and hold it out of the way during surgery (Fig 3).

Long hemostatic liver clamp—a nontraumatic slender clamp with a simple step-locking device at the distal end of the jaws, which can be easily adjusted according to the amount of liver tissue to be gripped (Fig 4). The convex shape of the "atraugrip" jaws conforms to the curvature of the liver. Apart from crushing the liver substance to enable closure of the raw liver edges, the jaws leave the capsule intact. The clamp is light, not cumbersome, and does not slip; more importantly, it facilitates complete hemostasis.

Small hemostatic liver clamp—mainly used for wedge resection.

Atraumatic "atraugrip" jaw vascular clamp.—specially designed for use in the clamping of hepatic veins and inferior vena cava (which require careful handling); it can also be used to occlude the vessels in the portal triad (Fig 5).

Long curved dissecting scissors (11 inch, 28 cm)—with slender tips and diamond-edged blades for easy detachment of the various ligamentous attachments of the liver.

Special suture materials—the raw edges of the liver are brought together with 3-0 metric green, Ethiflex-coated 75-cm polyester (Ethicon), with 90-cm curved, large, round-bodied needle with a sharp tip which does not damage normal liver tissue. These are reinforced by absorbable fibrin buffers made of stabilized ox fibrin (Biethium, Ethicon) (Fig 6).

Clinical Presentation

The 94 patients who underwent hepatic resection for trauma presented in one of three ways:

1. Seventy-nine patients with acute trauma were admitted directly to the Casualty Department at the General Hospital, Kuala Lumpur.

2. Nine patients were referred for definitive treatment from

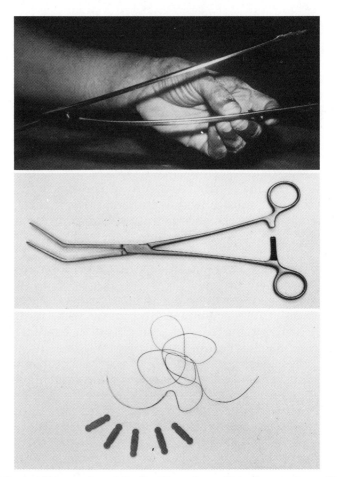

Fig 4 (top).—Closeup view of the long liver clamp. Note the curvature of the jaws and the adjustable step-lock device and atraugrip.

Fig 5 (center).—Close-up view of the atraugrip vascular occlusion clamp.

Fig 6 (bottom).—Biethium buffers and Ethiflex suture with special liver needles used for suturing the liver.

other institutions after laparotomy and temporary gauze packing to arrest the hemorrhage from a badly lacerated liver.

3. The remaining six were referred with late complications of an inadequately treated hepatic injury, such as subhepatic and hepatic abscesses, hemobilia, and biliary discharge.

Diagnosis

DIAGNOSTIC ACCURACY AND ASSESSMENT OF EXTENT OF INJURY

PENETRATING INJURIES.—Isolated penetrating wounds involving the liver posed little difficulty in diagnosis, especially when confined to the lower chest or upper abdomen. Assessment of the depth of injury was made by probing or by radiography following injection of contrast medium; anterior and lateral x-rays often helped determine the presence of a bullet or foreign body. In doubtful cases, exploratory laparotomy was performed.

High-velocity missile wounds were associated with multiple injuries to the upper abdominal organs, resulting in shock or hypotension in one third of the patients, and necessitated urgent laparotomy. These patients were in pallor with abdominal distension and marked tenderness or rigidity.

BLUNT INJURIES.—The mode of presentation in patients with blunt injuries always caused some concern, as the patients' condition varied from normotensive to hypotensive or frankly shocked.[13] Most of the 61 patients admitted directly to our unit had sustained such injuries from automobile accidents, particularly compression injury from the steering wheel, yet 20 had no fractures of the right lower ribs. Associated intraabdominal or concomitant head, chest, pelvic, and/or skeletal injuries often complicated the diagnosis. Suspicion of hepatic injury was often raised by upper abdominal bruising, hematoma, ecchymosis, steering wheel marks over the right upper abdomen and lower chest, tenderness, rigidity, and abdominal distension with hypotension or shock. Shock was present in 17 and hypotension in 28 of 61 patients and necessitated immediate laparotomy. Experience shows the importance of always excluding serious injuries to the organs above or below the diaphragm in every unconscious patient with severe head injury presenting with shock or hypotension.

In the remaining patients, despite a history of trauma, there were minimal physical signs to warrant a diagnosis of acute hepatic injury. Repeated examinations were required at frequent intervals to note changes in the abdominal signs, pulse rate, blood pressure, and central venous pressure. The conscious patient, unless intoxicated, invariably complained of progressive pain in the right upper quadrant of the abdomen, difficulty in breathing, and increased respiration.

Among the patients referred from other centers, the diagnosis was confirmed by the original laparotomy findings or the various investigations.

SPECIAL INVESTIGATIONS

A series of investigations may be required to determine the position and extent of the hepatic injury and its complications, although this is obviously not practicable in the acutely injured patient in shock or hypotension. Only the minimum of investigations must be performed in these patients. This includes blood and biochemical tests such as blood hemoglobin, packed-cell volume, serum amylase level, random blood sugar level, and renal profile. Other investigations may include abdominal paracentesis, erect plain x-rays of the abdomen, and/or chest and intravenous pyelogram (IVP) if there is hematuria suggesting possible renal injury.

Patients presenting with complications of hepatic injury were further investigated by gastroduodenoscopy, ultrasound, hepatic scanning, computerized axial tomography (CT), sinograms, and selective hepatic artery angiography.

ABDOMINAL PARACENTESIS.—Abdominal paracentesis helped confirm the presence of intra-abdominal bleeding when hepatic trauma was suspected.[14, 15] When carried out shortly after admission, abdominal paracentesis was positive in about 95% of patients in this series. A wide-bore, 14-gauge needle was used, in preference to a lumbar puncture needle. Paracentesis is performed in all four quadrants of the abdomen. Failure to aspirate any fluid should not be considered significant. Aspirated peritoneal fluid is observed for blood and analyzed for any elevation of amylase concentration.

PERITONEAL LAVAGE.—This method has proved to be a valuable diagnostic test. The primary indications for lavage are head injuries in unconscious patients, posttraumatic coma, and critical illness, when laparotomy would be a great risk. Lavage is performed by introducing a standard peritoneal dialysis catheter through subumbilical incision into the peritoneum. In the absence of peritoneal fluid aspirate, 1,000 ml of sterile saline is infused into the peritoneum with the patient in a slight

Trendelenburg position. After 15 minutes the returning fluid is observed for red blood cells; counts of more than 100,000 per mm^3 are considered evidence of intra-abdominal injury. The returning fluid is also analyzed for white blood cells, amylase concentration, bile, and the presence or absence of bacteria.

RADIOLOGIC STUDIES.—Plain radiographs of the abdomen and chest are essential and should be obtained simultaneously in the casualty ward. Plain abdominal radiographs have proved most valuable in diagnosing the acutely traumatized patient, because they reveal several important features: (1) raised right hemidiaphragm; (2) loss of clear definition of the hepatic outline and increase in the size of the hepatic shadow; (3) increased homogeneity and opacification of the upper abdomen, with or without loss of the gastric gaseous outline; (4) acute gastric dilatation with displacement of the gastric shadow; (5) duodenal paralytic ileus associated with right hypochondrial homogeneity; (6) relative intestinal paralytic ileus; (7) fracture of the right lower ribs; and (8) loss of clear outline of the right costophrenic angle, early pleural effusion, and right hemothorax/pneumothorax.

Other roentgenographic examinations are necessary in acutely injured patients only if they are likely to give further information about multiple trauma, e.g., blunt injuries to the head, chest, pelvis, and limbs. A careful analysis is of utmost importance in order to avoid time loss in carrying out unnecessary roentgenographic examinations in hypotensive or shocked patients.

Patients referred with additional complications were investigated by sinogram studies to display hepatic or biliary fistulas following mismanaged or inadequate initial treatment of the hepatic injury. Contrast medium was also introduced into the sinus to determine the position and extent of the tract and the rate of closure of the abscess cavity. This provides a comparative basis for assessing the response to treatment and the suitability of conservative management. Cavities that fail to reduce in size over a period of months require active surgical exploration. It also became necessary to intervene surgically in two patients who have persistent biliary fistulas.

Arteriography of the celiac and/or hepatic vessels is not a standard procedure in the management of acutely ill patients with hepatic injuries. However, it can be most informative when hepatic trauma results in the following conditions:[17, 18]

1. Subcapsular hematoma of the liver leading to constant pain and progressive hepatic enlargement: Leakage of contrast medium into the subcapsular region or the absence of vascular outline is indicative of such a lesion. Neely[19] has indicated extensive use of hepatic resections in cases of subcapsular hematoma of the liver when the central cavity is filled with blood and the traumatized liver has not undergone necrosis.

2. Intralobar rupture of the liver—diagnosed in two of the referred patients—causing progressive pain, pallor, and general signs of continuing hemorrhage. The contrast medium was observed to leak into the liver parenchyma.

3. Hemobilia. Although hemobilia is generally due to communication between the arterial and biliary systems, venobiliary communication has also been noted.

4. Liver abscess/necrosis. Arteriography outlines the abscess cavity and the necrotic liver tissue—information of great value in deciding between conservative or operative management.

Radioisotope studies.—These have little place as diagnostic procedures in acute liver trauma; they are time consuming and do not provide greater accuracy than alternative methods. Isotope scanning has, however, proved helpful in the diagnosis of liver abscess and in the localization of resolving subcapsular hematomas. Lung-liver scans are useful in the late phases of hepatic trauma to demonstrate the presence or absence of subdiaphragmatic collection of pus or blood.

CT.—CT was also used to investigate the late phases of hepatic trauma and proved helpful in identifying perihepatic and subdiaphragmatic abscesses. In polytraumatized patients with suspected liver injury, CT was helpful in excluding or locating the site and extent of intra-abdominal injury.[20]

Ultrasonography.—This method is relatively inexpensive, noninvasive, and less time consuming than CT but it has been rarely used in the preoperative diagnosis of acute hepatic trauma.[21]

INDICATIONS FOR INVESTIGATIVE PROCEDURES

Experience in the diagnosis of major hepatic injuries points to the following conclusions about the value of special investigations:

1. Immediate laparotomy is warranted in the presence of shock when there are signs of injury to the upper abdomen or lower chest. Shock is rarely present in patients with uncomplicated head injury.

2. Abdominal paracentesis and peritoneal lavage are helpful in determining the presence of hemoperitoneum and are particularly useful when the physical findings are equivocal or the patient is unconscious—either of which may divert attention from the abdomen. Sinograms are of value in assessing stab wounds.

3. Hepatic scanning, angiography, CT, and ultrasonography are of limited value in acute hepatic trauma, often leading to unnecessary delay in treatment. However, they do have a place in evaluating stable patients who have suspected liver trauma that may be obscured by head injury, subcapsular hematoma, or rupture of the central liver lobe. They may also help to exclude hepatic trauma in polytraumatized patients. These methods are extremely useful in the chronic phase of liver trauma when complications such as subcapsular hematoma, hemobilia, or intrahepatic abscesses are suspected.

Clinical Material

Major hepatic resection was performed on 94 patients between 1961 and 1982 at the General Hospitals of Seremban and Kuala Lumpur in Malaysia. Ten patients were younger than 25 years, 40 patients were aged 25–45 years, and the remaining 44 patients were aged 45–78 years. The youngest was 9 years old and the oldest 78 years. There were 14 female and 80 male patients. Analysis showed that the pattern of injuries varied with the severity and mechanism of the injuring force. Most injuries were the result of road accidents or civil violence; 61 patients sustained blunt trauma and 33 had penetrating injuries, in 26 cases due to high-velocity missiles.

All 61 patients with blunt trauma had extensive lacerations, tears, and subcapsular hematomas with intralobar rupture, including 10 patients with hepatic venous injuries that required major resection, mainly right-sided, hemi-, or extended hemi-resections. All but 7 of the 61 patients survived.

Of the 33 cases of penetrating wounds, 26 were due to high-velocity missiles in instances of civil violence. Twenty-six patients underwent resection and only three died. The remaining seven had stabbing injuries due to an unusual weapon used locally which often caused a churning internal motion, extensively damaging the liver. All underwent resection and survived. The types of hepatic resection performed are summarized in Table 2.

ASSOCIATED INJURIES

Associated and concomitant injuries were present in 24 patients. In instances of penetrating injuries caused by stabbing, the associated injuries were often high in the abdomen, whereas high-velocity missiles and motor vehicles caused both associated intra-abdominal and concomitant injuries of the head, chest, pelvis, and skeleton (Table 3).

Preoperative Assessment and Resuscitation

Three main groups of patients must be considered, according to the timing of their referral.

1. Acute trauma patients admitted directly to the casualty room were quickly and accurately assessed by the consultant surgeon or a senior member of the trauma team. Because most

TABLE 2.–SURGICAL MANAGEMENT OF HEPATIC TRAUMA

	TYPE OF TRAUMA		
TYPE OF REACTION	Blunt	High-Velocity Missile	Stab With Internal Shatter
Right hemihepatectomy	16 (3)*	5 (1)	2
Left hemihepatectomy	14 (1)	7	0
Right extended hemihepatectomy	18 (2)	9 (1)	2
Left extended hemihepatectomy	1	1	0
Left lateral segmental resection	3	2	0
Middle wedge resection	3	0	0
Right lobectomy	6 (1)	1	3
Combined right lobectomy and left lateral segmental resection	0	1 (1)	0
Total resections	61 (7)	26 (3)	7 (0)
Mortality	9.87%	11.53%	. . .

*Numbers in parentheses indicate postoperative deaths.

TABLE 3.—HEPATIC
RESECTION: ASSOCIATED
INJURIES IN 24 PATIENTS*

SITE	NO.
Spleen	6
Stomach	2
Pancreas	3
Cerebral	5
Thoracic	8
Kidney	1
Skeletal	14

*Several patients had two or
more organs involved.

patients with hepatic injury were admitted in shock, the first
priorities were immediate resuscitation and monitoring, notably:

Maintenance of the airway, by endotracheal intubation if
    necessary, with sucking out of any blood or secretion.

Insertion of a central venous pressure cannula into the right
    or left subclavian vein, through a subclavicular approach.

Administration of normal saline or Ringer's solution as
    quickly as possible through the central venous pressure
    line. The total volume transfused may be over 2L/hour. If
    the blood pressure remains low, human albumin and
    plasma protein fractionate including fresh frozen plasma
    are transfused as temporary plasma expanders.

A blood specimen is taken for a few preliminary investiga-
    tions and immediate grouping and cross-matching. In the
    event of hypovolemic shock not responding to the electro-
    lyte solutions and plasma expanders, group O Rh-negative
    blood is obtained urgently from the casualty ward. Fresh
    warm blood[22] is then rapidly transfused through second
    and third peripheral transfusion lines inserted in the an-
    tebrachial and/or cephalic veins. It is important to remem-
    ber that massive transfusion of stored cold blood can cause
    grave coagulopathies and nonmechanical bleeding. Moni-
    toring of the pulse rate and volume, blood pressure, central
    venous pressure, and blood gases is done at frequent inter-
    vals. Any metabolic acidosis is immediately corrected and
    the following measures are taken:

Rapid reassessment of vital signs to determine the response to treatment.

Detailed clinical examination to determine the extent of (a) head injury, (b) chest trauma, including rib features, and lung parenchymal injury with associated pneumothorax/hemothorax, (c) abdominal trauma, and (d) associated skeletal injuries.

Plain x-rays of the chest and abdomen. Views of the skull, pelvis, and skeleton may also be necessary to rule out associated injuries.

Insertion of chest tubes to decrease respiratory distress and collapse in cases of pneumothorax/hemothorax.

Prophylactic administration of broad-spectrum antibiotics.

Emergency laparotomy is then performed, without losing undue time on complicated tests, since delay may be to the detriment of the patient. An emergency laparotomy may sometimes need to be performed in the casualty theater as a life-saving measure.

2. Patients referred following initial resuscitation and laparotomy invariably continued to have mild to moderate anemia, due to blood loss, associated with roller-gauze packing of their hepatic injuries. They were assessed as above, and preliminary investigations were followed by administration of fluids, electrolytes, and colloids. Blood transfusions were given as required. Once stabilized, the patient was reexplored for definitive treatment as early as possible.

3. Patients referred with complications following initial treatment elsewhere were fully investigated before active surgical intervention. In the presence of nutritional depletion secondary to enteroenteric or enterocutaneous fistula, sepsis, or intraperitoneal abscess formation, it was imperative to support the patient by giving nutritional supplements consisting of intravenous fats, proteins, and dextrose, together with high doses of vitamins. Large doses of broad-spectrum antibiotics were essential and were started preoperatively.

Indications for Hepatic Resection

Following are indications for anatomical hepatic resection:

1. Extensive parenchymal damage to the liver (Figs 7 and 8)

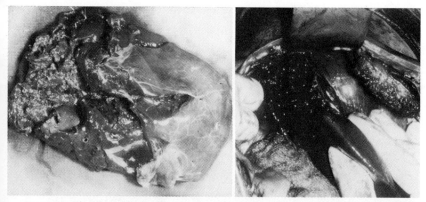

Fig 7 (left).—Resected specimen of a massive laceration of the right lobe of the liver. The 25-year-old patient sustained blunt injury and was admitted in a state of shock. An extended right hemihepatectomy was performed. Recovery was uneventful.

Fig 8 (right).—Laparotomy indicates an extensive injury to the lateral aspect of the right lobe in a 30-year-old patient admitted in an exsanguinated condition following a motor vehicle accident. A Balasegaram liver clamp was used to halt the bleeding, and a right lobectomy was performed.

in which a whole lobe of the liver is lacerated, with transections of intrahepatic branches of the larger vessels and bile ducts.

2. Excessive bleeding into the liver substance, with devitalization of the entire portion of a lobe.

3. High-velocity missile injuries of the liver that cause bursting or shattering injuries of a whole hepatic lobe. In addition to the obviously damaged wound, a zone of liver tissue around the missile tracks sometimes looks normal but may later undergo total necrosis. In the patients studied, these injuries were often caused by M16 or Chinese AK47 assault rifles. Their deceptive appearance is the result of damage to the liver cells by vibration, heat, and/or pressure waves.

4. Subcapsular hematomas of a hepatic lobe (Figs 9 and 10), with intralobar rupture and extensive devitalization and necrosis of the liver tissue extending to the principal plane or falciform ligament.

5. Injury to the hepatic veins or retrohepaticaval veins with wide parenchymal liver damage.

6. Gross damage to the hilar region with parenchymal de-

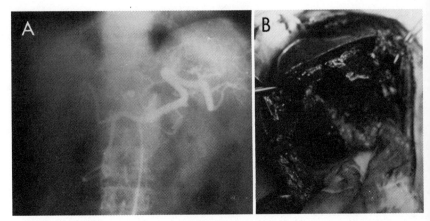

Fig 9.—A, celiac arteriogram of a patient who sustained a subscapular hematoma of the right lobe following a blunt injury to the right lower chest. Note the avascularity in the right superior and lateral aspects of the liver. B, laparotomy of the same patient a week after the injury shows necrosis and devitalization of tissue in the right lobe. The patient was initially treated conservatively, but an extended right hemihepatectomy was later performed because of problems with hypotension and septicemia.

struction of the medial segments of both lobes of the liver (Fig 11), coupled with injury to the portal vessels or bile ducts, often caused by blunt trauma from the steering wheel of a motor vehicle.

7. Stab injury to the liver with extensive churning of the right lobe due to a special type of weapon used in Malaysia (Fig 12).

8. Complications following improper treatment or undiagnosed initial hepatic injury.

Surgical Technique

ANESTHESIA

Since most anesthetic agents are metabolized in the liver, which is already injured in these patients, it is important to avoid using hepatotoxic drugs. Oxygen and nitrous oxide are adequate when coupled with muscle relaxants. Hypothermia is not advocated because it is too time consuming and may cause cardiac complications and adversely effect clotting mechanisms and metabolism.

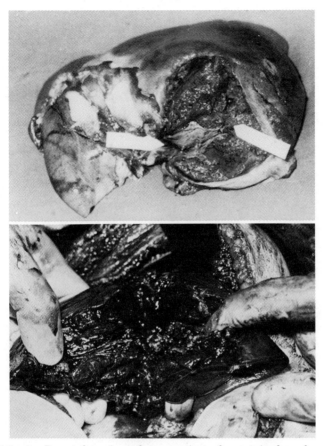

Fig 10 (top).—Resected specimen from a patient who sustained a subscapular hematoma indicates extensive intrahepatic injury to the right lobe. The arrows indicate rupture of the major vessels and ducts. The diagnosis was established at laparotomy by injecting methylene blue into the common bile duct.

Fig 11 (bottom).—Laparotomy in a 34-year-old patient who sustained blunt trauma from a steering wheel in an auto accident. Note the extensive damage to the hilar region and the large, deep rent in the upper aspect, which effectively splits the liver into two halves. The devitalized medial segments of the right and left lobes were resected and the lateral segments sutured. Postoperative recovery was uneventful.

INTRAOPERATIVE ASSESSMENT

As soon as the abdomen has been opened, the large amounts of blood in the peritoneal cavity (usually more than a pint or two) are immediately sucked out and all blood is scooped out with both hands. A quick examination is then made of the ab-

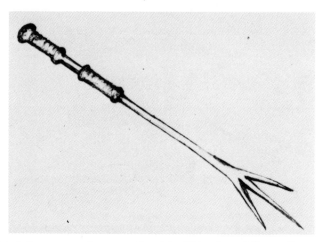

Fig 12.—A three-pronged weapon found in Malaysia and frequently used in civil violence. This lethal instrument often inflicts extensive damage to the liver due to the churning motion with which it is wielded. Patients who sustain such injuries are often candidates for hepatic resection.

dominal organs. First, the liver is inspected and then gently palpated. The extent of the injury to the hepatic parenchyma can be quickly and carefully assessed by visualization and bimanual palpation of the entire liver surface including the hilar region. Any subcapsular hematomas are noted, and in the case of penetrating injuries, the entry and exit wounds are identified. Lacerations of the hepatic veins are suspected in superior and posterior liver injuries close to the vena cava, particularly when a hematoma is present in the area or when excessive blood is seen coming from it. The dome of the liver is also inspected, especially its posterolateral aspect close to the attachments of the coronary ligaments, for it is in this region that severe injury may be hidden within the bare area of the liver and easily missed. Intraoperative resuscitation should be continued vigorously during this period of transfusing with fresh frozen plasma.

In the presence of an enlarged liver with subcapsular hematoma, intralobar rupture must be excluded. In such cases injection of aqueous methylene blue into the common bile duct is followed by extravasation of large amounts of the dye beneath the liver capsule. This technique has been found to be accurate and less time consuming than operative cholangiography, which calls for x-ray facilities in the theater. These hematomas require incision of the capsule, evacuation of the hematoma and examination of the extent of the parenchymal damage.

RIGHT OR EXTENDED RIGHT HEMIHEPATECTOMY

A wide subcostal incision is made from the midline to the lateral flank, thus avoiding a thoracotomy and the risk of consequent pulmonary complications postoperatively. If a paramedian incision has been made initially, it is extended subcostally. Adequate exposure is obtained by using the Balasegaram self-retaining liver retractor. Temporary hemostasis of the lacerated right lobe of the liver is achieved by manual compression with gauze packing over the site of the injury, and also by intermittent occlusion of the vascular inflow in the portal triad at the foramen of Winslow for 15–20 minutes at a time.[6] This occlusion can be performed with Balasegaram's lightweight "atraugrip" clamp, which does not crush the vessels. If these methods fail to control hemorrhage, a search should be made for the hepatic artery arising from the superior mesenteric, celiac, or gastric arteries, after excluding hepatic venous or caval injuries. Michels[23] found that in 25% of 200 dissections the left gastric artery gave rise to the left hepatic. The entire arterial blood supply comes from the superior mesenteric artery in about 12% of patients. In 17% there is an additional right hepatic artery branching from the superior mesenteric.

The duodenum, colon, and stomach are then displaced internally and downward with gauze packs to give good exposure of the liver. The various ligamentous attachments of the right lobe of the liver are now detached using the 11-in. (28-cm) curved dissecting scissors. This is done by first clamping and ligating the ligamentum teres with 0 silk, the lower edge of the liver being used for gentle traction. Next, the falciform ligament is cut as far from the liver as possible and kept intact to cover the raw liver segment at the completion of the operation. The coronary ligaments are divided and bleeding vessels are controlled by ligating with 3 metric (2-0) catgut or with diathermy.

The cystic artery and duct are next identified, ligated, cut, and ligatured with 2-0 silk. The porta hepatis is dissected to expose the portal structures, beginning at the hilum of the liver after incision of the peritoneum overlying the common duct. The hepatic artery is identified and followed to its bifurcation into the right and left branches. The right branches of the hepatic artery, bile ducts, and portal vein are quickly identified, dissected out, divided close to the porta hepatis, and ligated with 0 silk.

The specially designed adjustable blade is then attached to the main liver retractor. This enables the mobilized right lobe of the liver to be kept in position following rotation of the liver forward and to the left. Accidental slipping of the lobe is thus avoided.

The peritoneum overlying the inferior vena cava is incised to expose the right hepatic veins. The main right hepatic vein is first identified; it normally lies 2 cm below the diaphragm in the bare area of the liver and is covered by a tongue of liver or fibrous tissue. This tissue is carefully freed to avoid damage to either the inferior vena cava or the right hepatic vein, which is clamped firmly, close to the liver substance, with the angled "atraugrip" clamp, as these veins can easily be torn, resulting in severe hemorrhage. The cut distal end of the right hepatic vein is tied flush with the inferior vena cava using 0 silk, while the proximal end is sutured within the liver substance with 2-0 black silk. Using a MacDonald's dissector, the numerous accessory hepatic veins draining into the inferior vena cava from the liver are mobilized and ligated. If bleeding arises from the inferior vena cava due to tears or ligature slipping, the "atraugrip" vascular clamp is applied to the vein before the defect is sutured with 3-0 continuous silk.

The large Balasegaram hemostatic crushing liver clamp is then applied at the level of resection. Slipping of the clamp is prevented by applying it so that the liver tissue lies close to its handle and the step-lock device is well locked. In right hemihepatectomy the level of resection is from the gallbladder fossa to the right of the middle hepatic vein, while in extended right hemihepatectomy the level of resection is extended to include the middle hepatic vein and the area of the left lobe it drains. It is therefore mandatory to identify the middle and left hepatic veins before applying the clamp. Using the Balasegaram liver clamp makes it unnecessary to isolate the left segmental artery and the left segmental portal vein and duct, since these lie about an inch deep to the ligamentum teres.

The liver is resected at 0.5–1.0 cm beyond the clamp, using a scalpel. The larger blood vessels and bile ducts in the raw area, including the middle hepatic vein, are identified and ligated. Using the special 90-mm curve-bodied needle with a sharp tip, swaged to 75 cm of 3-0 metric green Ethiflex coated polyester, several mattress sutures are applied through the raw edges of the liver, brought together, and tied medial to the clamp. The clamp is removed, and small bleeding points are stopped with extra-long fine-jaw diathermy forceps. Any remaining necrotic tissues are removed. Recently, Biethium buffers[24] have been used in addition, to cover the raw edges before the hepatic wound is covered with falciform ligament. The common bile duct is not drained unless the major bile duct has been damaged, although Merendino and associates[25] have strongly advocated drainage. However, experience confirms an observation by Lucas,[33] who showed that drainage of the common bile duct increases the risk of intraperitoneal abscess formation, stress ulcers, and ascending cholangitis.

The abdomen is closed in layers after insertion in the subdiaphragmatic area of a polyethylene tube, which is brought out through the lower lateral flanks of the abdomen in the most dependent position and connected to an underwater seal. This drain is removed after 7–10 days. Multiple drainage tubes via a wide opening through the bed of the resected 12th rib are not advocated.

LEFT AND EXTENDED LEFT HEMIHEPATECTOMY

The operative procedure followed for left or extended left hemihepatectomy is similar to that for a right hemihepatectomy, namely, mobilization of the liver by ligamentous detachment of the left lobe, rotation of the lobe to the right, ligation of the portal vessels and bile duct, and application of the Balasegaram liver clamp. In left hemihepatectomy, the liver clamp is applied along the plane to the left of the middle hepatic vein; in extended left hemihepatectomy, it is applied to the right of the principal plant. In extended left hemihepatectomy, the right branch of the hepatic artery, portal vein, and bile duct are identified routinely before the left branches are ligated and the liver clamp is applied. The gallbladder is often removed as well.

Since in about 20% of patients the left lobe of the liver contains anomalous or accessory vessels arising from the left gastric artery or the celiac axis, and since the medial segment of the left lobe may be supplied by a branch of the right hepatic artery, time should be spent in searching for these arteries if bleeding continues. The raw cut surface is then treated as described above for right lobar resections.

Left Lateral Segmental Resection

For a left lateral segmental resection, the left lobe of the liver is first freed from the diaphragm by incising the left triangular ligament and the falciform ligament, care being taken to identify the left hepatic vein, which lies just posterior to the junction of these ligaments.

The hemostatic liver clamp is applied just to the left side of the falciform ligament and the liver is resected 0.5 cm beyond the clamp. The left hepatic vein is identified and ligated by slightly releasing the clamp. Individual dissection and ligation of the branches of the artery and duct are not required if the Balsegaram clamp is used since these structures can be identified and ligated in the raw surface of the liver.

Middle Wedge Resection

This is a difficult procedure that is used for extensive lacerations of the caudate lobe. It entails removal of the medial segments of both the right and left lobes of the liver.

The injury is first identified and the ligamentous attachments—the falciform ligament and the triangular ligament of the left lobe—are severed. Since important structures may be injured, splitting of the liver parenchyma at the hilar region is advocated, with careful dissection of the vessels and bile ducts, including identification of the right and left portal structures and the inferior vena cava. Hemostasis is achieved by ligating the segmental vessels supplying the medial segments of both lobes of the liver. The middle hepatic vein is then identified and ligated close to the inferior vena cava. It is important to do a choledochotomy before resecting the hepatic tissue. The devitalized liver tissue is excised using the small liver clamp, with the lateral segments of both lobes left free. They are then brought together and sutured using atraumatic Ethiflex sutures.

Hepatic Venous and Retrohepatic Caval Injuries

These venous injuries present a special problem because of their inaccessibility and severe hemorrhage. Temporary control of the active and profuse bleeding is the first priority and time is of the essence. Such injuries are treated first by manual compression over gauze packs, to permit blood volume restoration. The hepatic blood supply is then occluded by applying "atraugrip" clamps at the hepatoduodenal ligament. The simpler technique of vascular isolation is preferred to insertion of an internal veno-caval shunt.[26] Accordingly, the abdominal incision is quickly extended into the right chest through the 7th or 8th intercostal space and the diaphragm divided to reach the inferior vena cava. This incision permits wide exposure and ready access to the supradiaphragmatic and infradiaphragmatic vena cava and to the entire juxtahepatic venous area. A median sternotomy is not recommended, as our experience shows that it is time consuming and has no particular advantages, although other investigators strongly advocate it.[27, 28]

Vascular occlusion of the inferior vena cava is achieved by application of the Balasegaram atraugrip vascular clamp to the inferior vena cava above and below the diaphragm, the aorta being occluded above the celic axis. The injured veins are now quickly identified. Replacement of blood volume and correction of potentially lethal acidosis are carried out, and the patient is stabilized before the next step is undertaken. As most of the patients in this series had extensive hepatic and retrohepatic caval injuries, the liver was mobilized from the diaphragmatic attachments for ligation of the hepatic vein or repair of the injured inferior vena cava, followed by hepatic resection. Resection of the right lobe required ligation of the right and middle hepatic veins in twelve patients in the series, four of whom died postoperatively.

Postoperative Management

The postoperative management of patients after hepatic resection makes great demands on the support team.[29] The vital signs such as pulse rate, blood pressure, blood gases, and central venous pressure must be carefully monitored. Any acidosis revealed by the blood gas determination should be corrected promptly by intravenous administration of sodium bicarbonate. Similarly, the Ryle's tube is regularly aspirated and the urinary output carefully noted; an output of at least 30 ml of urine per hour is essential. If the output is less than this, mannitol 20% and Ringer's lactate are given until a satisfactory urine flow is obtained. Furosemide may also be used. The drainage tubes from the chest (if any) or abdomen are connected to underwater seals and the discharge volume recorded.

It is imperative to maintain a well-ordered system of support for the patient, including nutrition, calories, vitamins, and specific therapies to combat the imbalances of function that follow major trauma.

Sequential monitoring of the pulse rate and volume and of the blood pressure is vital, as these variables affect the quantity of blood lost after major hepatic resection—and consequently the postoperative morbidity and mortality. Antibiotic therapy is continued, giving 1 gm of cephalosporin every 6 hours combined with 80 mg of aminoglycoside every 8 hours, for 7–10 days, plus 10 mg of vitamin K. We have tried many types of analgesics, notably pethidine, pentazocine, and fentanyl. All are metabolized in the liver, but too much may kill the patient and too little will not result in sufficient analgesia. Entonox (a mixture of 50% oxygen and 50% nitrous oxide) and continuous epidural analgesia seem to be the answer.

Frequent estimations are made of the hemoglobin, packed cell volume, blood glucose, serum electrolytes, and renal profile. The liver function is estimated regularly, with emphasis on the serum proteins and bilirubin. Plain radiographs of the chest are obtained regularly. Severely traumatized patients with associated chest injuries needed to be maintained on the ventilator for a few days in the postoperative period. These patients require intensive management of the endotracheal tube with frequent tracheal clearance and coma nursing in the intensive care unit.

Nutritional balance and support to maintain a positive nitrogen balance[30] is also continued by daily intravenous alimentation, in the following protocol:

Infusion	Liters	Kilocalories
Intralipid 10%	1	1,100
Vamin 7%	1	650
Dextrose 10%	1	400
Dextrose saline 5%	0.5	100
Intermittent infusions of Dextrose 50%	20–50 ml/6 Hourly	2,250

Vitamins and supplements of serum albumin (25–50 gm/day) are given until the serum values stabilize. This regime is continued for 7–10 days, to allow the residual liver to regain its compensatory physiologic mechanisms and undergo regeneration. After extended resections, infusions should include fresh frozen plasma, platelets, and, if the blood sugar level is below 100 mg, 50% Dextrose. Liver failure is prevented by early detection and correction of metabolic derangements and hematologic deficits, to restore optimal blood volume and electrolyte balance, coupled with prevention and/or early treatment of sepsis.

Management of Late Complications

Postoperative complications following hepatic resection are listed in Table 4. Most of the respiratory complications, i.e., pneumonitis, pleural effusion, and basal atelectasis, were secondary to thoracic injury, usually with rib fractures and problems of ventilation, though some were associated with thoracoabdominal incisions. All were managed in the usual way—antibiotic therapy for wound infection with abscess drainage

TABLE 4.—POSTOPERATIVE
COMPLICATIONS

COMPLICATIONS	PATIENTS
Respiratory infections	10
Wound infections	7
Subphrenic or subhepatic abscesses	3
Prolonged biliary discharge	2
Hemorrhage	2
Jaundice	7
Bleeding diathesis	3

when necessary (as it was in seven patients). Large subphrenic abscesses required surgical intervention in three patients.

Prolonged biliary discharge presented a major problem in two patients, but had stopped spontaneously in all by 8–10 weeks. Continued hemorrhage from the abdominal drainage tube occurred in two patients; disseminated intravascular coagulopathy was suspected, and a full coagulation profile was carried out, including estimation of fibrinogen degradation products. A bleeding diathesis in three patients with hepatic venous injuries was attributed to massive blood transfusion and treated by administration of fresh blood, fresh frozen plasma, and replacement of clotting factors V and VII with platelet transfusions.

Jaundice was a transient feature in nearly all the patients who underwent major hepatic resections and was typically present for 1–3 weeks, with serum bilirubin levels rising to 3–4 mg/100 ml. Marked jaundice with serum bilirubin levels of 15–20 mg/ml indicated impending liver failure in ten patients, whose alkaline phosphatase and transaminase levels were abnormally raised. Treatment consisted of 10% dextrose intravenously, large parenteral doses of vitamins, oral neomycin, lactulose, and low molecular weight dextran (Rheomacrodex) infusions. One patient who had a marked rise in serum bilirubin with pyrexia but no abnormal transaminase or alkaline phosphatase levels was found to have subdiaphragmatic accumulation of bile, which was surgically drained. Early recognition of this complication is vital, since it demands immediate surgical intervention.

Hepatic resection was performed in the nine patients who were referred with existing complications. The five patients with hepatic and subdiaphragmatic abscesses had necrosis of the right lobe with exudation of fragments of devitalized and necrotic liver tissue. Hepatic artery ligation had been performed following the initial injury in two patients, the third had been treated by packing, while the fourth had undergone resectional debridement of the right lobe. Extended right hemihepatectomy was performed in all these patients.

Persistent biliary discharge necessitated resection in two of the patients referred with complications. One of these had a subcapsular hematoma, which was treated conservatively with drainage; the hepatic injuries, however, included intralobar rupture of the main vessels and the biliary duct in the right lobe, resulting in necrosis of the liver and persistent biliary discharge. The other had resectional debridement of a shattering injury to the right lobe but should have had resection, as the injury was very extensive.

Two patients had hemobilia of the right lobe. In both of them ligation and suture of deep lacerated injuries with parenchymal damage had led to accumulation of blood and bile, resulting in sepsis.

Two cases in this series are described in detail below.

CASE 1.—A 13-year-old Sikh boy was admitted to another surgical department on June 13, 1976, in a state of shock secondary to an intra-abdominal injury. Immediate aggressive resuscitation and laparotomy indicated: (1) an extensive laceration on the left lobe of the liver, (2) a tear of the portal vein, (3) complete transection of the left hepatic artery, and (4) leakage of bile from the porta-hepatis.

The portal vein was repaired, the left hepatic artery was ligated, and the liver wounds were sutured. He recovered postoperatively but discharge of pus and bile from the drainage tube began on the seventh day, associated with an intermittently spiking temperature.

A pleural effusion on the right side was drained by insertion of a chest tube. Liver scans showed a cold area in the entire left lobe of the liver suggestive of an abscess cavity. The patient's parents refused any further surgical intervention and the patient was discharged against medical advice.

He returned 2 years later. Repeated sinograms indicated a fistula communicating with the abscess cavity in the left lobe with extravasation of dye into the subdiaphragmatic area. The parents finally agreed to surgery, and the boy was referred to us. A laparotomy was performed on March 19, 1979, and we found the fistulous tract extending into the abscess cavity in the left lobe of the liver with subdiaphragmatic abscess formation. A left hemihepatectomy was performed, the abscess cavity in the subdiaphragmatic area was evacuated, and a T tube was inserted into the common bile duct. He recovered well postoperatively. The T tube was removed after 3 weeks (Fig 13).

Comments.—This patient had an extensive injury involving the left lobe of the liver and the vessels and ducts in the portal triad. Because of the poor general condition of the patient, the surgeon decided to suture the multiple injuries of the liver, although the left hepatic artery was ligated. Its complication could have been avoided if the left lobe of the liver had been resected initially. The common bile duct was drained because of extensive dissection in the portal region, requiring identification of the right hepatic duct by choledochotomy prior to resecting the left lobe.

CASE 2.—A 30-year-old man sustained bruises to the right lower chest and upper abdomen following a motor vehicle accident in April 1978. On admission the patient was in hypovolemic shock with multiple fractures of the sixth, seventh, and eighth ribs. Peripheral and central venous pressure lines (using the subclavian vein) were immediately set up and the patient was actively resuscitated. Emergency laparotomy revealed multiple lacerations of

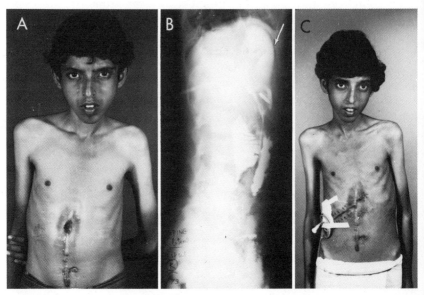

Fig 13.—Thirteen-year-old boy discussed in Case 1. **A,** preoperative photograph shows a chronically discharging fistulous opening at the upper end of the incision. Pus and bilious staining were discharged through this fistula. **B,** roentgenogram (lateral view) of the same patient following injection of contrast medium into the fistula. Note the abscess bordering the diaphragm and the left lobe (*arrow*), with dye in the duodenum. **C,** postoperative photograph of the same patient shows the subcostal incision used for resecting the left lobe. A left hemihepatectomy had been performed, with evacuation of the pus in the subdiaphragmatic area.

the right lobe of liver, extending from the anterior to the posterosuperior surface of the liver. The lacerations were sutured, hepatic artery ligation was performed, and a T tube was inserted into the common bile duct. Postoperatively the patient developed shock-lung syndrome and was effectively managed in the intensive care unit. He continued to develop disseminated intravascular coagulopathy, which was managed with repeated fresh blood and plasma transfusions together with administration of broad-spectrum antibiotics and parenteral nutrition. The sepsis was consequent to the development of a liver abscess, communicating with the common bile duct. Repeated sinograms through the drainage tube and cholangiograms via the T tube showed the abscess cavity still present after 3 months (Fig 14). The patient was referred to us and was reexplored. An extended right hemihepatectomy was performed. Recovery was uneventful.

Comment.—This case illustrates the complications following hepatic artery ligation in a patient who had extensive injuries to the right lobe of the liver. Devitalized tissue developed into abscess, resulting in severe complications, including pyobilia. In retrospect, this patient should have had an immediate hepatic resection performed on admission.

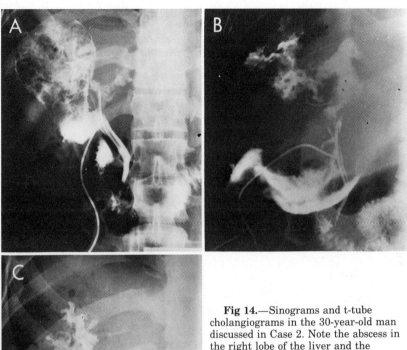

Fig 14.—Sinograms and t-tube cholangiograms in the 30-year-old man discussed in Case 2. Note the abscess in the right lobe of the liver and the subdiaphragmatic abscess that developed subsequent to hepatic artery ligation following multiple injuries to the liver. The patient eventually underwent an extended right hemihepatectomy. **A,** initial radiograph. **B,** 3 weeks after initial radiograph. **C,** 6 weeks after initial radiograph.

Overall Outcome of Hepatic Resection

In all, 29 patients had an extended right hemihepatectomy, 10 had a right lobectomy, 23 had a right hemihepatectomy, 21 had a left hemihepatectomy, 2 had an extended left hemihepatectomy, 5 had a left lateral segmental resection, 3 had a middle wedge resection, and 1 had combined right hemihepatectomy and left lateral segmental resection.

The mortality was 10.6% overall but slightly lower following blunt trauma (9.87%) and higher in high-velocity missile injuries (11.53%). There were no deaths from stab wounds, despite the "internal shatter" effect. Details of mortality for each type of trauma and resection were given in Table 2.

Of the ten patients who died, five did so of associated head, abdominal, and chest injuries, four of hemorrhage from hepatic venous and retrohepatic caval injuries (two of these died on the operating table). One patient, a 78-year-old male victim of civilian disorder, who had combined right hemihepatectomy and left lateral segmental resection following a high-velocity missile injury which caused shattering in both lobes of the liver, died in the third week of septicemia and hepatic failure.

Conclusion

The first hepatic resection was probably carried out for trauma in 1888 by Langenbach.[32] It was followed by hemorrhage requiring exploration, an event not uncommon today after nearly a century of surgical developments in hepatic surgery. Hepatic resection is still considered a formidable procedure, and the advisability of resection remains an issue of controversy.[33, 34, 35] The dilemma faced by surgeons has not changed since 1902, when Beck observed "that in cases of injury to the liver the Surgeon was often helpless in trying to check the bleeding by methods which would be applied to other organs." This remains the crux of the problem in treatment of liver trauma.[36]

Many methods and combinations for control of liver hemostasis have been proposed, yet there is little agreement among the handful of workers in this field. For this reason, we started our own investigative and therapeutic research on hepatic research for trauma in Malaysia. Based on our 18 years of experience we have proposed a unified surgical approach to hepatic resection.[37]

The 94 resections for hepatic trauma in this series represent 21.1% of 443 of the liver injuries seen. This is in marked contrast to recently reported series from the United States, where the frequency of resection varied from 2% to 13%.[38]

The criteria for hepatic resection must be very clearly defined. Essentially, hepatic resection is performed for severely injured patients with extensively lacerated liver tissue and for patients with major hepatic venous injury. This does not mean advocating formal hepatic resection as a preferred method of managing liver injuries,[39] nor should the indications be liberal. Why, then, should there be such wide disparity in the numbers of resections performed in different centers?

First, the nature and type of injuries sustained in different countries and even in different parts of a country are not identical; it is therefore impossible to compare two different series of patients without a common standard of assessment. For example, analysis of Walt's[34] series showed that only 40 patients (9.7%) had blunt trauma, compared with 206 (82.4%) with blunt injuries in our earlier series,[68] while Pachter and Spencer[40] reported that 64.7% of all hepatic injuries in their series were stab wounds, 25.8% were gunshot wounds, and only 9.4% were secondary to blunt trauma. Similarly, in Britain[41] and Australia[42] blunt liver trauma accounts for about 70% of local liver injuries, and it is inappropriate for us to compare our treatment with that of the American centers, where penetrating injuries are predominant.

Another major cause of controversy is that the overall operative mortality following emergency hepatic surgery differs widely. The figure of 10.6% of this series is close to the lower end of reported rates in industrialized countries, which range from 7% to 69%.[43-48] Reports of very high mortality have led to a progressive decline and an increasing tendency for surgeons who previously advocated resection to resort to nonresectional procedures. The disadvantages of these methods have been discussed in an earlier publication.

One of the reasons for high mortality may be that some resections described as emergency lobectomy are conducted in a less-than-emergency fashion. In severe liver trauma, resection must be carried out as quickly as possible, since bleeding is the main cause of death. The special Balasegaram liver instruments and the clamp technique[29] described earlier in this report are far better for controlling hemorrhage than the "finger fracture technique,"[49] where time is spent teasing and chiseling out blood vessels and bile ducts while the bleeding continues. Immediate hemostasis is vital; in many cases it can be reliably achieved only by acting promptly on precise indications for hepatic resection.[50, 51] Other techniques used range from blunt dissection using the handle of the knife to separate the liver tissue, cautery, guillotine resection, and, more recently, the sophisticated laser knife, the modified rubber catheter used like a knife using suction—and the latest gadget introduced uses a water jet![52-57]

Indications and contraindications also must be worked out for nonresectional methods of treating severe hepatic injuries—including multiple ligation, viable omental packing, hepatic artery ligation, "resectional debridement," hepatostomy and drainage, and temporary packing of lacerated wounds followed by a "second-look" operation 48–72 hours later.[58-61] Some of these may have a place, but all indications for treating hepatic injuries must take full account of the fact that hemorrhage is the immediate cause of death,[19, 47, 62] followed by sepsis, which is also the main complication, while retention of devitalized and necrotic liver tissue is the primary contributing factor in perpetuating hemorrhage, sepsis, and shock. The basic principles of controlling bleeding and removing nonviable tissue cannot be too strongly emphasized. Also, it is not sufficiently appreciated that hepatic artery ligation will *not* stop bleeding from the hepatic veins, though it can be useful for treating hemobilia or major deep arterial bleeding. The value of hepatic resection is compared with nonresectional methods in Table 5.

Major vascular injuries, especially tears of the hepatic and retrohepatic caval veins, can be effectively treated only by a specialized trauma team. Intubation of the inferior vena cava through the right atrium and shunting through balloon catheter carries a very high mortality,[26, 61, 63] whereas the direct approach by clamping and resecting the right lobe gives ready access to both hepatic and retrohepatic veins, enabling lacerations to be identified and appropriately treated by clamping and suturing or ligation. McNamara[64] advocates the latter procedure and described the experiences in Vietnam in "Rapid Right Hepatectomy."

The term "resectional debridement" is unsatisfactory. It may be better to distinguish clearly between debridement, in its accepted sense, and hepatic resection, using the points of differentiation outlined earlier.

Temporary packing is indicated when liver damage is unexpectedly encountered by a surgeon inexperienced in dealing with such injuries and without the facilities to cope with their complex "after-case." After packing and other resuscitative

TABLE 5.—VALUE OF HEPATIC RESECTION IN TRAUMA TO THE LIVER: COMPARISON WITH NONRESECTIONAL METHODS*

	PACKING	HEPATIC ARTERY LIGATION	"RESECTIONAL DEBRIDEMENT"	HEPATIC RESECTION
Onset of hemostasis	Delayed	Delayed	Delayed	Immediate
Method of hemostasis	Indirect local	Indirect distant	Indirect local	Direct local
Anatomical principles	None	Anomalies encountered	Nonanatomical	Sound anatomical principles
Devitalized liver tissue	Left behind	Left behind	Partly left behind	None left
Recurrent bleeding from raw surface of liver	Frequent	Frequent	Frequent	Rare
Postoperative infection and abscess formation	Common	Common	Common	Not common
Repair of biliary system and venous system	Not done	Not done	Partial anatomical	Complete anatomical

*Table from *Am. J. Surg.* (Reproduced by permission.)

measures, such patients should be transported to a major trauma center for definitive treatment. All other forms of packing for hepatic injuries are now contraindicated.

As regards drainage of the common bile duct, certain cases call for insertion of a T tube[61]—when there is a high risk of hemobilia, for example, or to facilitate cholangiography, when residual cavities might give rise to infection or bleeding. However, routine T tube insertion is not advocated for all cases of hepatic resection, and cholecystostomy offers no clear advantages as an alternative procedure.

Routine drainage of the subhepatic and subdiaphragmatic areas are mandatory in all patients following hepatic resections.[65, 66] More recently, angiographic embolization has been carried out radiologically in the treatment of hemobilia.[67]

From our experience, the prognosis following hepatic resection for trauma depends on the following factors:

1. Presence of gross intra-abdominal and concomitant head, chest, and pelvic injuries. The prognosis worsens if multiple organs are injured.
2. Hepatic or retrohepatic caval injuries. These carry a very high mortality, ranging from 25% to 80%.
3. The early arrival of the patient at the emergency treatment center.
4. Aggressive resuscitation and immediate intervention.
5. Delay due to multiple organ injury, leaving diagnosis in doubt.
6. An experienced surgical team.

Postoperative management is of paramount importance in view of the manifold functions of the liver. Patients who have had hepatic resections should have supplementary nutritional therapy in order to maintain a positive nitrogen balance. Such therapy consists of the transfusion of solutions containing carbohydrates, proteins, and fats in a well-balanced regime, including multivitamins and trace elements. The liver has a remarkable capacity to regenerate to its normal size and function. However, we stress the need for routine preoperative and postoperative administration of broad-spectrum antibiotics to prevent sepsis.

Hepatic resection is by no means a panacea for all liver injuries, but when it is correctly and promptly performed for clear indications, it can control hemorrhage, remove all devitalized tissue, and thus reduce the risk of all the major postoperative complications: exsanguination, sepsis, bile leakage, and abscess formation.[68-75] But how can these advantages, coupled with low mortality rates, be made available to the majority of patients with hepatic injuries? This problem is now exacerbated, paradoxically, by improvements in casualty evacuation using helicopters, military aircraft, and efficient ambulance services. The number of injured patients arriving nearly moribund at hospitals is already growing and likely to grow further. The answer must be to establish trauma teams staffed by experienced surgeons and ancillary staff in most major hospitals.[77]

Hepatic trauma can be minimized by the wearing of safety belts of the lap-and-shoulder variety, and by the enforcement of the 55 miles-per-hour speed limit. This policy has already been instituted in Malaysia.

Acknowledgment

I wish to express my grateful thanks to George F.B. Birdwood, M.D., Medical Director of Ciba-Geigy Foundation, for editing the manuscript, and to Dr. Devanand (FRCS. Ed), my Senior Registrar, for his assistance in the preparation of this manuscript. I am also indebted to Mrs. Siti Fatimah and Miss Ang Wai Lin for typing the manuscript and to Mr. Charles Abraham for the photographs.

REFERENCES

1. Defore W.W., Mattox K.L., Jordan G.L., et al.: Management of 1590 consecutive cases of liver trauma. *Arch. Surg.* 111:493, 1976.
2. Shires G.T.: *Care of the Trauma Patient.* New York, McGraw-Hill Book Co., 1966.
3. Beck C.: Surgery of the liver. *JAMA* 38:1063–1068, 1902.
4. Burckhardt P., cited by Deaver J.B., Ashurst A.P.C. 33, Zentrabe. *Chir.* 14:88, 1887.
5. Kousnetzoff M.E., Penski J.: Sur la resection partielle du foie. *Rev. Chir.* 16:507, 954, 1896.
6. Pringle J.H.: Notes on the arrest of hepatic haemorrhage due to trauma. *Ann. Surg.* 48:541, 1908.
7. Madding G.F., Lawrence K.B., Kennedy P.A.: Forward surgery of the severely injured. Second Aux. Surgical Group, 1:307, 1942–45.
8. Balasegaram M.: Hepatic surgery—Present and future. *Ann. R. Coll. Surg. England* 47:138, 1970.

9. Goldsmith N.A., Woodburne R.T.: The surgical anatomy pertaining to liver resection. *Surg. Gynecol. Obstet.* 105:310, 1957.
10. Healey J.E. Jr.: Clinical anatomic aspects of radical hepatic surgery. *J. Int. Coll. Surg.* 22:542, 1954.
11. Balasegaram M.: The use of natural rubber latex in the study of hollow systems of liver. *Br. J. Surg.* 58:902, 1971.
12. Joishy S.K., Balasegaram M.: Hepatic resections for malignant tumors of the liver: Essentials for a united surgical approach. *Am. J. Surg.* 139:360, 1981.
13. Balasegaram M.: Blunt liver injuries. *Ann. Surg.* 169:544, 1969.
14. Balasegaram M.: The surgical management of hepatic trauma. *J. Trauma* 16:141, 1976.
15. Thal E.R., Shires G.T.: Peritoneal lavage in blunt abdominal trauma. *Am. J. Surg.* 125:64, 1973.
16. Pachter H.L., Hofstetter S.R.: Open and percutaneous paracentesis and lavage for abdominal trauma: a randomised prospective study. *Arch. Surg.* 116:318, 1981.
16a. Jordan G.L.: The acute abdomen. *Adv. Surg.* 14:259, 1980.
17. Freeark R.J.: Role of angiography in the management of multiple injuries. *Surg. Gynecol. Obstet.* 128:761, 1969.
18. Lim R.C. Jr., Flickman M.G., Hunt T.K.: Angiography in patients with blunt trauma to the chest and abdomen. *Surg. Clin. North Am.* 52:552–565, 1972.
19. Flint L.M., Mays E.T., Aaron W.S., et al.: Selectivity in the management of hepatic trauma. *Ann. Surg.* 185:613, 1977.
20. Federle M.P., Crass R.A., Jeffery R.B., et al.: Computed tomography in blunt abdominal trauma. *Arch. Surg.* 117:645, 1982.
21. Gregory N.V., Ramon G., Kenneth J.W.T., et al.: Ultrasonic evaluation of hepatic and splenic trauma. *Arch. Surg.* 115:320, 1980.
22. Clagett G.P., Olsen W.R.: Non-mechanical hemorrhage in severe liver injury. *Ann. Surg.* 187:369, 1978.
23. Michels N.A.: Variational anatomy of hepatic, cystic and retroduodenal arteries: Statistical analysis of their origin, distribution, and relations to biliary ducts in 200 bodies. *Arch. Surg.* 66:20, 1953.
24. Balasegaram M., Capperauld I.: Biethium buffers in the control of liver haemorrhage. *Mal. J. Surg.* 3:139, 1977.
25. Merendino K.A., Dillard D.H., Cammock E.E.: The concept of surgical biliary decompression in the management of liver trauma. *Surg. Gynecol. Obstet.* 117:285, 1963.
26. Yellin A.E., Chaffee C.B., Donovan A.J.: Vascular isolation in the treatment of juxtahepatic venous injuries. *Arch. Surg.* 102:566, 1971.
27. Miller D.R.: Median sternotomy extension of abdominal incision for hepatic lobectomy. *Ann. Surg.* 175:193, 1972.
28. Fuellen W.D., McDonough J.J., Popp M.J., et al.: Sternal splitting approach for major hepatic or retrohepatic vena cava injury. *J. Trauma* 14:903, 1974.
29. Balasegaram M.: Modern concepts in the surgery of liver trauma. *J. R. Coll. Surg. Edinb.* 76:313, 1971.

30. McDermott W.V. Jr.: *Surgery of the liver and portal circulation*. Philadelphia, Lea & Febiger, 1974, p. 141.
31. Aronsen K.F., Ericsson N., Hagerstand I., et al.: Haemobilia after primary suture of deep liver rupture. *Acta. Chir. Scand.* 136:517, 1970.
32. Langenbuch C.: Resection of the left lobe of liver. *Lancet* 1:237, 1888.
33. Lucas C.E., Walt A.J.: Critical decisions in liver trauma: Experience based on 604 cases. *Arch. Surg.* 135:12, 1978.
34. Walt A.J.: The mythology of hepatic trauma, or Babel revisited. *Am. J. Surg.* 135:12, 1978.
35. Mays E.T.: Options in treating trauma to the liver. *Surg. Annu.* 12:103, 1980.
36. Beck C.: Surgery of the liver. *JAMA* 38:1063, 1902.
37. Balasegaram M., Joishy S.K.: Hepatic resection. Pillars of success built on the foundation of 15 years of experience. *Am. J. Surg.* 141:360, 1981.
38. Lewis F.R., Trunkey D.D.: Management of major liver trauma, in Carter D., Polk H.C. Jr., (eds.): *Surgery 1: Trauma*. Boston, Butterworths, 1981, pp. 99–109.
39. Carmona R.H., Lim R.C., Clark G.C.: Morbidity and mortality in hepatic trauma. *Am. J. Surg.* 144:88, 1982.
40. Pachter H.L., Spencer F.C.: Recent concepts in the treatment of hepatic trauma. *Ann. Surg.* 190:423, 1979.
41. Blumgart L.H., Drury J.K., Wood C.B.: Hepatic resection for trauma, tumor and biliary obstruction. *Br. J. Surg.* 66:762, 1979.
42. Little J.M.: Liver injuries in Australia. *Roy. Australas. Coll. Surg.*, Bulletin 2, July 1982.
43. Mays E.T.: Hepatic lobectomy. *Arch. Surg.* 103:214, 1971.
44. Mercardier R.J., Clot J.P., Cady J.P.: Right hepatectomy in the treatment of liver trauma. *Am. J. Surg.* 124:353, 1972.
45. McClelland R., Shires T., Poulos E.: Hepatic resection for massive trauma. *J. Trauma* 4:282, 1964.
46. McClelland R., Shires T.: Management of liver traums in 259 consecutive patients. *Ann. Surg.* 161:248, 1965.
47. Trunkey D.D., Shires G.T., McClelland R.: Management of liver trauma in 811 consecutive patients. *Ann. Surg.* 179:722, 1974.
48. Elerding S.C., Moore E.E. Jr.: Recent experience with trauma of the liver. *Surg. Gynecol. Obstet.* 150:853, 1980.
49. Lin T.Y.: Results in 107 hepatic lobectomies with a preliminary report on the use of a clamp to reduce blood loss. *Ann. Surg.* 177:413, 1973.
50. Arango A., Lester L.: Hemostatic suture of liver. *Arch. Surg.* 111:81, 1976.
51. Madding G.F., Kennedy P.A.: Trauma to the liver, in *Major Problems in Clinical Surgery*. ed. 2. Philadelphia, W.B. Saunders Co., 1971, pp. 163–181.
52. Quattlebaum J.K., Quattlebaum J.K. Jr.: Technique of hepatic lobectomy. *Ann. Surg.* 149:648, 1959.
53. Longmire W.P. Jr.: Hepatic surgery: Trauma, tumours and cysts. *Ann. Surg.* 161:1, 1965.
54. Brasfield R.D.: Right hepatic lobectomy. *Arch. Surg.* 84:578, 1962.

55. Brunschwig A.: The surgical treatment of primary and secondary hepatic malignant tumours. *Am. Surg.* 20:1077, 1954.
56. Hall R.R., Beach A.D., Hall J.D.W.: Partial hepatectomy using a carbon dioxide laser. *Br. J. Surg.* 60:141, 1973.
57. Papachristou D.W., Barters R.: Resection of the liver with a water jet. *Br. J. Surg.* 69:93, 1982.
58. Stone H.H., Lamb J.M.: Use of pedicled omentum as an autogenous pack for control of hemorrhage in major injuries of the liver. *Surg. Gynecol. Obstet.* 141:92, 1975.
59. Aaron S., Fulton R.L., May E.T.: Selective ligation of the hepatic artery for trauma of the liver. *Surg. Gynecol. Obstet.* 141:187, 1975.
60. Bengmark S.: *Liver surgery.* New York, 1968, pp. 1–59.
61. Lucas C.E., Ledgerwood A.M.: Prospective evaluation of hemostatic techniques for liver injuries. *J. Trauma* 16:442, 1976.
62. Lim R.C., Jr., Knudson J., Steele M.: Liver trauma: Current method of management. *Arch. Surg.* 104:544, 1972.
63. Schrock S., Blaisdell F.W., Mathewson C. Jr.: Management of blunt trauma to the liver and hepatic veins. *Arch. Surg.* 96:698, 1968.
64. Lim R.C., Lau G., Steele M.: Prevention of complications after liver hematoma. *Am. J. Surg.* 132:156, 1976.
65. Lewis F.R., Lim R.C., Blaisdell F.W.: Hepatic artery ligation: Adjunct in the management of massive hemorrhage from the liver. *J. Trauma* 14:743, 1974.
66. Madding E.F.: Injuries of the liver. *Arch. Surg.* 70:748, 1955.
67. Heimback D.M., Fergusson G.S., Harley J.D.: Treatment of traumatic hemobilia with angiographic embolization. *J. Trauma* 18:221, 1978.
68. Balasegaram M., Joishy S.K.: Hepatic resection: The logical approach to surgical management of major trauma to the liver. *Am. J. Surg.* 142:580, 1981.
69. Ackroyd F.W., Polland J., McDermott W.V. Jr.: Massive hepatic resection in the treatment of severe liver trauma. *Am. J. Surg.* 117:442, 1969.
70. Blaisdell F.W., Lim R.C. Jr.: Liver resection, in Madding G.F., Kennedy P.A., (eds.): *Trauma to the Liver.* (ed. 2) Philadelphia, W.B. Saunders Co., 1971, pp. 131–145.
71. Byrd W.M., McAffee D.K.: Emergency hepatic lobectomy in massive injury of the liver. *Surg. Gynecol. Obstet.* 133:103, 1961.
72. Donovan A.J., Turnill F.L., Facey F.L.: Hepatic trauma. *Surg. Clin. North Am.* 48:1313, 1968.
73. Foster J.H., Lawler M.R., Welborn M.B. Jr., et al.: Recent experience with major hepatic resection. *Ann. Surg.* 167:65, 1968.
74. Longmire W.P., Jr., Cleveland R.J.: Surgical anatomy and blunt trauma of the liver. *Surg. Clin. North Am.* 52:687, 1972.
75. Balasegaram M.: Hepatic resection. *Brit. J. Surg.* 55:168, 1968.
76. Balasegaram M.: The traumatised patient in large-scale civil disturbances with special reference to the pancreas liver. *J. Irish Coll. Physicians Surgeons* 4:47, 1974.
77. Aldrete J.S., Halpern N.B., Ward S., et al.: Factors determining the mortality and morbidity in hepatic injuries. *Ann. Surg.* 189:466, 1979.

Computed Tomography of the Abdomen

WILLIAM A. RUBENSTEIN, M.D., YONG HO AUH, M.D., AND ELIAS KAZAM, M.D.

Department of Radiology, The New York Hospital—Cornell Medical Center, New York, New York

IN THE LAST FEW YEARS, computed tomography (CT) has developed into a major imaging modality for the abdomen. With this procedure x-rays passing through the patient are recorded onto sensitive detectors, instead of the relatively insensitive x-ray film, and processed by computers to provide a cross-sectional image of the body. Scan time per section varies between 1.5 and 20 seconds. With faster scans there is less image degradation from motion artifact. Section thickness varies between 1.5 and 15 mm. The maximum radiation dose to the skin from a complete examination with sequential contiguous CT sections is 4–8 rad, comparable to the radiation dose from an intravenous pyelogram and much less than the dose from a barium enema.[1]

Opacification of the hollow viscera, usually with dilute oral contrast media, is essential to avoid confusion with pathologic masses and to aid in identification of mural and bowel-related lesions. Intravenous (IV) contrast media are helpful for opacifying the urinary tract and assessing the vascularity of parenchymal lesions.

In the last 7 years we have used combined body CT and ultrasound for sectional imaging of the abdomen.[2] Ultrasonography has been superior for imaging structures that are not ob-

0065-3411/84/0017-0171-0196-$04.00

scured by gas, fat, or bone. CT has been superior for imaging the deeper portions of the abdomen and for providing information on vascularity. Textural detail is generally better with sonography, and of course there is no ionizing radiation. Overall the thin, small patient is better imaged with ultrasound, whereas larger, more obese patients are better imaged with CT. This combined sectional imaging approach has reduced the need for more invasive procedures, such as angiography, at our institution.[2] Based on our experience, a summary of CT applications in the abdomen appears below.

The Liver:

For this organ the radionuclide colloid scan remains a primary imaging procedure. It is sensitive for focal lesions and provides valuable functional information. CT has been valuable for the following purposes:

1. Differentiating normal variants from pathologic masses. Normal anatomical variants such as the gallbladder fossa, interposed colon, or a congenitally small left lobe may mimic pathologic lesions on radionuclide scans but are easily diagnosed on CT. The left lobe may be elongated in the transverse dimension, wrapping around the anterior tip of the spleen. In such cases the left lobe, or lesions within it, may be confused with the spleen on radionuclide scans, but not on CT.

2. Determining the vascularity of a focal lesion. Using IV bolus injections of contrast media and rapid CT scans, the vascularity of liver lesions can be determined noninvasively. Characteristic patterns have been described for liver hemangiomas, which are often detected incidentally on sonography or CT (Fig 1).[3]

3. Demonstrating hepatoma superimposed on cirrhosis. Filling defects on radionuclide colloid scans of cirrhotic livers are not specific for neoplasms. Cirrhotic livers are also difficult to penetrate by ultrasound. In such cases focal lesions on CT corresponding to defects on radionuclide scans are strongly suspect for hepatoma. Morphologically, multicentric hepatoma is indistinguishable from metastases (Fig 2), although the relative rarity of metastases in a cirrhotic liver is helpful in the differential diagnosis. Multilobar involvement that is evident

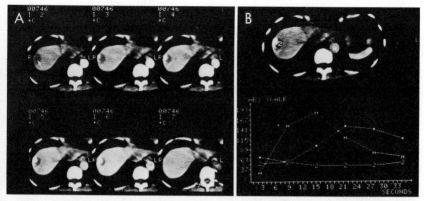

Fig 1.—Hepatic hemangioma. **A,** dynamic CT scan after IV bolus injection of contrast material. Sequential CT scans at 6-second intervals (images 2–6) and at 10 minutes (image 7) demonstrate progressive enhancement of hemangioma (*arrow*). The enhancement begins peripherally and progresses to the center of the lesion. At 10 minutes, (image 7) the hemangioma is invisible because it is isodense with normal liver. **B,** time-density curve of hemangioma during the first 35 seconds after IV bolus injection of contrast material. Cursors are placed over the enhancing lateral portion of the hemangioma (*small solid square*), over the nonenhancing medial portion of the hemangioma (2), and over the aorta (A). Time-density curves demonstrate early enhancement of aorta followed by progressive enhancement of the hemangioma. The medial portion of the hemangioma (2) enhanced on later scans (see Fig 1,A).

on CT may escape detection on radionuclide scanning or angiography.

4. Differentiating cystic from solid lesions. A simple cyst may be diagnosed on CT, though not as reliably as on sonography, when the lesion appears homogeneously lucent and has attenuation values between −20 Housefield units (HU) and +20 HU. Liver cysts are mostly benign and often noted incidentally. They may be congenital (predominantly in females), parasitic (the multiloculated echinococcal cysts), or associated with polycystic renal disease. Solid or mixed cystic-solid lesions appear inhomogeneous on CT and have higher attenuation values than cysts. We have been unable to distinguish abscesses from tumors on the basis of their CT appearance (Fig 3). Fatty tumors, which are rare in the liver, can be diagnosed definitively by CT.

5. Localization of lesions. The fissures for the ligamentum teres, ligamentum venosum, gallbladder, and falciform ligament are readily identifiable on CT. A lesion may then be lo-

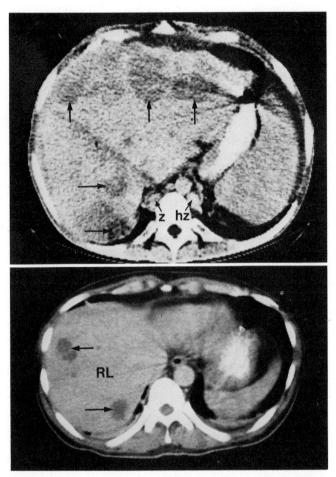

Fig 2 (top).—Multicentric hepatoma. CT demonstrates an enlarged liver with multiple low-density, noncystic masses *(arrows)* in both right and left lobes. The azygos *(z)* and hemiazygos *(hz)* veins are enlarged due to interruption of the retrohepatic inferior vena cava.

Fig 3 (bottom).—Multicentric pyogenic hepatic abscesses. CT demonstrates multiple low-density masses *(arrows),* one of which in the right lobe of liver *(RL),* appears multiloculated.

calized accurately to the left lobe (lateral segment), quadrate, caudate, or right lobe.[4] Accessory fissures and lobes are easily demonstrated. Although the right coronary ligaments are not visible on CT, their aproximate position can be estimated and lesions abutting the relatively inaccessible bare area can be identified. Visualization of the systemic hepatic veins, which is valuable for planning major resection, is possible on CT but easier on ultrasound. Extrinsic obstruction or major thrombosis of the systemic hepatic veins, portal veins, and retrohepatic vena cava is also easier to visualize on ultrasound. Venography is still necessary for demonstrating small thrombi.

Diffuse liver disease diagnosable by CT includes moderate or severe fatty infiltration, hemachromatosis, and glycogen storage disease.[5, 6] Traumatic lesions, including subcapsular and parenchymal hematomas, are well delineated on CT. Selective arteriography remains necessary for demonstrating arteriovenous or arteriobiliary fistulas.

Lesions that are isodense with surrounding liver can be missed on CT but diagnosed on ultrasound or radionuclide scanning. Some vascular lesions may become invisible on CT after IV contrast material is administered (see Fig 1). Ideally, liver lesions are best seen in the hepatic arterial phase following an IV bolus injection of contrast material,[7] but this procedure cannot be followed routinely for every section of the liver. Benign entities such as focal fatty infiltration and focal nodular hyperplasia may mimic neoplasm on CT and require radionuclide scanning for further evaluation. Superficial liver lesions readily visible at surgery are often missed on CT.

The Spleen

As with the liver, radionuclide colloid scanning remains a primary tool for imaging the spleen. Here the uses of CT parallel those outlined above for the liver. Normal variants due to splenic lobulation are easily distinguishable from pathologic lesions, such as subcapsular hematomas (Fig 4). Cystic and solid lesions can be differentiated, as in the liver. Splenic abscess, often occult and life-threatening, can be demonstrated on CT if it is larger than 1 cm,[8] but it may not be distinguishable from primary or metastatic tumors (Fig 5).

The Gallbladder

With the increasing availability of ultrasound equipment, especially of the real-time variety, sonography has replaced the x-ray gallbladder series as the primary imaging procedure in

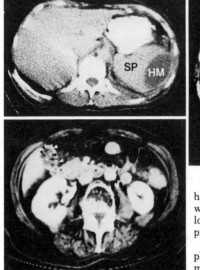
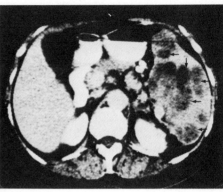

Fig 4 (above left).—Subcapsular splenic hematoma, an incidental finding several weeks after an automobile accident. CT shows low-density subcapsular hematoma *(HM)* compressing normal splenic parenchyma *(SP)*.

Fig 5 (above).—Splenic histiocytic lymphoma. CT shows multiple focal hypovascular masses *(arrows)* within an enlarged spleen.

Fig 6 (left).—Cholecystitis and cholelithiasis. CT demonstrates a thick-walled gallbladder *(white arrowheads)* containing calcified gallstones *(black arrows)*, and stones with internal gas-fissuring *(black arrowheads)*.

many institutions.[9] Its accuracy for detecting gallstones is 90%–95%. For suspected acute cholecystitis, a sonogram showing a distended, thick-walled, tender gallbladder with stones is diagnostic. Hepatobiliary scintigraphy with technetium iminodiacetic derivatives (Tc-IDA) is valuable for diagnosing cystic duct obstruction.[10]

CT is much less valuable for studying the gallbladder. Gallstones are visible on CT if they are calcified or have central gas fissuring (Fig 6). Otherwise gallstones are not detectable, since the CT attenuation value for cholesterol approximates that of surrounding bile. Biliary sludge appears dense on CT because of its high content of calcium bilirubinate crystals. This appearance may be mimicked by vicarious excretion of IV contrast media into the gallbladder lumen. The cystic duct is difficult to evaluate both on CT and on ultrasound. Occasionally a calcified cystic duct stone missed on sonography is visible on CT.

Because omental and peritoneal fat is well delineated by CT, gallbladder thickening (see Fig 6) is more reliably assessed with CT than with ultrasound. This is also true in patients with ascites, in whom the gallbladder may appear artifactually thickened on sonography,[9] and in patients with infiltrating gallbladder carcinoma. Calcium or gas in the gallbladder wall is also better shown on CT. Clinically, however, information on the gallbladder wall has not been as important as finding gallstones or localized tenderness on sonography or showing cystic duct obstruction on Tc-IDA scintigraphy. Furthermore, inflammatory gallbladder wall thickening is not distinguishable from neoplastic infiltration on CT.

The Bile Ducts

In the evaluation of the jaundiced patient, ultrasound is the initial procedure of choice.[2, 9, 11] Using the right anterior oblique view, dilation of the common hepatic duct and intrahepatic bile ducts can be demonstrated sonographically with 95% accuracy. Biliary dilation on sonography may precede elevation of the serum bilirubin level.[12] CT is useful as a supplementary procedure in the following instances:

1. To demonstrate distal common bile duct dilation or obstructing lesions. Although the common hepatic duct is routinely visible on ultrasound, the common bile duct and the overlying head of the pancreas may be obscured by gas or fat. With CT the common bile duct is often visible in normal patients, and it is consistently visible if dilated. As a result, the site and cause of obstruction are more often correctly identified on CT than on ultrasound (Fig 7).[9, 13] In early obstruction only the distal common bile duct may be dilated. If it is obscured by gas, sonography but not CT will be falsely negative.

2. To demonstrate common duct thickening. The fat in the hepatoduodenal ligament surrounding the common hepatic duct is well delineated on CT but not on ultrasound. Infiltration of this fat is more reliably demonstrable on CT, although inflammatory and neoplastic lesions cannot be differentiated.

3. To distinguish segmental obstruction of the left or right bile ducts from common duct obstruction. The major right and left intrahepatic bile ducts have constant relation to their corresponding portal veins, which make them easily demonstrable on ultrasound and CT. On CT they appear as lucent, closely

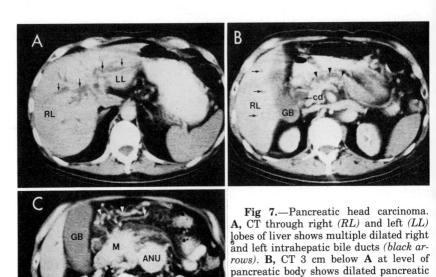

Fig 7.—Pancreatic head carcinoma. A, CT through right *(RL)* and left *(LL)* lobes of liver shows multiple dilated right and left intrahepatic bile ducts *(black arrows)*. B, CT 3 cm below A at level of pancreatic body shows dilated pancreatic duct *(black arrowheads)*, dilated common duct *(cd)*, and dilated gallbladder *(GB)*. C, CT 2 cm below B shows large pancreatic head mass *(M)*, the cause of common duct obstruction. The gallbladder *(GB)* is markedly dilated. Dilation of right and middle colic veins *(white arrowheads)* is due to obstruction of the superior mesenteric vein by the pancreatic mass, verified at surgery. *ANU,* aortic aneurysm.

branching tubular structures, in contrast to the opacified appearance of vessels after IV contrast material has been administered (Fig 8). Occasionally, mildly dilated intrahepatic ducts, particularly in the posterior right lobe of the liver, may be obscured on ultrasound by overlying ribs or gas. This is especially likely to occur in patients with small high livers, colonic interposition, ascites displacing the right lobe of the liver medially, and overlying surgical sutures. CT is therefore more reliable than ultrasound in differentiating obstruction of the left bile duct (see Fig 8) from obstruction of the common hepatic duct at the porta hepatis.

4. To show small amounts of air in the biliary tree (see Fig 8). These may be difficult to differentiate sonographically from the increased echogenicity of the portal triads that is seen in inflammatory disease and in some bile duct carcinomas.

The diagnosis of biliary obstruction on both ultrasound and

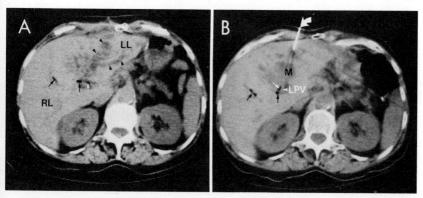

Fig 8.—Obstruction of the left hepatic ducts. Patient presented with fever and elevation of serum alkaline phosphatase level, but not of serum bilirubin level. **A,** CT shows patent right bile ducts *(black arrows)* and duct to caudate lobe *(white arrow),* filled with air from a choledochojejunostomy. The obstructed left bile ducts *(arrowheads)* are dilated and contain no air. **B,** CT 1 cm below **A.** Air is seen within the patent right bile ducts *(black arrows)* and main left bile duct *(white arrow).* A thin needle *(curved arrow)* has been inserted percutaneously to aspirate the low density mass *(M)* at the site of obstruction of the left bile ducts. *LPV,* left portal vein.

CT depends on ductal dilation. Fortunately, nonobstructive dilation in patients without previous gallbladder or biliary surgery is rare, although we have had two proved cases in elderly women. Obstruction without dilation is less rare and can be missed on CT if the ducts are uniformly narrowed by scirrhous neoplasm or sclerosing cholangitis. Endoscopic retrograde cholangiopancreatography (ERCP) or percutaneous transhepatic cholangiography (PTHC) may be needed to make the diagnosis.

While we have used 8 mm as the upper limit of normal for common duct diameter to reduce the number of false positive diagnoses, there is overlap between normal and mildly dilated ducts in the 6–9 mm range. Dilation of the common duct after a fatty meal has been used as a sign of obstruction in such patients.[14] Also, dilation up to 10–11 mm may be seen after cholecystectomy in the absence of common duct obstruction. Other studies such as hepatobiliary scintigraphy with Tc-IDA compounds or ERCP may be needed in such patients. Radionuclide scanning with Tc-IDA compounds has also been valuable for assessing biliary transit or anastomotic leaks in patients with choledochoenterostomy.

Nearly all stones in nondilated bile ducts, and one half to two thirds of stones in dilated common ducts, can be missed on ultrasound and CT. Again, ERCP or PTHC is necessary to make the diagnosis in such patients. IV cholangiography generally has not been helpful.[9] Overall, our approach to bile duct imaging in the jaundiced patient is based on ultrasound, with CT as a valuable supplement. Clearly, other tests may still be necessary, but in the last few years there has been a decrease in the number of invasive tests, such as PTHC, and in the number of diagnostic procedures with relatively high morbidity, such as IV cholangiography, performed in our institution.[2]

The Pancreas

CT is the initial procedure of choice for imaging the pancreas in the adult patient. The upper gastrointestinal series and barium enema are far less sensitive and less specific and are no longer performed initially.[2, 15] Radionuclide pancreatic scanning is obsolete. If the stomach, duodenum, and jejunum are well opacified the entire pancreatic bed can be visualized by CT in all cases. By contrast, part or all of the pancreatic bed is not visualized by ultrasound in 15% of patients in our experience.[2, 15]

The accuracy of CT for detecting pancreatic enlargement or masses in a series of surgically or autopsy proved cases was 90%, with a sensitivity of 88% and a specificity of 92%.[2, 15] In the same series the sensitivity of ultrasound was 66% and the specificity was 98%. When cases of nonvisualization were excluded, sonographic sensitivity rose to 76%. Our experience with pancreatic CT can be summarized as follows:

1. Tumors distorting the pancreatic contours, especially those larger than 3.5 cm in anteroposterior dimension, are easily visualized (see Fig 7). Extension into the lesser sac, mesocolon, and around the celiac axis and superior mesenteric arteries can be detected on CT if there is sufficient fat around these structures. Infiltration of this fat by tumor is a sign of nonresectability, although neoplastic and inflammatory causes of "dirty" fat are indistinguishable on the basis of CT scan appearance. Obstruction of the splenic or superior mesenteric veins can be diagnosed when enlarged short gastric, coronary, peripancreatic, or mesocolic venous collaterals are visualized (see Fig 7). The site of venous obstruction may be shown with rapid CT

scans obtained after bolus injection of IV contrast material. Tumors that do not distort the pancreatic contour have been missed on CT. These have varied from small islet cell tumors to unresectable scirrhous adenocarcinomas which produce no mass effect on CT.

2. Inflammatory pancreatic masses are usually more extensive than tumors. Cystic inflammatory masses are detectable on ultrasound and CT, whereas the solid infiltrative masses may be visible only on CT. Extension into the lesser sac, splenorenal space, mesocolon, and small bowel mesentery is best shown by CT (Fig 9). Pancreatic effusions in the superior recess of the lesser sac around the caudate lobe may mimic intrahepatic lesions[16] or may present as masses at the anterolateral aspect of the abdominal esophagus. These effusions can also spread readily through multiple perforations in the thin lesser omentum, from the lesser sac to the gastrosplenic space, where they may mimic left hepatic lobe lesions on CT. Air within these collections suggests pancreatic abscess (Fig 10), but air may also be seen after surgical or spontaneous drainage into the gastrointestinal tract.

3. Dilation of the pancreatic duct, whether due to tumor (see Fig 7) or inflammation, may be the only CT sign of pancreatic

Fig 9 (left).—Pancreatic pseudocyst. CT demonstrates a large pancreatic pseudocyst *(arrowheads)* surrounding the pancreatic tail *(pt)* and extending into the lesser sac *(LS)* and splenorenal recess *(SR)*. Ascites is present in the right subphrenic space *(SD)*. RL, LL, right and left lobe of liver; ST, stomach, SP, spleen.

Fig 10 (right).—Pancreatic abscess. CT shows a gas-containing abscess in the pancreatic head *(arrows)*. There is also a pseudocyst *(arrowheads)* anterior to the left kidney. *lcy*, left renal cyst.

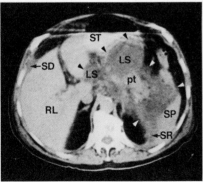
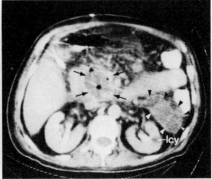

disease. Atrophy of the parenchyma surrounding the dilated pancreatic duct may be seen with tumors or chronic inflammation. Calcifications in and around the pancreatic duct and its branches are well seen on CT. These are usually visible on conventional x-ray films, though it may not be possible to localize them to the pancreas.

4. There are many normal variants that can be confused with disease. Irregularities of the pancreatic contours are seen normally on CT and should not be mistaken for disease. A prominent normal anterior convexity, the omental tuberosity, is often seen in the pancreatic body. Fat is normally interposed with the parenchyma in a linear, branching pattern. Occasionally this fat may form small islands that resemble focal lesions. An arcade of vessels surrounds the pancreatic head and should not be mistaken for lymph nodes.

The use of pancreatic CT at our institution has reduced the need for barium studies and invasive procedures, although these are occasionally needed, for example, in cases of duodenum inversum. Arteriography is still necessary to show small islet cell tumors, particularly insulinomas. ERCP has shown lesions obstructing the pancreatic duct that were missed on CT, or normal variants such as pancreas divisum that mimicked masses on CT. Sonography has been valuable in the thin or pediatric patient, or if there is motion artifact on the CT scans. With all these diagnostic procedures, there has been no improvement in the dismal survival figures for pancreatic carcinoma.

The Bowel and Mesentery

CT is ideally suited for imaging abnormalities of the bowel wall and mesentery in adults. Peritoneal or mesenteric fat and the mesenteric vessels are exquisitely demonstrated by CT. Men generally have a relative preponderance of intra-abdominal fat compared to women, and even thin men are good candidates for CT imaging in this area. If the bowel lumen is properly filled with air and dilute oral contrast material, and if glucagon is administered IV, the bowel wall can be delineated on CT against the surrounding mesenteric fat. We have found CT valuable in the following instances:

1. To image mural lesions of the hollow viscera. Because it

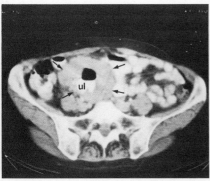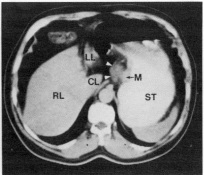

Fig 11 (left).—Small bowel lymphoma. CT shows a circumferential small bowel wall mass *(arrows)* with a posterior ulceration containing contrast *(ul)*. The mass displaces adjacent loops of small bowel.

Fig 12 (right).—Adenocarcinoma of stomach. Transverse CT through upper abdomen shows a flat mass *(M)* involving lesser curvature of stomach *(ST)*. Contiguous mass *(white arrowheads)* was thought to represent gastrohepatic ligament extension, but contained mucin and no tumor at surgery. *RL, LL, CL,* right, left, and caudate lobes of liver.

can show both the luminal and mesenteric sides of the bowel wall, CT is more sensitive than barium studies for focal or diffuse bowel wall thickening (Figs 11 through 14). Associated ulcerations may be seen if larger than 2 cm (see Fig 11). Unfortunately, neoplastic and inflammatory abnormalities are not distinguishable on the basis of their CT appearances. Thickening due to infiltrating carcinoma (see Fig 12) may be mimicked by peptic ulceration or granulomatous inflammation (see Fig 13). Abscesses due to perforated ulcers or diverticulitis (see Fig 14) may resemble those secondary to perforated carcinoma. Fistulas are better delineated by barium studies but may be inferred from the CT appearance if air is present in the noninstrumented urinary tract (see Fig 13), biliary tract, or subcutaneous tissues. Polypoid and ulcerating mucosal lesions may be missed on CT, particularly if there is hypersecretion or lack of bowel preparation.

2. Bowel obstruction may be localized on sequential CT sections to the level where discrepancy between distended and nondistended bowel is noted. In such cases oral contrast media may become diluted by the more lucent succus entericus. The dilated bowel loops then appear isodense with soft tissue and indistinguishable from masses. Therefore, we do not administer

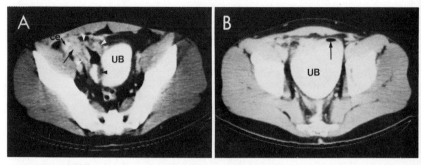

Fig 13.—Ileal-vesical fistula secondary to Crohn's disease, **A,** CT through upper pelvis shows gas- and contrast-filled ileum with thickened wall *(arrowheads)* adherent to urinary bladder *(UB)*. Associated soft tissue mass *(arrow)* indents cecum *(ce)*. **B,** CT through midpelvis shows gas *(arrowhead)* within the urinary bladder *(UB)*.

oral contrast material if bowel obstruction is suspected, unless the viscera have been suctioned. Intussusception has a characteristic CT appearance,[17] with the intussuscepted loop and mesentery surrounded by the wall of the intussuscipiens (Fig 15), although the leading lesion may not be visible.

3. Hernias may be more easily diagnosed on CT than on barium studies. Moderate to large sliding hiatal hernias are diagnosed when opacified stomach is seen in the mediastinum (Fig 16). Smaller sliding hiatal hernias can be diagnosed with certainty if the long axis of the posthiatal segment is inclined 40 degrees or more to the horizontal; the diagnosis can be excluded if the angle is less than 20 degrees.[18] Esophagogastric intussusception or prolapse is not uncommon in this region and may mimic masses on CT. Inguinal hernias are also easily

Fig 14.—Diverticular abscess. Lower abdominal CT shows a lobulated soft tissue mass *(M)* surrounding the opacified sigmoid colon *(black arrows)* with gas-containing diverticula *(black arrowheads)*.

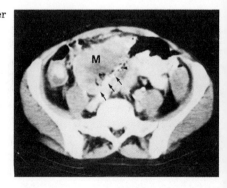

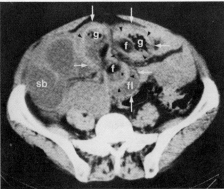

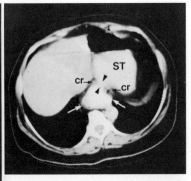

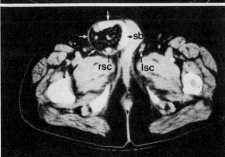

Fig 15 (above left).—Ileo-ileal intussusception. Lower abdominal CT shows intussuscipiens *(white arrows)* containing intussusceptum *(black arrowheads).* The intussusceptum contains gas-filled ileum *(g)* and mesenteric fat *(f).* A small amount of fluid *(fl)* separates the walls of the intussusceptum and intussuscipiens. *sb,* fluid-filled small bowel proximal to obstruction. A leading mass was not shown at surgery, but small bowel lymphoma was diagnosed histologically.

Fig 16 (above).—Hiatal hernia. CT shows herniated stomach *(white arrows)* in posterior mediastinum behind the crural margins *(cr)* of the esophageal hiatus, which compress the intrahiatal herniated stomach *(arrowheads).* ST, intra-abdominal stomach.

Fig 17 (left).—Right inguinal hernia. CT through lower ischia shows a right inguinal hernia *(white arrows)* containing opacified small bowel *(sb),* mesenteric fat, and vessels. The right spermatic cord *(rsc)* is displaced posteriorly. *lsc,* left spermatic cord.

shown (Fig 17), although the smaller hernias containing only omentum may be difficult to differentiate from lipomas of the spermatic cord. Associated urinary bladder herniation is readily visible. Other hernias demonstrable by CT include internal, umbilical, incisional, spigelian, Morgagni, and Bochdalek hernias.

4. Peritoneal and mesenteric masses. In the absence of previous surgery, linear or rounded densities within intra-abdominal fat are reliable CT evidence of inflammatory or neoplastic involvement. Such densities ("dirty fat") may be the only radiologic sign of what is palpated as a large mesenteric mass at surgery. Omental implants (Fig 18) and enlarged mesenteric

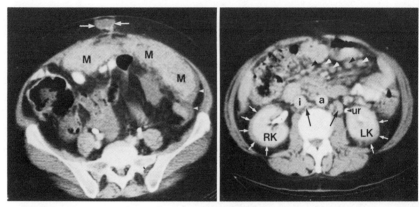

Fig 18 (left).—Metastatic adenocarcinoma involving greater omentum. Lower abdominal CT shows a solid omental mass *(M)* displacing bowel posteriorly and extending anteriorly to form a retroumbilical implant (Sister Mary Joseph nodule) *(white arrows)*. There is ascites *(white arrowheads)* in the left paracolic gutter.

Fig 19 (right).—Retroperitoneal and mesenteric lymphadenopathy due to lymphoma. Midabdominal CT shows extensive retroperitoneal *(black arrows)* and mesenteric *(arrowheads)* lymph node enlargement. The right *(RK)* and left *(LK)* kidneys are surrounded by lucencies *(white arrows)*, consistent with edema or lymphoma of the renal capsules. *i,* inferior vena cava; *a,* aorta; *ur,* ureter.

lymph nodes (Fig 19) are distinguishable from properly opacified viscera and blood vessels. In our experience, sonography plays a supplementary role to CT in evaluating the bowel wall and mesentery and is useful primarily to study the texture of masses identified on CT. An exception to this is the very thin or pediatric patient in whom the fat-depleted mesentery appears isodense with the abdominal great vessels on CT and can be mistaken for retroperitoneal lymph node enlargement.

Abdominal Abscesses and Fluid Collections

The search for abdominal abscesses is one of the most important radiologic procedures, as the disease is benign yet life-threatening. Here CT with its capability to delineate air, fat, and fascial planes is the initial procedure of choice (Figs 20 and 21; see also Fig 10). Sonography is less useful because collections may be camouflaged by overlying air or fat, fluid-filled adynamic bowel loops may mimic collections, and air-containing collections may be mistaken for bowel. As with other ab-

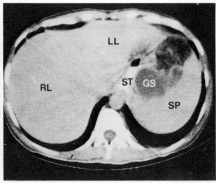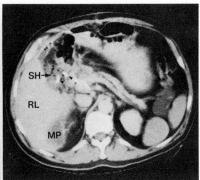

Fig 20 (left).—Left subphrenic abscess. CT through upper abdomen shows a lobulated collection under the left diaphragm in the gastrosplenic recess *(GS)*, indenting the greater curvature of the stomach *(ST)*. Abscess was proved at surgery. *SP*, spleen; *RL, LL*, right and left lobes of liver.

Fig 21 (right).—Subphrenic abscess after Whipple's procedure. Air-containing collection in anterior subhepatic space *(SH)* surrounds portions of T tube *(black arrowheads)* which fell out from common duct. *MP*, collection in Morison's pouch, or posterior subhepatic space. Note its marked posterior location in the abdomen.

dominal applications, opacification of the stomach and intestines is essential for proper CT diagnosis. Knowledge of the sectional anatomy of the abdominal spaces[16, 19] is important for distinguishing peritoneal from extraperitoneal or parenchymal collections.

Differentiation of abscesses from hematomas or lymphoceles is usually not possible on the basis of their CT appearances. Air within the collection is a good sign of infection if there has been no recent surgery, but this is seen in a minority of cases. Thin-needle aspiration with CT or ultrasound guidance is often valuable. Radionuclide scanning with gallium citrate or indium-labeled WBCs may also help in this differential diagnosis.

CT is less sensitive than sonography for the detection of small quantities of ascites. Multiloculation of ascites, high-density foci, peritoneal or mesenteric thickening (see Fig 18), focal hepatic lesions, and associated abdominal lymph node enlargement are signs that help distinguish complicated (malignant or infected) from serous ascites.[20] Differentiation between malignant and inflammatory ascites is not possible on the basis of CT and ultrasound appearances only.[20]

Retroperitoneal Lymphadenopathy

CT is the primary imaging procedure for suspected enlarged retroperitoneal and retrocrural lymph nodes (see Fig 19).[2] Opacification of the intestines with oral contrast material is essential. Infusion of boluses of IV contrast is helpful in differentiating normal vascular structures such as the gonadal veins, inferior mesenteric veins, duplicated inferior vena cava (Fig 22), and hypogastric vessels from enlarged lymph nodes. Similarly, enlarged splenorenal and peripancreatic venous collaterals due to portal hypertension or splenic vein obstruction must be distinguished from enlarged lymph nodes.

A major limitation of CT is its dependence on size (more than 1 cm in the retroperitoneum) to diagnose lymphadenopathy. Hyperplastic lymph nodes are indistinguishable from those enlarged by neoplasm. Metastatic lymphadenopathy without enlargement (for example, from epithelial pelvic tumors) is not detectable by CT. In such cases lymphangiography and CT-guided needle biopsies are valuable supplementary procedures. On the other hand, lymph nodes along the gonadal vessels, above the cisterna chyli, and occasionally along the hypogastric vessels are not opacified by lymphangiography. Intravenous pyelography (IVP), which formerly was often performed to detect ureteral deviation by enlarged nodes, is not needed after

Fig 22.—Duplication of the inferior vena cava. **A,** CT during infusion of intravenous contrast through a left leg vein shows enhancing vascular structure *(arrow)* to left of aorta *(a)*. The normal inferior vena cava *(i)* lies to right of aorta. **B,** on CT 3.5 cm above **A,** left-sided vessel *(arrow)* courses behind the aorta to join the normal inferior vena cava *(i)*. Duplicated inferior vena cava was verified during surgery. *ur,* ureter.

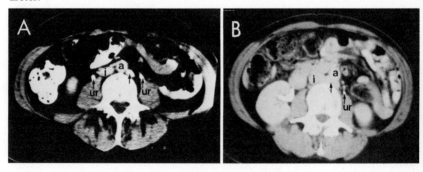

CT, as the opacified ureters can be identified on nearly every section (see Figs 19 and 22). Retroperitoneal fibrosis encases the abdominal great vessels and may mimic retroperitoneal adenopathy on CT. In most cases the flat appearance of the fibrotic tissue, its high attenuation values, and the marked enhancement of its extensive capillary network by IV contrast material help to distinguish it from enlarged lymph nodes.

Although semicoronal views of the abdomen improve sonographic visualization of the para-aortic and paracaval areas by avoiding anterior bowel gas,[2] only moderately to markedly enlarged lymph nodes can be detected reliably with this method. Ultrasound, therefore, remains a supplementary procedure to CT in this area. We have found it valuable in the very thin patient and occasionally for differentiating large collateral veins from lymph nodes.

Our approach to evaluation of abdominal lymphadenopathy, centered on CT as the initial procedure, has been associated with a decrease in lymphangiograms and an increase in the percentage of positive lymphangiograms at our institution.[2]

The Abdominal Aorta and Inferior Vena Cava

Sonography is the favored initial procedure for suspected abdominal aortic aneurysm.[2] Semicoronal sonograms of the flanks demonstrate the renal and common iliac arteries and their relation to the aneurysm, if any, in over 80% of cases. CT is used sparingly as a supplementary procedure to demonstrate the lower abdominal aorta or renal arteries if they are not seen on ultrasound, and in cases of suspected aneurysmal rupture to show associated retroperitoneal, mesenteric, or extrapleural hematomas.

The aneurysmal lumen can be opacified with IV contrast material and differentiated from mural thrombus by CT (Fig 23). Iliac artery aneurysms, occasionally obscured on sonography, are well delineated on CT (Fig 24). CT is valuable for delineating the infrahepatic vena cava and iliac veins, which are often poorly visualized or not visualized sonographically. Infusion of boluses of IV contrast material is necessary to demonstrate thrombi on CT. Duplication (see Fig 22), tumor, and displacement of the lower inferior vena cava can be easily delineated

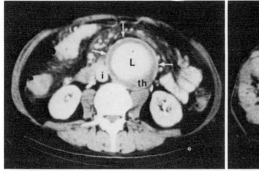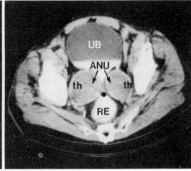

Fig 23 (left).—Abdominal aortic aneurysm. CT through lower poles of kidneys demonstrates abdominal aortic aneurysm *(arrow),* with a central patent lumen *(L)* and peripheral mural thrombus *(th). i,* inferior vena cava.

Fig 24 (right).—Internal iliac artery aneurysms. Pelvic CT shows bilateral internal iliac aneurysms *(ANU).* Low-density mural thrombus *(th)* is located peripherally. *UB,* urinary bladder; *RE,* rectum.

on CT. Sonography is superior for visualizing the retrohepatic inferior vena cava, which is poorly seen on CT because it is isodense with the liver.

Abdominal aortography is usually performed in our hospital only if an aneurysm is demonstrated on ultrasound and CT and if surgery is contemplated.

The Adrenal Glands

The cross-sectional configuration of the adrenal glands, with central, medial, and lateral rami, lends itself readily to CT evaluation. Perinephric fat surrounding these glands and interposed between their rami makes sonographic delineation difficult. This fat is easily penetrated by x-rays and helps in demarcating the adrenal from surrounding structures on CT. Since it may be isodense with the cholesterol-laden adrenal cortex, periadrenal fat may impair CT delineation of the peripheral cortical margins. For this reason, contralateral cortical atrophy in the presence of a functioning cortical tumor may be difficult to document on CT.

Adrenal hyperplasia causes diffuse enlargement of all adrenal rami on CT (Fig 25), in contrast to tumors, which cause focal enlargement of a ramus or part of a ramus. In our expe-

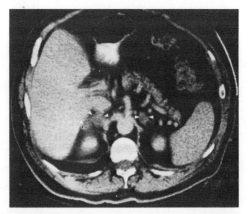

Fig 25.—Right adrenal hyperplasia. CT scan shows enlargement of lateral, central, and medial rami *(arrows)* of the right adrenal gland consistent with hyperplasia. This was verified at surgery. The low-density nodule in the left adrenal gland *(arrrowheads)* may represent focal hyperplasia or adenoma.

rience these criteria have been very useful for differentiating hyperplasia from tumors, except for rare cases of focal nodular hyperplasia which mimic adrenal adenomas on CT (see Fig 25). Granulomatous inflammatory disease, amyloid, hemorrhage, or metastases may all cause diffuse adrenal enlargement, mimicking hyperplasia. CT is the preferred initial imaging procedure for suspected adrenal hyperplasia or tumors in adults. Adenomas present as focal low-density lesions due to their cholesterol content. Functioning and nonfunctioning adenomas are not distinguishable on the basis of their CT appearance. Pheochromocytomas have higher CT densities than adenomas unless there has been internal hemorrhage with liquefaction. They are indistinguishable morphologically from primary carcinomas or metastases. In patients with clinically diagnosed pheochromocytoma, the CT search is continued into the remainder of the abdomen and pelvis and occasionally the chest if the adrenal glands appear negative.

Focal lesions less than 1 cm in diameter are difficult to distinguish from normal adrenal and are usually missed on CT. For this reason, adrenal venography with venous assay is recommended after a negative CT examination in patients with clinically diagnosed adenomas or pheochromocytomas. Iodocholesterol radionuclide scans after dexamethasone suppression have been used to differentiate autonomously functioning cortical tumors from nonfunctioning adenomas.[21]

Myelolipomas are benign adrenal tumors that can be diagnosed on CT by virtue of the islands of fat and occasional calcifications within them.[22] Adrenal metastases may appear as focal nodules (some of which calcify in response to chemotherapy), large necrotic masses, or diffusely enlarged glands. If the metastases are small enough the adrenals may appear morphologically normal on CT. In fact, in our experience, adrenal metastases are the cause of most false negative CT diagnoses.

The left adrenal gland is contiguous with the splenic vessels anteriorly and with the celiac nodes anteromedially. Segments of a tortuous splenic artery, enlarged splenorenal collateral veins, and enlarged celiac lymph nodes can silhouette the gland's contours and mimic primary left adrenal lesions on CT. There is a paucity of fat between the lateral right adrenal ramus and liver capsule, which may be adherent to each other. For this reason, right adrenal masses may mimic hepatic masses. Similarly, masses involving the medial right adrenal ramus may mimic retrocaval adenopathy.

Compared to other adrenal imaging procedures CT is relatively sensitive, though usually nonspecific. Its use has greatly reduced the need for extensive angiographic studies with injections of multiple vessels. It has also created diagnostic difficulties when unsuspected adrenal nodules are discovered incidentally. The great majority of these nodules have been followed by serial studies without surgery. In the thin or pediatric patient with no perinephric fat, we have found sonography more useful as the initial imaging procedure.

The Kidneys

For the evaluation of renal masses noted on IVP or of the nonfunctioning kidney, sonography is the initial imaging procedure.[2, 23, 24] It is better than CT for differentiating solid from cystic masses and it is more sensitive than CT for parenchymal abnormalities. Some observations on renal CT follow.

1. Renal cysts appear homogeneously lucent on CT with attenuation values between -20 HU and $+20$ HU, no visible wall, and no enhancement with IV contrast (see Fig 10). Occasionally, however, renal cysts may appear isodense with or den-

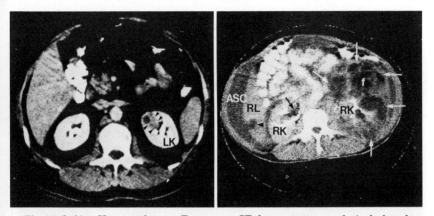

Fig 26 (left).—Hypernephroma. Transverse CT demonstrates a relatively low-density, heterogeneous, solid mass *(arrowheads)* in the upper pole of the left kidney *(LK)*.

Fig 27 (right).—Bilateral renal angiomyolipomas and hepatic fatty hamartoma in patient with tuberous sclerosis. CT shows large fat-containing angiomyolipoma *(white arrows)* involving left kidney *(LK)*. A smaller angiomyolipoma *(black arrow)* is present in right kidney *(RK)*. A fat-containing hamartoma *(arrowhead)* is seen in the right lobe of liver *(RL)*. *f,* fat within left renal angiomyolipoma; *ASC,* chylous ascites secondary to diffuse hamartomatous involvement of lymph nodes (autopsy proved).

ser than the kidney because of high levels of hemosiderin or minerals within the fluid. Renal cysts smaller than 1 cm are generally not resolvable sonographically, while cysts between 1 and 2 cm may be difficult to differentiate from small solid lesions sonographically. Rarely, the multiple cysts of polycystic kidneys are so small that they are visible on CT but not on ultrasound. Parapelvic cysts may mimic hydronephrosis or renal sinus lipomatosis on sonography. They are easily diagnosed on CT.

2. Renal carcinomas appear heterogeneous on CT with high attenuation values (Fig 26). Occasionally clear cell hypernephromas are markedly echogenic on ultrasound, mimicking angiomyolipomas.[2] These two entities can be differentiated on CT, which shows islands of fat within angiomyolipomas (Fig 27).[25, 26] Extension of malignant tumor through Gerota's fascia, into retroperitoneal lymph nodes, or into the renal veins may be clearly demonstrable on CT. Again, the CT findings are nonspecific. Perinephric hemorrhage or enlarged vessels may mimic tumor nodules, and hyperplastic nodes appear identical to metastatic adenopathy.

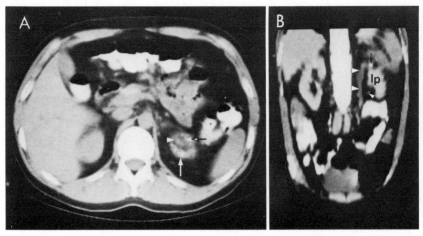

Fig 28.—Obstructed, pyelonephritic upper pole renal collecting system. **A,** CT through upper pole of left kidney shows a mass with internal lucencies *(arrowhead)* and calcifications *(arrows)* indistinguishable from hypernephroma. **B,** Coronal reconstruction of sequential CT cross sections shows dilated ureter *(large arrowheads)* leading to the calcified unopacified upper pole mass *(arrow)*. A nondilated ureter *(small arrowhead)* arises from opacified lower pole *(lp)* renal parenchyma. The diagnosis of duplex collecting system with obstructed nonfunctioning upper pole moiety was confirmed at surgery.

3. Hypertrophied renal column (Bertin's column) can be definitively differentiated from tumor with rapid-sequence CT sections obtained after infusion of a bolus of IV contrast material.

4. Renal abscess is classically necrotic centrally with an enhancing ring of renal parenchyma. Focal areas of inflammation without cavitation may be easier to visualize on CT—appearing as low-density defects within the opacified renal parenchyma—than on ultrasound.

5. The renal nephrogram, a valuable indicator of parenchymal function, is assessed much better with CT than with conventional methods.

6. The ureters are seen much better on CT than on ultrasound. Hydroureters can be followed by sequential CT sections to the site of obstruction, where the extent of the lesion can be determined. Calcification at the site of obstruction is strongly in favor of calculi, even if the abdominal film is negative, and may preclude the need for radical surgery. Obstructed nonfunctioning upper pole moieties may be differentiated from tumor

when the associated hydroureter is visualized on CT (Fig 28). The use of ultrasound supplemented by CT for evaluating the kidney has been associated with a decrease in invasive procedures such as arteriography and retrograde pyelography at our hospital.

Summary

The CT applications described above are based on our experience with an integrated ultrasound-CT approach, tailored to the patient and aimed at reducing radiation and invasive diagnostic procedures. This approach is not presented as the ideal example to be followed by all. Rather, it is only a sample of the many possible uses of CT. Though there may be many disagreements with our approach, there can be no doubt that CT has revolutionized diagnostic abdominal imaging, to the benefit of all concerned.

REFERENCES
1. Whalen J.P., Balter S.: *Radiation risk associated with diagnostic radiology. DM* 28:2–96, 1982.
2. Whalen J.P.: Radiology of the abdomen: Impact of new imaging methods. *AJR* 133:585, 1979.
3. Araki T., et al.: Dynamic CT densitometry of hepatic tumors. *AJR* 135:1037, 1980.
4. Cantlie J.: On a new arrangement of the right and left lobes of the liver. *J. Anat. Physiol. (London),* vol. 32, 1898.
5. Royal S.A., et al.: Detection and estimation of iron, glycogen and fat in liver of children with hepatomegaly using CT. *Pediatr. Res.* 13:408, 1979.
6. Chapman R.W.G., et al.: Computed tomography for determining liver iron content in primary hemochromatosis. *Br. Med. J.* 280:440, 1980.
7. Moss A.A., et al.: Dynamic CT of hepatic masses with intravenous and intra-arterial contrast material. *AJR* 138:847, 1982.
8. Davis J.M., et al.: Diagnosis of splenic abscess: Recent advances. *J. Infect. Surg.* 2:90, February 1983.
9. Schneider M., et al.: Ultrasonography and computed tomography in the evaluation of biliary tract disease, in Thorbjarnarson B. (ed.): *Surgery of the Biliary Tract.* Philadelphia, W.B. Saunders Co., 1982.
10. Freitas J.E., et al.: Cholescintigraphy in acute and chronic cholecystitis. *Semin. Nucl. Med.* 7:18, 1982.
11. Behan M., Kazam E.: Sonography of the common bile duct: Value of the right anterior oblique view. *AJR* 130:701, 1978.
12. Weinstein D.P., et al.: Ultrasonography of biliary tract dilatation without jaundice. *AJR* 132:729, 1979.
13. Baron R.L., et al.: A prospective comparison of the evaluation of biliary

obstruction using computed tomography and ultrasonography. *Radiology* 145:91, 1982.
14. Mueller P.R., et al.: Observations on the distensibility of the common bile duct. *Radiology* 142:467, 1982.
15. Katz R.J., et al.: Sonography and CT of the pancreas. *Semin. Ultrasound* 1:209, 1980.
16. Rubenstein W.A., et al.: CT and ultrasound of the perihepatic spaces. Unpublished manuscript.
17. Donovan A.T., et al.: Computed tomography of ileocecal intussusception: Mechanism and appearance. *J. Comput. Tomogr.* 6:630, 1982.
18. Govoni A., et al.: Hiatal hernia: A new look. Exhibition at the 68th meeting of the Radiological Society of North America, Chicago, November 1982.
19. Kazam E., Whalen J.P.: Anatomy of computed tomography, in Margulis A.R., Burhenne H.J. (eds.): *Alimentary Tract Radiology*. St. Louis, C.V. Mosby Co., 1979, vol. 3., pp. 72–122.
20. Khanuja A.K., et al.: Personal observations.
21. Sarkar S.D.: Clinical applications of radionuclide adrenal scanning. *Appl. Radiol.*, to be published.
22. Behan M., et al.: Myelolipoma of the adrenal: Two cases with ultrasound and CT findings. *AJR* 129:993, 1977.
23. Behan M., et al.: Sonographic evaluation of renal masses: Correlations with angiography. *Urol. Radiol.* 1:137, 1980.
24. Behan M., et al.: Sonographic evaluation of the nonfunctioning kidney. *J. Clin. Ultrasound* 7:449, 1979.
25. Pitts W.R., et al.: Ultrasonography, computerized transaxial tomography and pathology of angiomyolipoma of the kidney: Solution to a diagnostic dilemma. *J. Urol.* 124:907, 1980.
26. Behan M., Kazam E.: The echographic characteristics of fatty tissues and tumors. *Radiology* 129:143, 1978.

Arthroscopic Knee Surgery

ROBERT W. METCALF, M.D.

Division of Orthopedic Surgery, University of Utah School of Medicine,
Salt Lake City, Utah

NEARLY EVERY surgical specialty has developed an endoscopic technique that allows atraumatic examination of various parts of the body. Although diagnostic examination was the initial aim of these "oscopies," surgeons have discovered therapeutic applications as well. Ingenious endoscopic surgical techniques have been developed that have permitted converting many open operations to closed procedures.

Orthopedic surgeons have now joined other specialty surgeons in adopting such an endoscopic procedure. Arthroscopy, the examination of joints with a rigid endoscope, is rapidly becoming an alternative to arthrotomy for many knee operations, such as meniscectomy (Figure 1), and is also being used to examine other joints of the body, including the shoulder, elbow, hip, and ankle.

History

Even though the greatest advances in surgical arthroscopy were made in the past 6 years, arthroscopy itself is a relatively old technique dating back over 50 years to the work of Takagi of Japan,[1] who in 1918 examined a knee joint with a rudimentary cystoscope. He coined the term "arthroscope" and designed a specific instrument for the knee. Bircher of Switzerland, in 1921, reported using arthroscopy on 21 patients, and in the United States in the 1930s there were various reports of endoscopic examination of the knee, elbow, shoulder, and ankle by

0065-3411/84/0017-0197-0240-$04.00

Burman, et al.[2, 3] However, the technique did not catch the interest of orthopedic surgeons in the United States. The Japanese continued to investigate its use. Takagi's student, Watanabe, and co-workers developed a series of arthroscopes and in 1953 published a color atlas of arthroscopy[4] containing beautiful photographs of the interior of many joints throughout the body, primarily the knee joint. Jackson reintroduced the technique to North America in 1968 and a few scattered reports began to appear in the literature in the early 1970s,[5–8] claiming that arthroscopy had distinct advantages for improving diagnostic accuracy for knee problems.

The Watanabe No. 21 arthroscope, which utilized a tungsten bulb apparatus, had very clear optics and an excellent photography system, but it was large and cumbersome to use and the tungsten bulb could easily be broken within the knee joint. Needless to say, this was a significant deterrent to most orthopedic applications and the technique was not widely accepted.

The introduction of fiberoptics to arthroscopy helped solve these technical problems and by 1974 there was a surge of interest in diagnostic arthroscopy. Johnson[9] introduced a 1.7-mm needle arthroscope, and O'Connor,[10] Casscells, McGinty,[11] Joyce, and others began lecturing on the technique at various orthopedic seminars in North America. In 1974, at a postgraduate course in diagnostic arthroscopy held in Philadelphia, the International Arthroscopy Association was formed, with 50 members. At that time probably fewer than 100 orthopedic surgeons were utilizing these techniques in their knee practice. In 1983, there are an estimated 3,000 orthopedic surgeons in the United States and Canada who use arthroscopy for diagnosis and surgery. This dramatic increase has had a significant impact on knee surgery. Most knee arthrotomies are now preceded by diagnostic arthroscopy, and the list of knee operations that have been converted to an endoscopic technique is growing.

Learning a New Technique

Orthopedic surgeons are finding that arthroscopy is an entirely new type of technique. Previously, orthopedic operative experience was oriented to open techniques requiring dexterity in skeletal reconstruction through large incisions, by means of tools such as osteotomes, mallets, curettes, and rongeurs. In arthroscopic surgery very small instruments are used; these are manipulated while the surgeon is looking into a tightly confined compartment through a rigid monocular telescope.

Because arthroscopy is such a new and different technique, the learning process can be frustrating; it demands much time and patience. There have been few experienced arthroscopists to train other surgeons. Most training has taken place in postgraduate courses, including hands-on laboratories using knee joint simulators for endoscopic practice. Self-teaching is still the cornerstone of endoscopic instruction, but one-to-one instruction at the residency and fellowship levels is increasing.

The training process is not difficult unless it is rushed. The most important prerequisites are patience and persistence. Those who assume they can quickly learn this technique often become discouraged and discover that a graduated, step-by-step development of skills is necessary before they can really enjoy, and become proficient in, these procedures.

PROGRESSION OF SKILLS

There is an order in the development of arthroscopic skills that can be listed as follows:

1. *Diagnostic arthroscopy.* A surgeon must first learn how to examine the knee joint endoscopically. This involves familiarizing himself or herself with various portals of entry, solving problems of visualization, maintaining good joint distention and adequate flow rate of saline during the procedure, and understanding angled optics (Fig 1). Once there is confidence that all parts of the joint can be clearly seen, the surgeon is ready to try the simpler surgical techniques, gradually progressing to more complicated operations.

2. *Use of a probe.* During diagnostic examination surgeons should also learn to manipulate a blunt angled probe within the joint. The arthroscope is monocular and everything is magnified and two-dimensional, making depth perception a matter of experience. By palpating with a probe brought from another angle across the joint, depth perception is enhanced and the surgeon begins to get the feel of manipulating and maneuver-

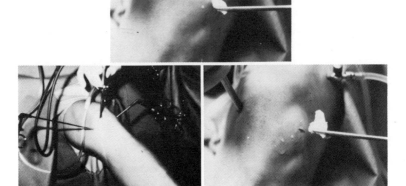

Fig 1 (top).—Right knee. A torn fragment of medial meniscus has been resected and is being teased from the small medial skin incision. Note the barrel of the 5-mm arthroscope inserted in a similar lateral incision.

Fig 2 (bottom).—Grasping and cutting instruments are inserted on opposite sides of the knee, with the viewing arthroscope positioned centrally. This triple-puncture approach facilitates triangulation.

ing an instrument within the joint cavities. Palpation of internal knee structures also adds to diagnostic accuracy.

3. *Triangulation.* In time the surgeon learns to position the probe at a desired place inside the joint. This requires a kind of stereoscopic sixth sense that is developed only with experience. Once it is learned, the surgeon can accurately bring the probe, and later a cutting or resecting instrument, to a location within the joint. This triangulation soon becomes an automatic skill. Eventually two or even three instruments might be brought to one point in the knee to grasp or cut a specific structure, such as a piece of meniscus deep within the joint (Fig 2).

4. *Multiple punctures.* The arthroscope is usually inserted anterolaterally at the jointline level and a probe is inserted anteromedially. About 90% of the joint can be examined in this manner. It may be necessary to switch the arthroscope from a lateral to a medial position for a better viewing angle. The posterior compartments of the knee joint can be examined by passing the arthroscope through the intercondylar notch or by making a direct posteromedial or posterolateral puncture. The area

of the patella is often better examined from an additional suprapatellar puncture. Once familiarity is gained with these different insertions of the arthroscope, various combinations of triangulation with the probe or other instruments can be tried so that all areas of the knee joint can be observed and manipulated.[12]

In the early days of diagnostic arthroscopy, workers spoke of "blind spots" within the knee joint, primarily the posterior horns of the menisci. With the use of angled optics and multiple punctures, there are no longer any such unvisualized areas. A skilled arthroscopist can view every compartment of the knee joint with confidence.

5. *Use of angled optics.* Most diagnostic arthroscopy is done using a rigid arthroscope that has a tip angle of 30 degrees. When the arthroscope is rotated a wider field comes into view and there is also some ability to "look around corners." This angle still allows a sense of looking straight ahead, which is very important for maintaining orientation within the knee joint.

The arthroscopist next becomes familiar with the 70-degree angle arthroscope, which makes it possible to look through the intercondylar notch onto the posterior horns of the menisci. With the 70-degree arthroscope inserted in the suprapatellar pouch, the anterior horns of the menisci and the joint surfaces in the intercondylar notch can be better seen. This different angle of perspective is often helpful. As the angled arthroscope is rotated, a wide field of view is obtained, but this can be confusing to the beginner, and these angled arthroscopes should not be used until later in one's experience. There is also a 120-degree angled rigid arthroscope that allows a "look backward." Some surgeons have become quite adept at using this type of arthroscope, especially for viewing the anterior horns of the menisci.

6. *Use of hand equipment.* There is now available a variety of hand-held cutting instruments ranging from 3 to 5 mm in diameter, including scissors, knives, and cutting forceps. Using these hand instruments while looking through a viewing arthroscope is the next skill that is developed. Care must be taken not to scuff or cut into the normal articular surfaces of the joint or force these instruments beneath joint surfaces.

7. *Motorized instruments.* Motorized devices are available

that can grind and morselize soft and hard tissues within a joint and suction the pieces away (Fig 3). These instruments are even more capable of damaging normal structures and obviously require practice to use properly.

8. *Operating arthroscopes.* In 1975 O'Connor introduced an operating arthroscope designed to guide a cutting instrument down inside the knee joint. This arthroscope is 8 mm in diameter and consists of a viewing lens, a channel for passage of a 3-mm instrument, fiberoptic fibers, and a channel for irrigation (Fig 4).

The operating arthroscope is no longer used as much as it was 4 or 5 years ago. Today, most surgery is done using a television camera attached to the viewing arthroscope. The resecting instrument is brought in from a different angle. Attaching a television camera to the operating arthroscope is quite cumbersome, which may account for its decreased use. However, the operating arthroscope is still a very accurate instrument for some types of meniscal resection.

It should be stressed again that there is a step-by-step progression to the learning of arthroscopic skills. Rushing this process is counterproductive. Unfortunately, many orthopedic surgeons feel compelled to learn these techniques quickly because their patients are requesting this less-invasive type of surgery. Attempts to master arthroscopic skills rapidly sometimes produce so much frustration that the technique is eventually abandoned.

Indications for Arthroscopy

Arthroscopy is a helpful diagnostic technique but should not be used indiscriminately. A thorough history, physical examination, and biplane x-ray films are still the foundation for diagnosis of knee disorders. Arthrography can delineate meniscal tears with 80%–90% accuracy,[13] but it is not as helpful for ligament injuries or chondral defects. Arthroscopy is indicated in acute knee injuries if the diagnosis is unclear, particularly when there is question of a chondral fracture[14] or tear of the anterior cruciate ligament. When an arthrogram is normal and symptoms of a meniscal tear persist, arthroscopy can solve the dilemma and also provide the means for resection of the tear, if one is encountered.

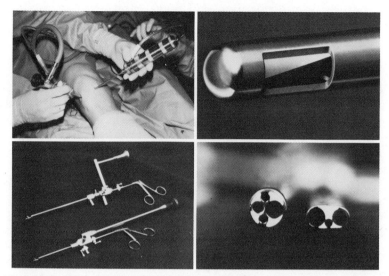

Fig 3 (top).—Motorized shaving device is used to trim away synovium. *Insert* shows the 4-mm tip of the instrument with the inner blade rotating across the window of the outer sheath.

Fig 4 (bottom).—Left, two examples of operating arthroscopes with a cutting instrument inserted through the central channel. **Right,** tips of the two arthroscopes, one round and one oval. Both have interspersed fiberoptic bundles around the operating channel and lens. There are also irrigating channels for flushing debris out of the view of the arthroscope.

Whenever conservative treatment has failed and "internal derangement" is the diagnosis, any contemplated arthrotomy should be immediately preceded by diagnostic arthroscopy (at the same anesthetic). An unnecessary arthrotomy may thus be avoided or the proposed operation may be revised or changed to another. Keene and Dyreby[15] have shown that arthroscopy has little value prior to varus or valgus osteotomy, and the same is likely true before total knee arthroplasty. In some cases of mild-to-moderate degenerative arthritis, however, there is benefit in using arthroscopy to plan the best operation or even to debride or lavage the joint for temporary relief.

To summarize, diagnostic arthroscopy is indicated in any knee disorder that has not responded to conservative treatment and in which there is diagnostic uncertainty. It is also an essential part of arthroscopic surgery to confirm the diagnosis and rule out other causes of symptoms. It is well known that disorders in the knee can mimic one another (e.g., chondromalacia patella can mimic meniscal tears), and arthroscopy is the most accurate way of ascertaining the correct diagnosis.

Advantages

REDUCED MORBIDITY.—In comparison to an arthrotomy, the immediate benefits of knee surgery done arthroscopically are impressive. Reduction in postoperative pain, immediate postoperative ambulation, significant reduction of complications, and rapid return to work or sports activities are all benefits of this procedure.

OUTPATIENT SURGERY.—Most arthroscopic surgery is now done on an outpatient basis. This has two advantages: first, there is no cost for overnight hospitalization, and second, patients have a much different attitude toward surgery when they can walk into the operating room and 2 or 3 hours later walk out of the outpatient center. Traditionally, patients have had a dread of knee surgery, anticipating much pain and a prolonged rehabilitation requiring physical therapy and at least 4–6 weeks away from work. Friends and relatives who have had open knee surgery often instill in the patient a high degree of anxiety prior to an arthrotomy. With endoscopic techniques, there is no need for this type of apprehension, because of the reduced morbidity mentioned above.

COST REDUCTION.—By eliminating 3–5 days in the hospital, the total bill for a meniscectomy performed with arthroscopic technique can be reduced by 50% or more.[16] Outpatient surgery charges are also generally less than hospital-based fees. There is a savings to the patient and his or her employer because of reduction in time lost from work. Average time for return to work of our patients is 2 weeks, compared to 6–8 weeks after the same procedure done with an arthrotomy.

MORE ACCURATE SURGERY.—The etiology of knee joint symptoms can be obscure. One problem may mimic another in the knee joint. For example, chondromalacia and subluxation of the patella almost exactly simulate a torn meniscus. If a thorough diagnostic arthroscopy is done, the exact cause of the knee problem can be discovered and unnecessary surgery can be avoided. Performing the correct surgery for the knee problem the first time can eliminate multiple knee operations.

POSSIBLE PREVENTIVE ASPECT.—Because patients are much

more amenable to having their knee problem taken care of by arthroscopy than by an arthrotomy, the development of chronic problems can sometimes be prevented by early intervention. For example, a torn meniscus can cause further damage to the articular surfaces of the joint if it continues to catch or lock into the joint. If the torn segment of meniscus is removed atraumatically at an early stage, degenerative changes within the joint can be reduced. Removal of loose bodies, realignment of the patella by lateral release, synovectomy, and joint debridement in the arthritic knee may all forestall or even eliminate the need for more extensive operations later on.

RAPID REHABILITATION.—Because there is usually no need to immobilize the knee joint or to use strong analgesics, the patient can start an immediate program of muscle exercises and range of motion exercises of the joint after arthroscopic surgery. Patients still need guidance in the type of exercises they must do to rehabilitate the knee, but the need for extensive physical therapy is considerably reduced with this type of surgery. Immediate ambulation also helps prevent thrombophlebitis and enhances overall joint function.

Disadvantages

ARTHROSCOPY CANNOT MANAGE ALL KNEE PROBLEMS.—The advanced arthritic knee still requires a total joint prosthesis or osteotomy, and major ligament injuries must be repaired by direct suture or reconstructive procedures. Neither kind of procedure is feasible with current arthroscopic methods. However, repair or prosthetic replacement of the anterior cruciate ligament has been attempted and may be a future possibility.

EQUIPMENT IS EXPENSIVE AND FRAGILE.—This is not a major disadvantage but must be considered both in structuring fees and in training operating room personnel to care for the new types of equipment. The average cost of a typical set of arthroscopic instruments, including television, is approximately $40,000.

TEACHING IS DIFFICULT.—As mentioned earlier, one-to-one teaching is the best way of learning endoscopy. Television has greatly enhanced this method of instruction.

ARTHROSCOPY TAKES TIME AND PATIENCE TO LEARN.—This factor seems to be the main disadvantage that most orthopedic surgeons are experiencing. It is a new technique and largely self-taught. The skills involved in endoscopic surgery are unlike those in which we have previously been trained. These skills cannot be rushed but are developed gradually in a sequential manner.

Use of a Knee Model in Learning Endoscopic Skills

Because endoscopic knee surgery is largely a self-taught technique, it is essential to have some way to practice these skills. Several types of knee simulators have been developed that utilize replaceable plastic menisci with premolded practice tears. Joint surfaces have a thin coating of white paint to show scuff marks. The most recent models have a constant flow of saline so that motorized devices can be used. This type of knee trainer can be used to simulate an actual endoscopic operation closely enough that it is valuable for training oneself or residents (Fig 5).

The knee simulator can be brought into an operating room during evening and weekend hours and all of the equipment used for surgery set up exactly as in surgery. A television camera can be attached to the arthroscopes so that the surgeon can practice hand-eye coordination by looking at a television monitor while manipulating instruments inside the joint. Sweeney, who developed this knee simulator model, points out that simulated practice teaches the surgeon to avoid damage to the joint and allows much more rapid transition to becoming skilled in both diagnostic and operative techniques.[17]

Equipment

ARTHROSCOPES

The arthroscopes currently in use are straight and rigid and come in varying diameters and angles of view. The most commonly used arthroscope is 4–5 mm in diameter and has a 30-degree tip angulation, which allows an 80-degree angle of view within the joint. The lens system is in fixed focus from 1 mm to infinity. The diameter of arthroscopes ranges from 1.7-mm needle arthroscopes to 8.0-mm operating arthroscopes. The viewing lens angulations come in orientations of 10, 30, 70, and

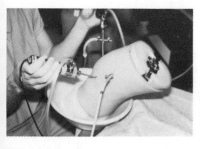

Fig 5.—Arthroscopic surgery simulator used for practice with a motorized shaver and television camera. The surgeon can gain a feel for actual surgical techniques using this knee model.

120 degrees at the tip. Flexible scopes have been tried but are not useful because of the difficulty in manipulating them about the knee joint.

HAND-HELD INSTRUMENTS

Most arthroscopic surgery is done with hand-held instruments, including knives, grasping forceps, scissors, and single- and double-jaw cutting forceps. The latter are often called "basket" forceps because the first models had a fixed lower jaw with bars across the base that would catch each piece of meniscus as it was cut. It was soon found that this design clogged easily, often breaking the upper jaw of the instrument. The current design allows the cut segment of meniscus to fall freely through the lower jaw, thus allowing multiple "bites" of meniscus or other tissue to be taken. These pieces are later washed and suctioned out of the joint.

Knives include disposable and fixed varieties. Improved metallurgy allows maintenance of a very sharp edge. Some knives are retractable into a sheath so as to protect articular cartilage until the sharp blade is needed for cutting. Knives and scissors come in a wide variety of curves and angles at the tip and different handle designs.

MOTORIZED DEVICES

The first motorized device was developed in 1978 by Johnson[18] and consists of an outer sheath with a rectangular window near its rounded tip and a rotating inner hollow sheath with a similar-sized window (see Fig 3). Suction is generated down the center of the two sheaths. Tissue is thus drawn into the window system and clipped off as the edge of the inner window shears across the fixed edge of the outer window. The small piece of tissue cut off is then suctioned out through the instrument.

This design has been retained in all of the motorized devices available at this time from various manufacturers, with only minor variations in power source, window size, and configuration. The original shaver was used for smoothing the patella. Now the tip has been opened up near the end and sharpened in a way to allow meniscal resection as well. There are also heavy-duty motorized burrs that allow smoothing and resecting of bony surfaces within the joint.

USE OF TELEVISION

Beginning in 1978, a 5-lb camera was attached to the arthroscope to produce videotapes for teaching. Although the image obtained was very sharp and clear, the manipulation of the arthroscope with the heavy camera attached was so cumbersome that television was used only for making teaching films. By 1980, endoscopy cameras were reduced in weight to 8 oz, a significant advance that made it possible to use television routinely for each surgery case. The intra-articular image is viewed on a television monitor at the side of the operating table (Fig 6). Solid-state cameras (Fig 7) became available in 1982 at a reduced weight of about 4 oz, allowing the surgeon to

Fig 6 (left).—Surgeon viewing the interior of the knee on a small television monitor at the head of the table. One assistant is holding the television camera to free the surgeon's hands; another assistant is stressing the knee open for better visualization. This is the author's standard operating setup. The operating table is angled 90 degrees at knee level.

Fig 7 (right).—New solid-state television camera attached to an arthroscope. Camera weighs 4 oz and can be soaked in disinfectant.

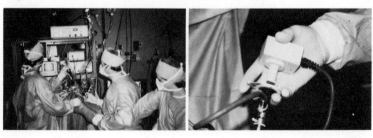

maneuver the arthroscope-camera unit freely. These solid-state cameras can also be soaked in disinfectant, which permits them to be transferred from one size of arthroscope to another without contaminating the sterile field. The disadvantage to the use of solid-state cameras is some loss of image detail compared to the image obtained with the tube-type cameras. However, the videotapes obtained are still adequate for teaching purposes.

The use of television during arthroscopic surgery allows others to observe what is being done, which is a great help in training other surgeons in the technique and in keeping operating room personnel interested and involved in the case. The surgeon can stand or sit while viewing the monitor, which relieves the fatigue associated with standing over and looking directly into an arthroscope. In addition, a videotape record can be kept of interesting cases (or all cases, if desired). This record provides a dynamic documentation that is very helpful in studying such problems as the tracking alignment of the patella during knee motion or the action of a meniscal tear as it is being probed. Thirty-five-millimeter photographs are also taken through the arthroscope and used for documentation and teaching.

There are some disadvantages to the use of television. The expense may not be justifiable unless there is a fairly large volume of knee work being done. A television system can cost $18,000–$20,000. The view obtained with television is not as clear and color-accurate as that obtained by looking directly through an arthroscope. The use of television also adds time to each case and the surgical technique is different because manipulation of instruments within the knee is done in one location while looking across the table at another angle to view the monitor. This requires considerable practice. In the beginning, operative arthroscopy skills are developed faster without the use of television.

Outpatient Routines

A patient having an arthroscopic meniscectomy typically arrives at our outpatient surgical center 1 hour before operating time. The anesthesiologist takes a history and does a physical examination to confirm the patient's suitability for a general anesthetic. The hematocrit is determined and urinalysis performed. Patients over age 14 are also required to have a chest x-ray and ECG. No preoperative medications are given. The patient walks into the operating room. Sodium brevitol is used for anesthetic induction. Narcotics are rarely used. After surgery the patient is transferred to a recovery room until fully awake and able to do straight-leg lifts. Then another period of observation is carried out in the postoperative lounge where the patient sits in a chair to avoid orthostatic hypotension. By 1–2 hours after surgery the patient is ambulatory, has received postoperative instructions, and may leave the surgical center. Postoperative nausea has been kept at a minimum with these techniques.

GENERAL VERSUS LOCAL ANESTHESIA

While it is possible to do both diagnostic and operative arthroscopy using local anesthetic agents, I prefer the light general anesthetic technique mentioned above. With local anesthesia there is more patient apprehension and the thigh muscles are not as well relaxed, making it more difficult to stress open the knee compartments for adequate visualization. Also, a tourniquet is needed in some operations and it is difficult for patients to tolerate the tourniquet for more than 30 minutes under local anesthesia.

Regional and spinal anesthesia can be used but do prolong the postoperative recovery time because patients may take several hours to regain use of the lower limbs.

OPERATING ROOM ROUTINE

Arthroscopic knee surgery is best done with two persons scrubbed besides the surgeon. A surgical technician (or scrub nurse) is in charge of the instruments, including sterilization between cases, protection from damage, organization and passage to the surgeon during the operation, storage, etc. This person also must be knowledgeable about the television cameras, various motorized units, fiberoptic light cables and light sources, and other photography equipment.

A second person, designated a surgical assistant, has the primary responsibility for manipulating the limb during the operation and stressing the joint open to give the surgeon good access into various knee compartments. This assistant may also hold the television camera during times when the surgeon is maneuvering the joint. The surgeon and surgical assistant must learn to work as a team while both are viewing the television monitor at the head of the table.

The circulating nurse is the third member of the endoscopic surgery team. This person has primary responsibility for keeping the irrigation flow constant by changing the bottles of irrigating saline as needed. The circulating nurse must also be familiar with operation of fiberoptic light generators, motorized power sources, and television equipment.

INSTRUMENT STERILIZATION

Steam autoclaving can damage fiberoptic cables and arthroscopes and dulls the small, sharp instruments used for meniscal resections. Therefore, gas autoclaving or a 10-minute cold soak in activated glutaraldehyde (Cidex) is used in most operating rooms for sterilizing arthroscopy instruments.

Gas autoclaving provides completely safe, bactericidal sterilization but is an overnight process, which precludes multiple arthroscopic surgical operations in succession on a given day. If gas sterilization is used and multiple operations are to be done, then multiple sets of equipment must be purchased, which adds greatly to the cost of the procedure.

The cold-soaking method, such as is used for urologic endoscopy instruments, allows rapid turnover of instruments between cases. However, cold soaking in glutaraldehyde does not kill spores or hepatitis virus. Because of this, some operating-room committees have not allowed activated glutaraldehyde to be used for arthroscopy procedures. Nevertheless, most arthroscopists favor activated glutaraldehyde as a safe and effective method of instrument disinfection. Johnson et al.[19] reported performing 10,000 diagnostic and surgical arthroscopy operations using Cidex, with an infection rate of 0.4%. None of the infections were attributable to the instrument sterilization method.

Since 1974, we have used Cidex as a 10-minute soak in approximately 3,500 arthroscopy procedures, with no deep infections to date. The remarkably low incidence of infections following arthroscopy procedures is probably related to the continuous irrigation of the joint during the procedure. An average of 4–8 L of saline flows in and out of the joint during a typical arthroscopic procedure. Any contamination that might occur is quickly washed away by this copious and continuous washing of the joint.

Diagnostic Arthroscopy Technique

The patient lies supine with knees flexed to 90 degrees over the end of the operating table. A general anesthetic is given. A tourniquet is placed on the upper thigh and then a thigh-holding device is applied just distal to the tourniquet to provide a fulcrum for leverage to open the joint spaces. The limb is devascularized with a rubber bandage wrap from toe to tourniquet and the tourniquet is inflated to approximately 400 mm Hg, varying according to thigh size. Skin preparation consists of applying a 2% tincture of iodine paint, which is left on the skin to dry. Hair about the knee is removed the night before surgery, using a depilatory cream (Surgex).

After placement of standard sterile knee drapes, a 12-gauge needle cannula is inserted into the suprapatellar pouch laterally and the joint is distended with 60–80 cc of saline. A 1-cm transverse skin incision is made adjacent to the lateral border of the patellar tendon and 1.5 cm above the palpable anterior edge of the tibial plateau. The joint capsule is pierced with a sharp trocar, then the sheath of a 5-mm diagnostic arthroscope is passed into the joint, using a blunt obturator for entry through the synovium and into the intercondylar notch region.

The 5-mm-diameter, 30-degree tip angle arthroscope is then inserted into the sheath (Fig 8). An irrigation system is established, with the saline entering the joint through the sheath of the arthroscope and exiting through the cannula in the suprapatellar pouch. A tube is attached to the outflow cannula and empties by gravity into a bucket on the floor. Two 2-L bottles of saline are hung from an IV pole and connected by Y tubing. Both bottles are left open and the IV standard is raised to approximately 4–5 feet above the level of the knee, which insures a good flow rate and enough pressure to keep the knee joint distended. This is very important for good visualization. If joint distention is not adequate, the synovium tends to collapse

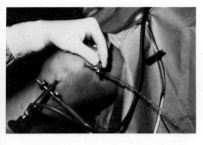

Fig 8.—Saline flows into the knee through the sleeve of the arthroscope, here inserted in the anterolateral portal. Note the flow exiting the knee through the suprapatellar cannula. The knee joint is constantly distended and irrigated during both diagnostic and surgical arthroscopy procedures.

around the tip of the arthroscope, making it difficult to see clearly.

The knee joint is then examined from this inferolateral portal. The different parts of the joint are examined in set order, insuring a complete examination. The order is as follows:

1. Suprapatellar pouch
2. Medial patellar gutter and medial synovial shelf
3. Lateral patellar gutter
4. Articular surface of the patella
5. Patellar tracking studied while flexing and extending the joint
6. Articular cartilage of the patellofemoral groove
7. Articular cartilage of the medial femoral condyle
8. Medial meniscus (anterior two thirds) and medial tibial plateau
9. Lateral femoral condyle
10. Lateral meniscus and lateral tibial plateau
11. Intercondylar notch, including fat pad and anterior cruciate ligament (occasionally, the posterior cruciate ligament can be seen from this approach)
12. Posterior one third or medial meniscus

To help visualize the medial meniscus, the knee is flexed about 20 degrees and a valgus stress is applied. The tibia is placed in external rotation by rotating the foot. For visualizing the lateral compartment and lateral meniscus, just the opposite stress is applied: varus and internal tibial rotation.

Often the posterior one third of the medial meniscus cannot be visualized from the initial lateral jointline portal and an alternative approach must be used. First, the arthroscope is changed to a medial anterior portal (adjacent to the patellar tendon and 1.5 cm above the tibial plateau). If the posterior meniscus is still not clearly seen, the 5-mm arthroscope is replaced with a 2.7-mm-diameter arthroscope which can be passed beneath the femoral condyle to look at the posterior horn of the meniscus directly. Two other alternative approaches to the posteromedial compartment include a direct posteromedial puncture or a view with a 70-degree arthroscope inserted through the intercondylar notch.

PROBING

During the diagnostic examination it is helpful routinely to probe various parts of the knee while simultaneously observing. The probe has a right-angled, 4-mm-long tip which is rounded smooth. Use of this type of probe avoids scratching the normal articular surfaces of the joint. Using a probe also has the additional advantage of training the surgeon to manipulate an instrument inside the joint, thus developing the skill of triangulation to a precise location.

Before long this probing technique becomes second nature, and the surgeon gains a great deal of information about the normal knee that can then be compared with any abnormalities encountered. For example, the anterior cruciate ligament may look normal, but testing with a probe may show it to be elongated and somewhat loose because of an interstitial tear. Or a meniscus might appear intact but when probed the tip will fall into a small tear posteriorly, and, on traction, the mobile torn segment of the meniscus can be pulled into the more central part of the joint. Articular cartilage of the patella sometimes looks normal but when probed will have a softened, mushy character, indicating early smooth and pressure damage from malalignment.

During the diagnostic examination, the surgeon can either sit or stand at the lateral side of the knee joint with the arthroscope in one hand and the probe in the other. An assistant maneuvers the knee against the thigh-holding device, going from full extension to examine the patella and suprapatellar pouch to slight flexion for the menisci or even 90 degrees of flexion for examining the anterior cruciate ligament or various portions of the femoral condyles. The operating table is flexed to 90 degrees at the knee level. The limb that is not being examined hangs in dependent fashion over the end of the flexed table and is wrapped with an elastic bandage from toe to groin to prevent hemostasis or thrombophlebitis.

ALTERNATE METHODS OF ARTHROSCOPIC KNEE JOINT EXAMINATION

In 90% of cases, the anterolateral and anteromedial jointline entries of the arthroscope, as just described, are adequate for complete examination of the knee joint. But if the posterior horns of the menisci are not well visualized, or if additional views of the suprapatellar or patellar regions are needed, the surgeon should not hesitate to make additional incisions (portals) to examine the joint. Facility in using these accessory portals greatly enhances the surgeon's confidence that all parts of the joint have been examined. Several accessory portals and their uses are described below.

SUPRAPATELLAR PORTAL.—To study the dynamics of patellar tracking or to look more thoroughly for a medial synovial shelf, a lateral suprapatellar portal is helpful. The incision is made 1.5 cm beyond the superolateral border of the patella. A similar incision can be made superomedially. These portals are also used for doing a synovectomy for rheumatoid arthritis.

Patel describes a midpatellar lateral portal which he recommends for routine diagnostic examination.[20] This portal and the more proximal suprapatellar portals give an excellent view of the anterior horns of the menisci, often very helpful in some types of meniscal resection.

CENTRAL PATELLAR TENDON PORTAL.—Gillquist and Hagberg from Sweden first described this approach and use it routinely for all of their diagnostic and surgical arthroscopic procedures.[21] The arthroscope is inserted 1 cm above the tibial plateau in the anterior midline of the knee and passed through the patellar tendon. The advantage to this approach is that the arthroscope stays in a stationary central location, and, by rotating the 30-degree angled tip, most of the knee joint can be visualized without changing from one portal to another. Also, accessory portals for instruments can be made on either side of the joint, which can be helpful if a segment of meniscus needs to be grasped and cut at the same time. This technique is also known as the "triple puncture" technique.

Disadvantages to this approach include problems viewing the undersurface of the patella and some congestion and difficulty in maneuvering instruments in the anterior part of the joint. The latter is only a minor annoyance that can be overcome with experience. Those who use this approach routinely like it very much. Fibers of the patellar tendon are not cut. Rarely, a mild patellar tendinitis will develop postoperatively, but usually this portal of entry is well tolerated by the knee joint.

INTERCONDYLAR NOTCH PORTAL.—Using either the central patellar tendon approach just described or an inferolateral portal adjacent to the patellar tendon, an arthroscope with a 70-degree view at the tip can be passed across the intercondylar notch into either the posteromedial or posterolateral compartment. A direct view is thus obtained of the posterior meniscal horns, the posterior compartments, and the posterior cruciate ligament.[22]

POSTEROMEDIAL PORTALS.—When the joint is well distended and the knee flexed at 90 degrees, the posteromedial capsule will bulge and a direct puncture can be made at the posteromedial corner. The posteromedial capsule is pierced with a sharp trocar and a 5-mm arthroscope is inserted. With this approach the entire posteromedial compartment can be examined for loose bodies or additional meniscal tears. Capsular tears of the meniscus in particular are well visualized. Also, the posterior cruciate ligament can be examined and avulsion of this ligament from the tibia can be discovered. When surgery is done in the posterior compartments, an additional posteromedial portal can be made 2 cm superior and anterior to the first puncture site for introduction of a grasping instrument, scissors, or motorized device (Fig 9).

ACCESSORY JOINTLINE PORTALS.—An incision can be made anywhere along the anterior jointline from the level just adjacent to the medial collateral or lateral collateral ligaments. These entries are sometimes made to introduce a small grasping or cutting forceps for meniscal surgery and are especially helpful in a knee joint that is very tight and resistant to opening with stress.

MULTIPLE PORTALS.—The postoperative morbidity from multiple punctures is not a function of or multiplied by the number of incisions. When it has been necessary to make five or six punctures, these patients have not complained of any more dis-

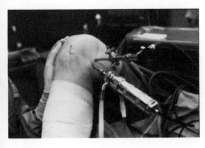

Fig 9.—Both a motorized meniscal cutter and a 5-mm arthroscope have been inserted directly into the posterolateral portal to remove a tag of the medial meniscus that could not be reached from anterior approaches.

comfort than did those in whom one or two punctures have sufficed. These incisions are very small (1 cm), and the entry through the tissues is atraumatic. Occasionally, with multiple punctures, saline will flow into subcutaneous spaces and cause swelling, but this subsides 24–48 hours after surgery.

With all of these punctures, especially the posteromedial and central portals, care must be taken not to force an instrument toward the neurovascular structures in the popliteal area. Damage to these structures during arthroscopy is very rare but has been known to occur.[23]

Normally, two or three punctures are all that are required to complete both diagnostic and surgical arthroscopy. But depending on the particular surgical case, multiple portals may be needed, and various combinations of these portals can be helpful, particularly for meniscal resection. There should be no hesitancy on the part of the arthroscopist to bring the arthroscope in from another angle of direction to achieve a better perspective on a particular part of the knee joint. This multiple puncture approach avoids any blind spots within the tightly fitting knee joint and allows manipulation of instruments from various angles and locations.

ARTHROSCOPIC MANAGEMENT OF SPECIFIC KNEE LESIONS

Types of Lesions Treated and Order of Difficulty

Once proficiency is gained in diagnostic arthroscopy, the surgeon is ready to start doing the various therapeutic procedures. There is an order of difficulty in the types of knee lesions that can be managed by arthroscopic surgery. The more difficult procedures, such as suture of a torn meniscus, should not be attempted until confidence is gained in the management of the easier procedures. If a more complicated problem is encountered during diagnostic arthroscopy than was anticipated during clinical examination, it is much better to proceed with open knee surgery rather than struggle with an endoscopic procedure.

The following arthroscopic procedures and knee lesions are arranged in order of progressive difficulty. The list may serve as a guide to developing arthroscopic surgery skills.

1. Synovial biopsy
2. Excision of a medial synovial shelf
3. Removal of a loose body or foreign body in the suprapatellar pouch area
4. Patellar shaving and lateral patellar release
5. Excision of a "flap" tear, middle third, either meniscus
6. Bucket handle tear, either meniscus
7. Loose body or foreign body, posterior compartments
8. Posterior and anterior horn tears, lateral meniscus
9. Posterior and anterior horn tears, medial meniscus
10. Abrasion, curettage, or drilling of chondral defects, femoral condyles, and tibial plateaus
11. Synovectomy
12. Placement of crossed fixation pins in an osteochondritis dissecans fragment; femoral condyles
13. "Total" meniscectomy
14. Endoscopic suture of peripheral meniscal tears

TECHNIQUES FOR SPECIFIC KNEE LESIONS

It is not the purpose of this general review to describe in detail the technique of each knee operation that can be performed with arthroscopic technique. Texts and instruction manuals are available which give this information.[10, 19, 24–26] However, a description of each procedure, its indications, and achievable results should be helpful as an overview of what is possible with these new endoscopic surgical procedures, which have changed so dramatically the way knee surgery is done today.

SYNOVIAL BIOPSY.—There are many causes of synovitis in the knee joint. After inspection with the diagnostic arthroscope it is helpful to take biopsy samples for a more specific diagnosis by the pathologist. With the viewing arthroscope inserted in one of the anterior jointline portals, a single- or double-jaw biopsy forceps is introduced through a superolateral portal. Three to five pieces of tissue are usually taken to give adequate specimens for sectioning. Sometimes representative samples are taken from different quadrants of the knee joint and so labeled. A compressive cotton padding dressing is worn for 24 hours and the patient is allowed immediate ambulation. This dressing gives good hemostasis, and there have been no problems associated with this procedure. It is really a diagnostic rather than a therapeutic procedure, but it does require familiarity with arthroscopic instruments.

MEDIAL SYNOVIAL SHELF.—The medial synovial shelf, or plica, is found, normally, in 20%–50% of knees.[27] It is a longitudinal fold of synovium which runs from the suprapatellar level to insert distally into the infrapatellar fat pad.[28] Normally, this fold of synovium is asymptomatic, thin, and pliable, measuring about 2–5 mm in width. The pathologic shelf becomes thickened, fibrotic, and wider than 5 mm and begins to get caught between the patella and femur (Fig 10). This can occur from direct trauma to the medial side of the knee or from unknown causes. The result of the pathologic medial synovial shelf is chronic irritation manifested by pain, catching, giving way, and swelling in the knee of the patient. It can almost exactly simulate a torn medial meniscus or chondromalacia and subluxation of the patella.

It is difficult to establish the diagnosis of pathologic medial synovial shelf by clinical means. Occasionally there is point tenderness along the medial border of the patella or a palpable subluxation of a rigid tissue across the femoral condyle as the patient flexes and extends the knee, but usually symptoms are vague and the diagnosis is established during diagnostic arthroscopy.

Sometimes the pathologic shelf is so large that it protrudes more than halfway across the patellofemoral joint, with a great deal of surrounding synovitis and hypertrophy of the infrapatellar fat pad. Usually, though, the shelf is just thickened and can be observed to sublux across the medial border of the femoral condyle as the knee is flexed and extended while the surgeon is looking with the arthroscope in the lateral suprapatellar portal.

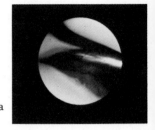

Fig 10.—Arthroscopic view of a medial synovial shelf or plica. Tip of probe is touching the shelf; patella is seen above, femoral condyle, below.

If a patient has symptoms that correspond to an enlarged medial synovial shelf and no other cause of these symptoms can be found, resection of the shelf is indicated. The shelf is a non-essential structure in the knee, probably vestigial. There is no harm in removing this synovial fold, but it should not be done indiscriminately.

The pathologic shelf is removed by first dividing it in two or three places with a scissors or basket forceps. Then a motorized cutter is used to remove all of the shelf and also the adjacent synovium about 2 cm anterior and posterior to the shelf. This partial synovectomy reduces the chances of the shelf re-forming. There may also be an associated fringe of synovitis around the medial patella border, which is removed. If the infrapatellar fat pad is hypertrophied, a partial resection of this structure is also done in the same manner.

Postoperative bleeding is controlled with a compression pad made of sponge rubber, and measuring $10 \times 10 \times 3$ cm. The patient keeps this pad against the medial side of the knee joint for 3–5 days, using an elastic bandage. Immediate ambulation is permitted and active range of motion is encouraged as soon as possible.

Sometimes this procedure brings about immediate relief of pain, but more often general synovitis in the knee takes 6–8 weeks to subside. Jackson et. al. reported that 70% of 69 patients achieved significant improvement or complete relief of symptoms.[29] They recommend arthroscopic resection as simple and effective.

LOOSE BODIES.—So-called joint mice were once extremely difficult to remove from the knee joint. Sometimes it was necessary to open the knee medially, laterally, and posteriorly to locate the elusive, cartilaginous loose body, which often seemed to move from one compartment of the joint to another, just ahead of the surgeon's search. With arthroscopic technique, locating the loose body is much easier and does not require disruption of normal muscle and fascial layers. Most loose bodies are lodged in the suprapatellar pouch or the intercondylar notch. These can be easily visualized, secured by piercing with a percutaneous needle,[30] and then grasped with a multitoothed clamp and withdrawn through a very small stab wound, all under arthroscopic visualization and control (Fig 11).

Loose bodies in the posterior compartments can be located with a 70-degree angled arthroscope inserted through the intercondylar notch. They are then withdrawn with a grasping clamp inserted directly posteromedially.

Arthroscopic technique also has the advantage of using suction. Suction can be attached directly to the sleeve of the arthroscope so that loose pieces within the joint are drawn toward the view of the lens. Articular debris, which occurs with chondromalacia or chondral fractures, can also be washed out of the knee joint through an 8-mm-diameter cannula. This flushing technique is used after an arthroscopic meniscectomy to help remove any debris that might have been left.

Motorized instruments draw loose bodies into their cutting mechanism, grind them up, and suction them out of the knee joint.

FOREIGN BODIES.—Needles, bullets, toothpicks, thorns, and even broken arthroscopic instruments have been removed from the knee joint by arthroscopy. When broken instruments must be removed, metal foreign body retrievers that have a magnetized tip are used. The techniques and principles for foreign body removal are similar to those for removal of loose bodies.

PATELLAR SURGERY. When the patella is malaligned and rides

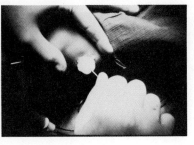

Fig 11.—Large loose body is removed through a small incision after being located and secured under arthroscopic control.

over the femoral condyle laterally, the central facet of the patella becomes compressed and begins to develop chondromalacia, or fibrillation and fragmentation of normally smooth articular cartilage. This syndrome has been called "patellar
compression syndrome,"[31] "malalignment syndrome,"[32] and
"excessive lateral facet syndrome."[33] It is a knee problem that
is seen commonly in female patients and begins in the early
teenage years, usually secondary to rotational malalignment of
the tibia and femur. If untreated, the chondromalacia can become severe, and even in 14- and 15-year-old patients extensive
breakdown of the patellar articular cartilage can occur.

Typically, the young patients complain of peripatellar intermittent aching pain, especially related to bent-knee types of
activities such as jumping and going up and down stairs. Clinical examination reveals tenderness around the patella and
palpable crepitation throughout the range of motion. Roentgenograms taken with the knees flexed at 30–45 degrees give evidence of lateral patellar subluxation.

Sixty to seventy percent of these teenage patients respond to
nonsurgical management, which includes rest, salicylates, and
isometric exercises.

For patients who do not respond to conservative treatment
and who show progressive signs of chondromalacia patella, a
realignment operation is indicated to try to reduce the compressive stress forces on the patella. Traditionally, alignment
surgery has been a major procedure involving a lengthy incision, transfer of the patellar tendon, release laterally, and im-
brication and advancement of the medial quadriceps musculature. For a young teenage female this is a formidable operation
with a long recovery time, and various reports indicate a high
complication rate. Complications include the need for revision,
disturbance of bone growth, keloid formation, infection, and,
most importantly, failure to relieve symptoms.[34-36]

The development of arthroscopic surgery has enabled operative management of this patellar problem with a significant reduction in morbidity and complications. The procedure consists
of lateral release of the contracted lateral retinaculum, synovium, and insertion of the vastus lateralis muscle under arthroscopy. The latter is part of the problem because there is an
overpull of this muscle which shifts the vector of pull by the
quadriceps muscle on the patella to a more laterally oriented

direction. If a portion of the vastus lateralis is released, the vastus medialis can be strengthened by postoperative exercises and thus dynamically pull the patella over into the center of the patellofemoral groove, where it belongs.

If chondromalacia of the patella is present and has progressed to the fibrillated, fragmentation stage, these strands of damaged articular cartilage can be debrided with an arthroscopic shaving device (see Fig 9). It is not possible to make the patella perfectly smooth again, but the debridement procedure does reduce or eliminate the feeling of crepitation. If lateral subluxation is also present, realignment with a lateral release should help prevent further roughening of the patellar articular cartilage.

This arthroscopic procedure offers an alternative to major patellar realignment surgery that is cosmetically pleasing and involves significant reduction in morbidity. Several series of lateral release show a success rate of 80%–85%.[37-39]

The technique of lateral release is relatively simple. Under arthroscopic control, a scissors or knife is used to divide the tight structures along the edge of the patellar tendon, the lateral border of the patella, and up into the vastus lateralis musculature (Fig 12). Synovium is also divided. Once all tight structures have been divided, the tracking of the patella can be immediately checked by having the patient flex and extend the knee and watching the patella glide in its proper location rather than being subluxated laterally.

Electrocutting is used for release, and bleeding vessels are cauterized as they are encountered. Distilled water, glycine, or carbon dioxide gas must be used instead of saline for irrigation during electrosurgery.

If electrosurgery is not used, postoperative bleeding can be a

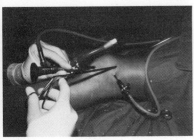

Fig 12.—Two-puncture method for arthroscopic release of the subluxating patella. Scissors superior to the arthroscope are cutting the tight fascial and synovial layers that have tethered the patella laterally.

problem. However, a snugly fitting sponge rubber compression pad, worn for 7 days after surgery, reduces the likelihood of bleeding to about 10%. A closed suction drainage system can also be left for 48 hours if bleeding has been difficult to control.

This procedure is done routinely in an outpatient surgery center. Patients may ambulate with full weight-bearing as soon as they can tighten their quadriceps muscle and do straight-leg lifts, often the same day as surgery. A compression pad and wrap are worn for 7 days to prevent bleeding. Range of motion exercises are started within the first week, and by 2 weeks the patient is doing more vigorous isometric and even isotonic exercises. Recovery from lateral release and patellar shave takes 6–8 weeks, but during this time the patient is ambulatory and is not wearing any cast or brace. Much of the success of the operation depends on the patient's willingness to exercise and regain quadriceps muscle strength.

There are two types of patellar subluxation that cannot be managed with just an arthroscopic release. The first is patella alta (a high-riding patella), which subluxes superiorly as well as laterally. This type of knee usually has a very shallow patellofemoral groove and a small patella. Advancement of the patellar tendon, combined with a lateral release, is needed to bring the patella down into proper position. The second type of knee that requires open surgery has severe chondromalacia involving wear down to subchondral bone over at least 50% of the surface area. In these knees, a lateral release will relieve pressure but improvement is only temporary and the patella continues to give pain because of the loss of articular cartilage. For these patients, a patellectomy is a better method of treatment.

Arthroscopic Meniscal Surgery

The best and most common therapeutic application of arthroscopy in the knee is in the treatment of a torn meniscus. The goal is to preserve as much normal meniscus as possible, thus helping to retain joint stability and some meniscal function. Only the damaged portion of the meniscus is removed.

Johnson and Kettlecamp showed that long-term results from open total meniscectomy have been discouraging, with as high as 68% unsatisfactory results on long-term follow-up.[40] Tapper and Hoover found that only 43% of patients were completely relieved of pain at 10-year follow-up after total meniscectomy.[41] Once the meniscus is totally excised, very little, if any, regeneration occurs. Instead, these patients begin showing osteophytic spurring and other roentgenographic changes of degenerative arthritis in the compartment of the knee that has had a total meniscectomy.

The meniscus is now recognized as an important structure in the knee joint. Meniscal functions partially or totally lost after total meniscectomy include load transmission between the femur and tibia during weight-bearing, joint congruity, joint stability, joint lubrication from even distribution of synovial fluid, and shock-absorbing capabilities to the perimeter of the joint.[42]

The knee is encased in a cuff of fibroelastic tissue which helps stabilize the joint. The meniscus has longitudinal fibers at its periphery that are an integral part of this capsular support. When a total meniscectomy is done, it is difficult to avoid cutting into this fascial cuff. With the meniscus gone and the capsule loosened, joint friction and wearing increase and degenerative sequelae occur over a period of time.

ADVANTAGES OF ARTHROSCOPIC MENISCAL RESECTION

Using the arthroscope, the meniscus can be approached at its inner margin where tears begin rather than cutting through the outer capsular layers, as in an arthrotomy. Because only tiny punctures are made there is no disruption of surrounding muscle layers. The resection is begun at the most damaged area (the inner margin) and then carefully advanced toward normal meniscal cartilage, making it possible to accurately define a limited meniscal resection, especially with the magnification and illumination possible with current optical and fiberoptic technology.

Arthroscopic surgery is therefore much more accurate for meniscal lesions than open surgery. We carefully classify the exact type of tear, and the method of arthroscopic resection is carried out according to this classification. This is an important distinction between arthroscopic meniscectomy and open total meniscectomy, for in the latter method the meniscus was removed entirely, regardless of the type of tear.

Classification of Meniscal Tears

Using a probe, the meniscal tear can be carefully delineated before arthroscopic resection is begun. Four basic patterns of tear are found and are demonstrated in Figure 13. Table 1 indicates the incidence of each of these basic patterns in a study of 258 meniscal tears.

The medial meniscus was torn about three times more commonly than the lateral. Bilateral tears occurred in 7% of knees in our series. Over 95% of tears were in the posterior one half of the meniscus, with isolated anterior horn tears being least common. This latter observation is explained by the combina-

Fig 13.—Four basic patterns of meniscal tears. **A,** vertical longitudinal (bucket handle tear). **B,** vertical transverse (radial) tear. **C,** vertical horizontal ("fish mouth") tear. **D,** oblique (flap or "parrot beak") tear.

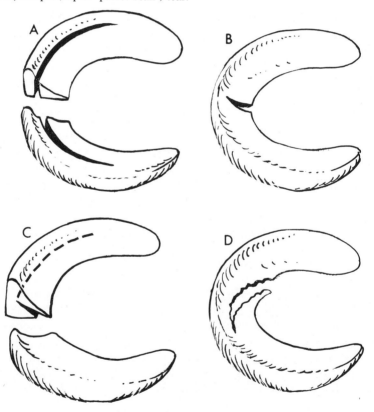

TABLE 1.—CLASSIFICATION OF 258
MENISCAL TEARS

Oblique tears (flap or "parrot beak")	117 (45%)
Vertical longitudinal tears (bucket handle)	92 (35%)
Multiple-plane tear (degenerative and complex)	30 (12%)
Vertical transverse (radial)	12 (5%)
Horizontal	4 (2%)
Miscellaneous (discoid, cysts)	3 (1%)

tion of rotatory and sliding action of the femoral condyle on the tibial plateau during weight-bearing, which produces a shearing action across the posterior horn of the meniscus. Torn fragments are thus easily caught in the joint interface, producing further tears. The anterior meniscal horns, however, are not subjected to these shearing stresses but instead act like "bumper stops" during knee extension, receiving mainly compressive forces and thus seldom tearing.

Bucket Handle Tear

This vertical longitudinal tear produces a large, mobile fragment that keeps catching in the center of the joint, producing giving way, locking, and pain in the knee. Arthroscopic meniscal resection of the bucket handle fragment is relatively easy because only these two attachment points (anterior and posterior) must be cut.

After the bucket handle fragment is removed, it is important to identify and further resect any secondary tears of the remaining posterior peripheral rim. Associated tears of the opposite meniscus occur in 20% of cases and must also be resected.

The following step-by-step approach illustrates how an arthroscopic partial meniscectomy proceeds (Fig 14). The description is for a bucket handle tear of the medial meniscus. Two portals (incisions) are made for diagnostic arthroscopy (one on each side of the patellar tendon, 1.5 cm superior to the tibial

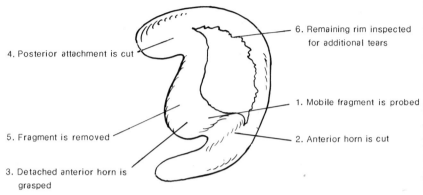

4. Posterior attachment is cut

6. Remaining rim inspected
for additional tears

1. Mobile fragment is probed

5. Fragment is removed

2. Anterior horn is cut

3. Detached anterior horn is grasped

Fig 14.—Diagram of a bucket handle tear with numbers showing location of the six steps of resection (see text).

plateau) and are referred to as the anterolateral and antero-medial portals in this description.

STEP 1: PROBING.—With the surgeon using the diagnostic arthroscope to look across the joint from the anterolateral portal, a probe is introduced anteromedially and the exact location of the anterior attachment of the bucket handle fragment is identified. Often there is hypertrophied synovium that obstructs the view of the anterior horn; this is removed with a motorized shaver.

STEP 2: CUTTING THE ANTERIOR HORN.—A 3.0-mm knife or scissors is inserted anteromedially and the fragment is detached along a line that will leave an even contour to the remaining rim.

STEP 3: GRASPING THE FRAGMENT.—The free end of the torn fragment is grasped with a forceps inserted anterolaterally. The viewing arthroscope is switched to the anteromedial portal. Tension is put on the fragment, the posterior attachment is inspected and the line of resection is determined. Rotating the fragment 180 degrees often helps visualize this posterior tibial attachment.

STEP 4: CUTTING THE POSTERIOR HORN.—A third incision is made along the medial jointline just anterior to the medial collateral ligament and a 3-mm scissors or knife is passed beneath the femoral condyle to cut the attachment directly. An alternate technique involves use of an operating arthroscope placed anterolaterally. This scope has a central channel through which the resecting instrument is used, thus giving a straight-line view of the cut and avoiding the need to triangulate across the joint.

STEP 5: REMOVING THE FRAGMENT.—The fragment is carefully twisted and teased out through the lateral portal while the surgeon watches with the arthroscope to make sure the fragment doesn't become loose in the joint.

STEP 6: INSPECTING AND TRIMMING THE REMAINING RIM.—The rim is probed for additional tears. A posteromedial puncture or intercondylar notch approach can be used for direct inspection of the posterior rim. Sometimes there is a secondary or even tertiary bucket handle tear in the remaining rim which is removed by repeating steps 1–6, above. The probe helps to determine when the remaining rim is stable so there are no further loose fragments to catch in the joint.

This bucket handle resection takes an average of 45 minutes, including the diagnostic examination and operating time. Arthroscopic techniques have been criticized as too time-consuming, compared to doing the same procedure with an arthrotomy. This is not a valid criticism. Our average operating time for all arthroscopic meniscectomies has been 55 minutes (range, 15–120 minutes), which compares very closely to the time required for a meniscectomy done with an arthrotomy. And of course, the postoperative recovery time is significantly shorter with arthroscopy.

Oblique (Flap) Tears

This most common meniscal tear, sometimes termed a "parrot beak" or "flap" tear, is an oblique tear that usually occurs at the junction of the middle and posterior thirds of the meniscus. A small tag is produced that protrudes toward the central part of the joint. This tag gets caught during weight-bearing and the tear extends, making a progressively larger "flap," until eventually there is a pedunculated piece of tissue that catches and locks into the joint. The patient then has symptoms of giving way, localized pain, and catching or locking.

These flap tears are quite easily resected with arthroscopic technique (Fig 15). The flap is grasped and stretched and the base is cut with a knife or scissors, then the rim is trimmed with a motorized meniscal cutter. As with the bucket handle

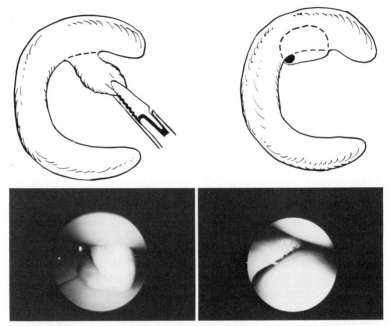

Fig 15.—Diagram showing a meniscus tear in which the flap was tucked under the meniscus. **Top left,** the clamp puts the base on the tag on stretch; **top right,** arthroscopic scissors will then transect the torn segment at the level represented by the *dotted line.* **Lower left,** an arthroscopic appearance of a typical flap tear. This small nubbin of cartilage is enough to continually catch the joint. Pain is quickly relieved after resection. **Lower right,** the meniscal rim left after such a resection. Most of the meniscus is still intact and functional.

tear, it is very important to inspect the peripheral rim for any further tears. By resecting just the damaged portion and then reprobing it is possible to determine the integrity of this remaining meniscal rim. Great care must be taken to avoid cutting across the meniscocapsular junction. If this does occur, the remaining peripheral rim will be unstable and a total meniscectomy will be necessary.

Discoid Meniscus

A good example of the advantages of arthroscopic partial meniscectomy is seen in the discoid meniscus. Children can develop a limp and loss of knee extension from such a thickened disc of lateral meniscus. Total excision of the meniscus would almost certainly leave the growing knee vulnerable to later degenerative changes. With arthroscopic technique, only the central portion of the meniscus is removed, leaving a remaining rim of normal width (Fig 16). This rim eventually smooths and retriangulates. At second-look arthroscopy, the meniscus looks normal.

Degenerative Meniscal Tears

Patients over the age of 60 can develop fragmented tears of the meniscus that produce sharp pain and catching along the joint line. Arthroscopic removal of these degenerative tears is often combined with lavage of the joint and debridement of chondromalacic articular cartilage. This procedure can give significant relief of symptoms in the older population. It is not curative for osteoarthritis, but the low morbidity and early ambulation make this procedure a good alternative to arthrotomy. If there is extensive loss of articular cartilage or angular deformity of the knee, then arthroscopic procedures are of little value. But for the mild to moderate symptomatic degenerative arthritis, arthroscopic surgery can help.

Other Meniscal Tears

All types of meniscal tears can now be managed arthroscopically and it is seldom necessary to do an arthrotomy to complete a meniscal resection. Even a total meniscectomy can be done by nipping away progressive bites of meniscal tissue with a cutting rongeur or making a circumferential cut with a knife inserted from two or three portals around the periphery of the meniscus, as described by Gillquist and Oretorp.[43]

MENSICAL REPAIR

When the meniscus is torn at or near its capsular junction and the remainder of the meniscus is intact, it is possible to suture this tear and have it heal. These vertical longitudinal capsular tears usually occur in the posteromedial or posterolateral horns of the menisci. Hughston has emphasized the importance of repairing this type of tear to salvage the meniscus. Open repair is done through a posteromedial incision. Recently,

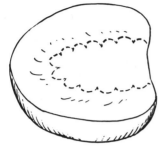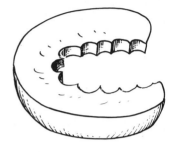

Fig 16.—Method of central excision of a discoid meniscus.

however, techniques have been developed that allow arthroscopic repair of the meniscus. Long needles are used to pass an absorbable suture across the meniscal capsular junction. The suture is then tied in horizontal mattress stitches on the outside of the skin over a dental roll (Fig 17). The knee is immobilized in a cast for 6 weeks. This is a technically difficult procedure. Results are preliminary, but second-look arthroscopy at 6–12 months shows healing to be secure. Hamburg et al. recently reported 50 open repairs of both new and old peripheral meniscal tears, of which 84% had clinically apparent healing at mean follow-up of 18 months.[44] Twenty-seven repeated arthroscopic procedures showed complete healing in all cases. It is likely this will be a common procedure in the future.

Postoperative Management

At the completion of the arthroscopic meniscectomy, the joint is lavaged thoroughly to remove loose pieces. A compressive cotton dressing is worn for 24 hours. Immediate ambulation is allowed and encouraged. Range of motion exercises are also started immediately. Most patients are able to return to sedentary work within 1 week, some within 2 days. More vigorous activities are not allowed until the patient's knee has acquired full range of motion and good quadriceps strength, and there is no swelling and pain. This usually occurs in an average of 2–3 weeks. Well-trained athletes have been able to return to competition, midseason, within 1–2 weeks after arthroscopic meniscectomy.

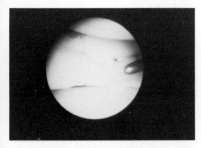

Fig 17.—Arthroscopic view immediately following intra-articular repair of a peripheral meniscal repair. The two absorbable sutures pass through the meniscus and capsule and are tied over a dental roll on the outside of the knee. The tear was first freshened with a motorized burr to promote vascularity. This tear will heal in about 6 weeks, preserving the important functions of the meniscus.

RESULTS OF ARTHROSCOPIC PARTIAL MENISCECTOMY

We recently reported our 5-7 year results of partial arthroscopic meniscectomy.[45] In 148 patients with an age range of 12–67 years (mean, 32 years) there was an 84% overall incidence of good and excellent results. Weight-bearing x-rays in 74 patients showed significantly fewer degenerative changes than would be expected after total meniscectomy. The best results were found with bucket handle and flap tears. In 37 knees with no preexisting chondromalacia or anterior cruciate ligament instability, 36 (97%) had an excellent result. Shybut et al. reported 85% satisfactory overall results at 3 years after arthroscopic meniscectomy.[46] Complications are markedly reduced. Our patients had no postoperative infections or thrombophlebitis.

Arthroscopic management for meniscal tears is not yet the standard of care. As more and more surgeons become skilled with these techniques, it appears likely that all meniscal tears will either be resected or repaired arthroscopically.

SYNOVECTOMY

Current arthroscopic motorized instruments can effectively morsalize and remove the synovial lining of the knee joint. The capacity to perform a synovectomy through six small punctures rather than a large arthrotomy has significantly reduced the morbidity associated with this operation and essentially eliminated such serious complications as loss of knee motion and the poor wound healing so common in rheumatoid patients.

In addition to these advantages, synovectomy can be done in an outpatient center and the patient can ambulate with full weight-bearing in 3–5 days, in marked contrast to the prolonged hospitalizaton and extensive physical therapy required to regain motion after an open synovectomy. Cost savings are greater in this arthroscopic procedure than in any other.

Finally, arthroscopic synovectomy is more thorough than an open synovectomy. Full-thickness synovium can be removed not only from the entire suprapatellar pouch, but also from hard to reach areas such as the intercondylar notch, around the fringes of the meniscus, and in the posterior compartments.

The indications for synovectomy are a matter of coordination with rheumatologists. Synovectomy has come in and out of vogue more than once in the past 3 decades, but with the advancements and reduced morbidity possible with arthroscopic surgery, we are hopeful that the indications will be broadened. Patients with juvenile rheumatoid arthritis might derive special benefit from this procedure, in terms of prevention of joint erosion and deformity. Currently, prospective studies are under way with such patients.

A six-portal technique is used for arthroscopic synovectomy. These portals are made medially and laterally in the posterior, anterior, and suprapatellar compartments. The procedure is done with tourniquet control. Because of the 90-minute limit of tourniquet time, the arthroscopist must proceed in an expeditious manner to have enough time to complete the procedure. Motorized instruments with a large window opening have recently been developed which greatly facilitate this operation.[47]

A cotton batting compressive dressing is kept in place for 48 hours. Postoperative hemarthrosis has not been a problem. Active range of motion exercises are started immediately so that by 1 week, there should be 90 degrees of motion in the knee. In our series of 16 knees, good or excellent results were seen in 15 at 28 months' mean follow-up after arthroscopic synovectomy. No patient required a knee manipulation, and all regained at least their preoperative range of motion. The series included patients with rheumatoid arthritis, pigmented villonodular synovitis, synovial chondromatosis, and gout.

OSTEOCHONDRITIS DISSECANS

Osteochondritis dissecans of the knee usually heals in the young patient (ages 10–14) with rest and limitation of activities for 4–6 months. However, patients in their late teens and early 20s, with even a moderately large lesion, have difficulty getting the avascular segment to heal. In these unhealed lesions, surgery is indicated to try to promote vascularity and stability for healing. This surgery has usually consisted of curetting and drilling the base of the avascular crater and then fixing the loose segment back into this crater with crossed pins or smooth-headed nails—all done with an arthrotomy.

Guhl has developed methods for doing the same procedure using arthroscopic technique, and he reports that 20 of 25 knees healed within 9 months.[48] Four patients required a repeat of the arthroscopic drilling and one patient required a bone graft to the segment to promote healing.

One definite advantage to arthroscopy in this lesion is the ability to accurately identify and evaluate the osteochondritic segment. A probe can determine the amount of loosening of the fragment and the amount of chondral damage. Sometimes just a diagnostic arthroscopy is done and then repeated in 4 months to determine the progress in healing. Rigid fixation of the osteochondritic segment can be obtained with crossed pins inserted under arthroscopic control. The pins are removed percutaneously in 6 weeks. Smaller lesions (less than 1.5 cm in diameter) are treated by excision if the fragment is already loose. The base of the defect is then curetted and drilled to stimulate bleeding and the patient uses crutches for 6 weeks to protect the joint from full weight-bearing. During that time, vigorous, active range of motion exercises are carried out, which according to Salter et al.[49] may stimulate formation of new fibrocartilage. This has been a successful method of treatment. Unfortunately, most osteochondritic lesions are too large to justify doing an excision.

DEGENERATIVE ARTHRITIS

Lavage of the arthritic joint is an effective means of temporarily relieving symptoms of pain and giving away. Small flecks of loose articular cartilage debris are flushed out of the joint. This procedure often produces improvement for 6–12 months.

A generalized debridement of the joint can also be done with arthroscopic methods. Small rongeurs were originally used to remove osteophytic spurs, but now there are motorized burrs which efficiently do this and suction the bone fragments out through the hollow center of the instrument. Torn fragments of meniscus are excised, and in general all loose debris is removed and roughened areas are smoothed off as much as possible.

Areas of the joint with full-thickness loss of articular cartilage can be treated by abrading the cortical bone to promote blood supply and formation of fibrocartilage. The best results are seen in defects that are less than 2 cm in diameter. Johnson has advocated this technique and emphasized that it is not necessary to curette to cancellous bone to stimulate this healing process.[50] He recommends using this technique even when there is a varus malalignment and reports 75% satisfactory results at 2 years, with some knees showing increased joint space radiographically. Biopsy specimens show the abraded area of bone to be covered with fibrocartilage. However, others have emphasized the need to obtain relief of pressure on the worn-down medial compartments by doing a valgus osteotomy.[51–52]

At present, arthroscopic management of osteoarthritis is somewhat controversial. At best, prognosis after an arthroscopic debridement is guarded, and results of abrasion arthroplasty are still preliminary. As a temporary measure, lavage and debridement may help the patient bridge a period of time until a more definitive procedure such as a total knee replacement or an osteotomy could be considered.

ACUTE KNEE INJURY

The sports medicine physician, who is often confronted with perplexing knee problems in high-performance athletes, finds arthroscopy an invaluable aid. An accurate diagnosis can be made using the arthroscope, which might then alter significantly the course of treatment. Often arthrotomy and prolonged recovery can be avoided in the athlete. Some meniscal tears can be resected arthroscopically so that the patient can return to competition midseason. Much research is currently being done on artificial ligaments, and it may one day be possible to install these with arthroscopic control.

Future Developments

As in all endoscopic surgical fields, the frontiers of arthroscopic surgery are being continually expanded. Other joints besides the knee are being treated. For example, tears of the glenoid labrum in shoulders of athletes such as baseball pitchers can be debrided with arthroscopic surgical methods. Loose bodies have been removed from the elbow and ankle.

Some workers are using carbon dioxide instead of saline as an insufflation medium for endoscopic knee surgery. Eriksson and Sebik[53] report much better visualizaton, with clearer optics and a wider angle of view, when using carbon dioxide. Eliminating the constant flow of saline allows structures being resected to stay in a fixed position. However, use of carbon dioxide does not permit flushing out loose debris or the use of motorized cutting devices that require suction.

Some high-energy devices have been experimented with. Electrosurgery for lateral patellar release has already been mentioned and is now being used for meniscal resections. High-speed cutters which rotate at 70–80,000 rpm have also been tried within the joint and are effective for cutting hard tissue such as bone and articular cartilage but are not as effective with soft tissue such as meniscus and synovium. Use of these instruments carries an increased risk because they can readily damage the normal articular surfaces of the knee joint.

Research is also being done on the use of lasers to ablate tissue within the knee joint. The argon laser has little value for meniscal resection, as its energy absorption occurs best in red tissue. The constant-wave yttrium-aluminum-garnet laser can produce high wattage down a fiber, making it easier to deliver the beam through an arthroscope, but its energy pattern tends just to "cook" the meniscus and produces thermal burns to surrounding tissues more readily. The pulsed-waved carbon dioxide laser appears best at this time for resecting meniscal tissue. It is still experimental and is more costly, more dangerous, and less efficient than current hand-held and motorized arthroscopic instruments. Laser does have one advantage of being able to totally ablate tissue. We have been doing in vitro research the past 2 years at the University of Utah but to date have not used the laser clinically.

Summary

Endoscopic knee surgery, like other endoscopic procedures in other specialties, takes considerable time and patience to learn. But once the technique is learned, the noninvasive, nondestructive nature of endoscopy lends itself well to many types of knee operations, and we are beginning to see results at 4 and 5 years that are at least equal to those achieved by the same operation done with an arthrotomy, and with a marked reduction in complications and morbidity.

Patient acceptance of these endoscopic knee procedures is very high because of the small scars, minimal postoperative discomfort, rapid rehabilitation and return to work, and avoidance of a lengthy and costly hospitalizaton.

The challenge to arthroscopic surgeons is to perform these operations without damaging normal structures within the knee joint. The use of television has greatly enhanced the ability to teach residents and carry on postgraduate instruction. The coming years should bring an ever-increasing utilization of arthroscopy in managing most knee problems, as well as some limited use in other joints.

REFERENCES

1. Takagi K.: The arthroscope. *J. Jpn. Orth. Assoc.* 14:359, 1939.
2. Burman M.S.: Arthroscopy or direct visualization of joints: An experimental cadaver study. *J. Bone Joint Surg.* 13:669, 1931.
3. Burman M.S., Finkelstein H., Mayer L.: Arthroscopy of the knee joint. *J. Bone Joint Surg.* 16:255, 1936.
4. Watanabe M., Takeda S., Ikeuchi H.: *Atlas of Arthroscopy*, ed. 1. Tokyo, Igaku Shoin, Ltd., 1956.
5. Jackson R.W., Abe I.: The role of arthroscopy in the management of disorders of the knee: An analysis of 200 consecutive cases. *J. Bone Joint Surg.* 54B:310, 1972.
6. Casscells S.W.: Arthroscopy of the knee joint. *J. Bone Joint Surg.* 53A:287, 1971.
7. DeHaven K.E., Collins H.R.: Diagnosis of internal derangements of the knee: The role of arthroscopy. *J. Bone Joint Surg.* 57A:801, 1975.
8. Dandy D.J., Jackson R.W.: The impact of arthroscopy on the management of disorders of the knee. *J. Bone Joint Surg.* 57B:346, 1975.
9. Johnson L.L.: *Comprehensive Arthroscopic Examination of the Knee Joint.* St. Louis, C.V. Mosby Co., 1978.
10. O'Connor R.L.: *Arthroscopy.* Philadelphia, J.B. Lippincott Co., 1977.
11. McGinty J.B., Matza R.A.: Arthroscopy of the knee: Evaluation of an outpatient procedure under local anesthesia. *J. Bone Joint Surg.* 60A:787, 1978.

12. Whipple T.L., Bassett F.H.: Arthroscopic examination of the knee: Polypuncture technique with percutaneous intra-articular manipulation. *J. Bone Joint Surg.* 60A:444, 1978.
13. Korn M.W., Spitzer R.M., Robinson K.E.: Correlations of arthrography with arthroscopy. *Orthop. Clin. North Am.* 10:535, 1979.
14. Gilley J.S., Gelman M.I., Edson M., et al.: Chondral fractures of the knee: Arthrographic, arthroscopic, and clinical manifestations. *Radiology* 138:51, 1981.
15. Keene J.L.S., Dyreby J.R.: High tibial osteotomy in the treatment of osteoarthritis of the knee. *J. Bone Joint Surg.* 64A:36, 1983.
16. Rosenberg T.D., Wong H.: Arthroscopic knee surgery in a free-standing outpatient surgery center. *Orthop. Clin. North Am.* 13:277, 1982.
17. Sweeney H.: Teaching arthroscopic surgery at the residency level. *Orthop. Clin. North Am.* 13:255, 1982.
18. Johnson L.L.: *Arthroscopic Surgery of the Knee and Other Joints.* St. Louis, C.V. Mosby Co., 1981.
19. Johnson L.L., Shneider D.A., Austin M., et al.: Two per cent glutaraldehyde: A disinfectant in arthroscopy and arthroscopic surgery. *J. Bone Joint Surg.* 64A:237, 1982.
20. Patel D.: Superior lateral-medial approach to arthroscopic meniscectomy. *Orthop. Clin. North Am.* 13:299, 1982.
21. Gillquist J., Hagberg G.: A new modification of the technique of arthroscopy of the knee joint. *Acta Chir. Scand.* 142:123, 1976.
22. Lysholm J., Gillquist J.: Arthroscopic examination of the posterior cruciate ligament. *J. Bone Joint Surg.* 63A:363, 1981.
23. Mulhollan J.S.: Symposium: Arthroscopic knee surgery. *Contemp. Orthop.* August 1982, p. 79.
24. Metcalf R.W.: *Operative Arthroscopy of the Knee.* Instructional Course Lectures, Chicago, American Academy of Orthopedic Surgery, 1981, vol. 30, p. 357.
25. Dandy D.J.: *Arthroscopic Surgery of the Knee.* Edinburgh, Churchill Livingstone, 1981.
26. Metcalf R.W.: *Instruction Manual: Arthroscopic Surgery of the Knee.* Salt Lake City, Press Publishing, 1980.
27. Hughston J.C., Stone M., Andrews J.R.: The suprapatellar plica: Its role in internal derangement of the knee. *J. Bone Joint Surg.* 55A:1318, 1973.
28. Patel D.: Arthroscopy of the plicae: Synovial folds and their significance. *Am. J. Sports Med.* 6:217, 1978.
29. Jackson R.W., Marshall D.J., Fujisawa Y.: The pathologic medial shelf. *Orthop. Clin. North Am.* 13:307, 1982.
30. McGinty J.B.: Arthroscopic removal of loose bodies. *Orthop. Clin. North Am.* 13:313, 1982.
31. Larson R.L., Cabaud H.E., Slocum D.B., et al.: The patellar compression syndrome: Surgical treatment by lateral release. *Clin. Orthop.* 134:158, 1978.
32. Insall J., Falsvo K.A., Wise D.W.: Chondromalacia patellae: A prospective study. *J. Bone Joint Surg.* 58A:1, 1976.
33. Ficat R.P., Hungerford D.S.: *Disorders of the Patello-Femoral Joint.* Baltimore, Williams & Wilkins Co., 1977.

34. Crosby E.B., Insall J.: Recurrent dislocation of the patella: Relation of treatment of osteoarthritis. *J. Bone Joint Surg.* 51A:9, 1976.
35. Fielding J.W., Liebler W.A., Urs D., et al.: Tibial tubercle transfer: A long range follow-up study. *Clin. Orthop.* 144:43, 1979.
36. Hampson W.G.J., Hill P.: Late results of transfer of the tibial tubercle for recurrent dislocation of the patella. *J. Bone Joint Surg.* 57B:209, 1975.
37. Metcalf R.W.: An arthroscopic method for lateral release of the subluxating or dislocating patella. *Clin. Orthop.* 167:9, 1982.
38. Merchant A.C., Mercer R.L.: Lateral release of the patella: A preliminary report. *Clin. Orthop.* 103:40, 1974.
39. Chen C., Helal B., King J., et al.: Lateral retinacular release in chondromalacia patellae. *Int. Rev. Rheumatol.* 33:35, 1976.
40. Johnson R.J., Kettlecamp D.B., et al.: Factors affecting late results after meniscectomy. *J. Bone Joint Surg.* 56A:719, 1974.
41. Tapper E.M., Hoover N.W.: Late results after meniscectomy. *J. Bone Joint Surg.* 54A:517, 1969.
42. Krause W.R., Pope M.H., Johnson R.J., et al.: Mechanical changes in the knee after meniscectomy. *J. Bone Joint Surg.* 58A:599, 1976.
43. Gillquist J., Oretorp N.: The technique of endoscopic total meniscectomy. *Orthop. Clin. North Am.* 13:363, 1982.
44. Hamburg P., Gillquist J., Lysholm J.: Suture of new and old peripheral meniscal tears. *J. Bone Joint Surg.* 65A:193, 1983.
45. Metcalf R.W., Coward D.C., Rosenberg T.D.: Arthroscopic partial meniscectomy: A five-year follow-up. Read before the annual meeting of the American Academy of Orthopedic Surgeons, Anaheim, Calif., March 1983.
46. Shybut G.T., Altman B.R., McGinty J.B.: Extended results of endoscopic meniscectomy. Read before the annual meeting of the American Academy of Orthopedic Surgeons, Anaheim, Calif., March 1983.
47. Highenboten C.L.: Arthroscopic synovectomy. *Orthop. Clin. North Am.* 13:399, 1982.
48. Guhl J.F.: Arthroscopic treatment of osteochondritis dissecans: Preliminary report. *Orthop. Clin. North Am.* 10:671, 1979.
49. Salter R.B., Simmonds D.F., Malcolm B.W., et al.: The biological effect of continuous passive motion on the healing of full thickness defects in articular cartilage: An experimental investigation in the rabbit. *J. Bone Joint Surg.* 62A:1231, 1980.
50. Johnson L.L.: Arthroscopic abrasion arthroplasty. Read before the annual meeting of the American Academy of Orthopedic Surgeons, Anaheim, Calif., March 1983.
51. Insall J.N., Shoji H., Mayer V.: High tibial osteotomy: A five-year evaluation. *J. Bone Joint Surg.* 56A:1397, 1974.
52. Coventry M.B.: Upper tibial osteotomy for gonarthrosis: The evaluation of the operation in the last eighteen years and long-term results. *Orthop. Clin. North Am.* 10:191, 1979.
53. Eriksson E., Sebik A.: Arthroscopy and arthroscopic surgery in a gas versus a fluid medium. *Orthop. Clin. North Am.* 13:293, 1982.

Staples and Staplers

MARK M. RAVITCH, M.D.* AND FELICIEN M.
STEICHEN, M.D.†

*Department of Surgery, University of Pittsburgh School of Medicine and
Montefiore Hospital, Pittsburgh, Pennsylvania †Department of Surgery,
New York Medical College and Lenox Hill Hospital, New York, New York

CERTAINLY THE USE of staples to replace conventional sutures in surgical operations received its greatest impetus from the work of the Scientific Research Institute for Experimental Surgical Apparatus and Instruments in Moscow. Beginning in 1950 with Gudov's[1] stapling instrument for vascular anastomoses, several entire families of instruments have been successfully devised for applying metal staples, first of tantalum and then of stainless steel, in vascular anastomoses, and in the operations of gastrointestinal, thoracic and pulmonary surgery, with some side excursions into experimental stapling instruments for bone surgery, ophthalmic surgery, etc. Our own interest in stapling, apart from an amateurish attempt in 1942 to use an ordinary paper stapler for closure of portions of the alimentary tract, arose from a visit to Kiev in 1958. On that occasion, we were enormously impressed at the performance by N. M. Amosov of a pneumonectomy, in which, with one application of the instrument, he stapled the pulmonary artery, both pulmonary veins, and the bronchus, amputating the lung on the stapler and applying no further sutures to the bone-dry stumps. We were able to secure one of the instruments by purchase in Leningrad a week later, and began the laboratory and clinical studies which have occupied much of our interest in the 25 years since. In fact, the use of stapling instruments was al-

0065-3411/84/0017-0241-0280-$04.00

ready almost a half a century old before the work at the institute in Moscow began. And as might be expected, there was a
history, going back for the best part of the previous century, of
numerous mechanical contrivances devised by surgeons to
make bowel anastomosis possible. In the days before anesthesia, let alone the modern day of cadaveric relaxation, when
lighting was poor, when suction to clear the field of blood and
intestinal juice had not yet been brought into play, when most
surgeons tended to employ rather gross needles and heavy
thread, and when the principles of intestinal suture were not
understood, successful intestinal closure or anastomosis was
rarely performed and surgeons eagerly explored the possibili-
ties that might be offered by mechanical devices. We have dealt
with that story in considerable detail elsewhere,[2, 3] and here
provide only one or two highlights.

The first device to be proposed, and one of those for which we
have records of successful clinical use, was that of Denans,[4]
who in 1827 described the device pictured in Figure 1. The instrument consisted of one long cylinder and two shorter ferrules. The shorter ferrules were inserted into the ends of bowel
to be anastomosed, the bowel ends inverted in the ferrules, and
then the longer cylinder, slightly smaller in diameter than the
ferrules, slipped snugly inside the two ends as the ferrules were
pushed together to abut the bowel ends against each other. The
basic principle, of an apparatus that provided a lumen for passage of gas and bowel content until such time as pressure necrosis released it, the anastomosis having by that time become
secure, was to be used in many subsequent instruments.

In 1826, Henroz,[6] of Liège, Belgium reported in a doctoral
thesis successful animal experiments with two slender, articulated rings armed with alternate pins and holes. The rings
were slipped around the bowel ends, the bowel ends *everted*
over them and caught by the pins, and then the two rings
snapped together, pins and holes engaging, producing a mucosa-to-mucosa everting anastomosis (Fig 2). This was in the
very year that Antoine Lembert[7] established what has since
been regarded as one of the surgical verities, that the safety of
intestinal anastomosis depends upon a serosa-to-serosa union
and hence that all anastomoses and closures must be inverting.

It is no surprise, therefore, that in 1893, Nicholas Senn,[8] airily ignoring the fact that Henroz had, in fact, claimed that his

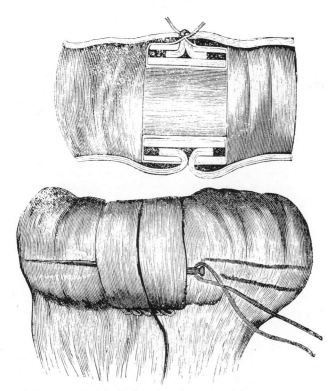

Fig 1.—Samuel D. Gross (1843),[5] in the book on the technique of intestinal suture, upon which he set so much store, shows a method of passing the suture to hold the Denans rings in place. (From Gross S.D.)

method had succeeded, and had been awarded a doctorate for his effort, said ". . .union was effected with the mucous membrane turned outward, consequently it must have proved a failure even in experiments on the lower animals." Senn was a critical student of surgical problems who conducted a very large number of systematic and careful investigations on healing of all kinds and was particularly interested in surgery of the intestines, so that it is a little unusual that he did not put this statement to the test of the laboratory.

Benjamin Travers, Astley Cooper's most distinguished student and long his colleague and co-author, published a book in 1812[9] dealing with the healing of sutured intestine and the performance of intestinal anastomosis, showing very clearly

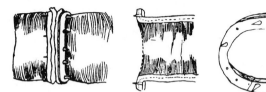

Fig 2.—Nicholas Senn (1893)[8] provided illustrations of Henroz' technique but, airily ignoring the fact that Henroz had, in fact, claimed his method had succeeded, said, ". . . union was effected with the mucous membrane turned outward, consequently it must have proved a failure even in experiments on the lower animals," ignoring Travers' statement[9] ". . . the absolute contact of the everted surfaces of a divided intestine in their entire circumference is requisite . . . it is therefore necessary to include such a portion of the everted lip, as will ensure this contact . . . the eversion is permanent." (From Senn N., *J.A.M.A.*, 1893.)

that everting anastomoses in the dog would heal quite satisfactorily. It is difficult to say to whom we owe the misconception that Travers said just the opposite. Ironically, it may be to Lembert[7] himself, who in his important paper referred to *"les belles experiences"* (the lovely experiments) of Travers, without actually spelling out their findings, leaving it to the reader to assume that they confirmed his own opinion. The assumption is that Lembert and Senn either never read Travers' paper themselves or, unaccountably, misunderstood the very clear illustrations and his very clear statements. In spite of the fact that there are now numerous references in the current literature documenting what Travers actually had demonstrated, it is still common to see statements that Travers demonstrated the necessity for inverting anastomoses.[10]

Henroz would have been delighted to see, a century and a half after he obtained his doctorate, the appearance of an anastomosing instrument basically composed, like his, of two articulated half rings in a modern stapler for creating mucosa-to-mucosa everting anastomoses. The staples in this instrument having been driven in, the articulated rings are opened and removed[11–14]—the modern evolution of Henroz' simple device.

A number of individuals proposed the use of cylinders, the ends of which either had alternating pins and holes or were made of a soft material, so that the pins could be driven into the substance. The cylinders were inserted in the lumen of the two bowel ends which were drawn over the pins and the two ends then compressed together.[15]

The most widely used indwelling anastomotic device was certainly that of John B. Murphy of Chicago, the Murphy button, introduced in 1892.[16] By this time, anesthesia had long been available, lighting was reasonably good, and instruments had been refined. More to the point, William S. Halsted,[17] in Baltimore, had already demonstrated the feasibility and effectiveness of what was to be the standard technique of intestinal anastomosis and closure, a minimally inverting suture with fine needle and thread engaging the submucosa. Halsted made a point of saying that previous writers on the subject had ignored the importance of the submucosa, the sole layer strong enough to hold sutures. Murphy's button (Fig 3) consisted of two metal mushrooms with hollow stems which telescoped into each other. The mushroom cap of each end being secured in the bowel by a purse-string suture around the hollow stem, the stems were telescoped, compressing the mushroom caps together, and with them the purse-stringed bowel ends. In a later model, the compression was augmented by an internal spring which acted on a free cylinder within the button. The lumen of the bowel remained open by virtue of the channel through the caps and stems. Compression necrosis of the edges of bowel included between the two halves of the button allowed the button to be passed, by which time healing was secure. The button was widely used throughout the world and reports of its use came from the great surgical figures of the day—Willy Meyer,[18] Marwedel,[19] Czerny,[20] and others—and often, as in Czerny's case, they had manufactured modifications of their own. For that

Fig. 3.—J.B. Murphy's anastomosis button, 1892.[16] The cutaway section of the button in place shows the two bowel ends purse-stringed around the stems of the buttons and the buttons compressed against each other. The button was soon modified to have an internal ring that would be compressed upwards by a coiled spring to make more certain the production of necrosis of the bowel ends. (From Murphy J.B., *Medical Record,* New York and Chicago, Medical Record, 1892.)

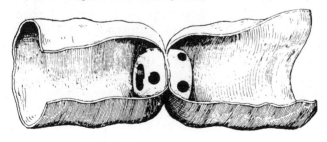

matter, Adalbert Ramaugé,[21-23] professor of surgery of the School of Medicine in Buenos Aires, not only described an elegant button of his own, but pretty clearly had done it independently of Murphy and before Murphy's first publication, but not before Murphy's own experiments and first operations.

In more recent times, the principle of the Murphy button has been applied to esophagogastric and esophagojejunal anastomoses by Boerema,[24, 25] who described his device as a modification of the Murphy button. His buttons were egg-shaped, made of plastic, and were operated by a long, slender, detachable handle, so that they could be slid up to the esophagus from the stomach or jejunum which was being attached to it. The instrument was also used for the treatment of esophageal varices, much as modern stapling instruments are, except that the Boerema instrument, like the Murphy button, relied upon compression necrosis to create the anastomosis and permit the button to pass. For that matter, as late as 1968, Prioton, of Montpellier,[26] used actual Murphy buttons for control of esophageal varices. With a ligature, the undivided esophagus was tied between the halves of the button inserted from below through a gastrotomy. Ton and associates,[27] in The Netherlands, devised an ingenious button for rectal anastomoses.

The difficulty of the low rectal anastomosis, like the difficulty of esophageal anastomoses, has been recognized as presenting a special problem. William S. Halsted,[28] in 1910, presented before the American Surgical Association one of a number of techniques with which he was to experiment over the next decade in an attempt to solve the special problem of rectosigmoid anastomosis by one or another "bulkhead" method. His final paper on the subject was published in 1922, the year of his death.[29] The purse-string closed ends of the colon and rectum were sutured together. To restore intestinal continuity through the closed ends, an assistant passed through the anus a sheathed knife which the surgeon then guided through the joined ends of colon and rectum, following this then with dilators from below. In the light of current instrumentation (the EEA), it is interesting that Halsted said in his 1910 paper, "To eliminate this diaphragm [of the abutted purse-string closed ends of colon and rectum], I devised a sharp-edged punch, with the idea of introducing it at a higher point in the bowel through a lateral opening, slipping down to the diaphragm and

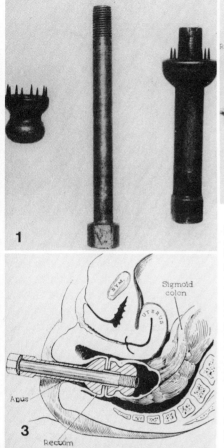

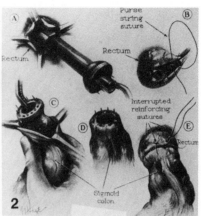

Fig 4.—1, apparatus devised by Sugarbaker[31] for his colorectal anastomosis technique. **2,** in the Sugarbaker technique, both ends were inserted from within the pelvis, the distal end sutured (pursestring) over the protruding end, the two halves snapped together, and the anastomosis reinforced by sutures. **3,** sagittal section of instrument in place. The tubular element is threaded to engage the button in the proximal bowel and has a flange (not well shown) that presses against the bottom of the distal button. This keeps the buttons in closer and closer apposition as the clamp is tightened. Sugarbaker reported successful clinical use of the instrument. (From Sugarbaker E.D., Wiley H.M.: *Surg. Gynecol. Obstet.* 93:597, 1951. Used with permission.)

pressing it through this obstruction and into a cork introduced per anum, to withdraw both cork and punch by means of a thread attached to the former. This method was not tested." It will be recognized that this is the principle involved in the low rectal anastomosis when the EEA instrument is inserted from above, as preferred by Nance[30] and others.

The recurrence of the perception and application of principles, often in combination, in anastomotic devices—surely without awareness of the preceding experiences—is seen in the device of Sugarbaker[31] for rectocolic anastomoses (Fig 4). It involved the Murphy button principle with the pins-and-holes retention mechanism, which Henroz had described in 1826 (for his everting anastomosis), and which Bonnier, in 1885, employed in the ends of cork, metal, and ebony ferrules for inverting anastomoses, devised before Murphy. In Sugarbaker's device, a hollow stem, threaded at its upper end, and long enough to protrude from the rectum, compressed the halves of the Murphy button analogues. The two halves were first loosely compressed, and compression was increased on the third and sixth days by twisting the external portion of the device, avoiding the risk that necrosis and separation would occur before healing was secure. When the inverted bowel flanges necrosed and the instrument came loose, it was withdrawn, usually by the tenth day.

Other instruments to achieve the same purpose were devised by Hallenbeck, Judd, and David at the Mayo Clinic in 1963,[32] and Brummelkamp in Holland in 1965.[33] Most recently Jansen and colleagues,[34, 35] from Utrecht, have proposed a still further modification of this principle. The ends of rectum and colon are inverted over metal rings containing powerful magnets. The bowel ends are held by pins in the metal rings. An applicator passed per rectum guides the two ends together. The magnetic compression of the inverted ends, not otherwise attached to each other, causes the flanges of bowel to necrose.

For the actual introduction of stapling instruments in surgery, we are indebted to Humer Hültl,[36] of Budapest, who in 1908, at the Second Congress of the Hungarian Surgical Society, presented an instrument for use in gastrectomy (Fig 5). The instrument placed two double rows of fine steel wire staples, similar to those used today, so that the stomach or duodenum could be transected, leaving a double row of staples on either side of the section. The staples closed in the B-shape that has been the standard staple closure ever since. Although the instrument was fairly widely known and Willy Meyer[37] and others made reference to it and pictured its use in their papers, it was a massive instrument, weighing 3.5 kg, and had numerous parts so that it was tedious to assemble. It was completely supplanted by the instrument of Aladar von Petz, a former student of Hültl's, that was presented in 1921 at the Eighth Annual Meeting of the Hungarian Surgical Society.[38, 39] The instrument was essentially a giant Payr clamp, the upper jaw of

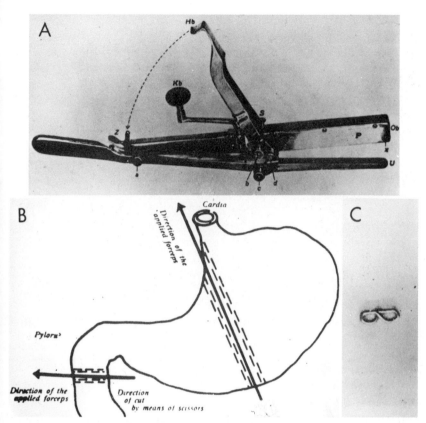

Fig 5.—The first stapling instrument (Humer Hültl, 1908). **A,** as in all of the stapling instruments, the required degree of compression was created by first closing the device; the staples were then driven through the fixed tissue. Turning the crank advanced a rod that sequentially drove in the staples. **B,** this diagram from the original manufacturer's brochure shows how the instrument, which employed fine wire staples, could be used to place four staggered rows, permitting the operator to divide the viscus, leaving two rows on either side. The closure was always inverted by manual sutures. **C,** the staples closed in the B-shape, which has been standard ever since. (From: *Manufacturer's Brochure,* 1908.)

which had slots for the insertion of flat German silver staples, while the lower jaw had recesses, or anvils, to form the staples in the B-shape that Hültl had introduced. For the next 30–40 years, in most clinics stapling meant the use of the von Petz machine, which, like the Hültl, was used only to seal the viscus temporarily, the stapled closure always being turned in (Fig 6).

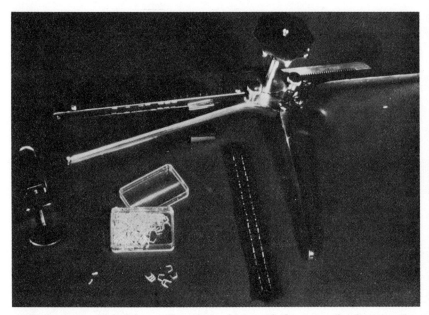

Fig 6.—Late model of the von Petz clamp shown with the coarse, flat German silver staples, the two Indian-file rows of staples applied to a sheet of felt, and on the left the screw clamp to secure the nose of the instrument. The instrument shown is now in the collection of the Smithsonian Institution. For almost three decades, stapling in surgery meant the von Petz clamp. (From Steichen F.M., Ravitch M.M.: *Stapling in Surgery.* Chicago, Year Book Medical Publishers. In press.[3])

We have described elsewhere in some detail[3] the variety of other instruments that were introduced in Europe and in Japan, of which the most interesting is perhaps that of Friedrich of Ulm (Fig 7).[40] That instrument was simple to operate, since one squeeze of a handle approximated the jaws, a release was thrown, and a second squeeze of the handle drove in the staples, which were of the same coarse German silver type as von Petz had introduced. A principal advantage to Friedrich's instrument was the provision of interchangeable staple magazines, so the same instrument could be used repeatedly in a single operation.

From the time of Hültl, all of the stapling instruments operated in two phases. In the first, the tissues were approximated to the required degree of compression and in the second, the staples were driven in. This avoided the unregulated trauma of

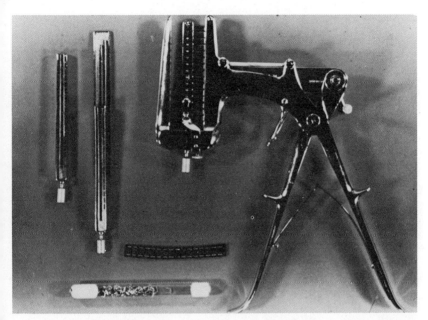

Fig 7.—Gastrointestinal stapler of H. Friedrich, 1934.[40] Model of the instrument owned by Dallas Phemister at the University of Chicago, and now at the Smithsonian Institution. Division of the bowel after stapling resulted in only a single staple line which was then always manually inverted, but the operation of the instrument was infinitely simpler than that of the von Petz and Hültl instruments, and the interchangeable cartridges represented a real advance. (From Steichen F.M., Ravitch M.M.: *Stapling in Surgery*. Chicago, Year Book Medical Publishers. 1984.[3])

the slam-bang closure of a powerful instrument, and at the same time held the tissues immobile so that the sharp staples passed through without tearing.

The Russian vascular anastomotic instruments, the first instruments to emerge from the Scientific Research Institute for Experimental Surgical Apparatus and Instruments, were models of ingenuity and produced mathematically perfect circular anastomoses both end-to-end and end-to-side. They were complicated, had a large number of moving parts, required considerable lengths of vessel and for all practical purposes could be used only with normal vessels.[1] Their weight and complexity presented problems, particularly in use deep within body cavities. In general, it could be said of the Russian instruments that they were extremely well made, but tended to be complex.

Three general families of instruments emerged from the Russian experience. The first type of instrument is a series of linear staplers (US equivalents, TA 30, TA 55, TA 90) usually applying a double-staggered row of staples. Numerous instruments were devised to modify slightly in one way or another the pattern of the staple lines, or to provide techniques for inverting or covering over a first row of staples with a second row, without having to remove the instrument, as in transection of the stomach or pulmonary parenchyma. Our own studies have persuaded us that the standard double-staggered staple line serves for almost all purposes and that two sizes of staples, in terms of length of the leg, suffice for the range of tissues to be sutured in most circumstances. In suturing the pulmonary vessels and the proximal end of the portal vein, we do rely on a special cartridge with finer, shorter staples, closer together. The instruments of this family consist essentially of two sliding Ls; in the upper short limb of the L is the staple cartridge and in the lower limb, the staple-forming anvil. All of these ordinarily produce mucosa-to-mucosa closure of bronchus or bowel, which we do not reinforce with sutures. Under special circumstances, a portion of an intestinal closure can be made serosa-to-serosa with these instruments.

The second type is a linear anastomosing instrument (US equivalent, GIA). The two 5-cm limbs of the instrument are inserted into the loops of bowel to be anastomosed, the one containing the four rows of staples, a knife, and two staple-pusher bars, and the other the anvils. When the instrument halves are mated and locked, and the knife assembly pushed home, four rows of staples are driven in and the knife divides the approximated tissues to within one and one-half staples of the end of the staple line, leaving two rows of staples on each side of the cut. The instrument is then removed and the site of insertion closed either manually, serosa-to-serosa, or with staples, mucosa-to-mucosa.

And finally, there exists a third type of instrument, a tubular, end-to-end or end-to-side, minimally inverting anastomotic device (US equivalent, EEA). This instrument has a sigmoidoscope-like barrel with an obturator which is beyond the end of the cylinder. That obturator-like nose cone contains the anvils to form the staples. In the end of the "sigmoidoscope" are the staples.

These three basic patterns have been radically refined by the

American manufacturers,* whose instruments are here under discussion. [At this writing, there has appeared in this country only one other visceral stapler—a tubular instrument for end-to-end anastomoses.** We have had no experience with it and thus far have seen no published experience with its use.] In addition to making the instruments lighter and more elegantly balanced, the cartridges have been made disposable, preloaded with staples, sterilized, and readily inserted into the instruments. The most dramatic change made by the American manufacturers is the transfer to the disposable cartridge of the small moving parts needed to drive in the individual staples. The result has been to convert the basic instrument simply into the power train. This has simplified cleaning and maintenance and, in the case of the instruments of the latter two families, obviously provides a new knife for each use. There has also been devised in this country an instrument (LDS) for ligature of omental and mesenteric vessels, cystic duct, etc., that simultaneously applies two clips and divides the tissue between them. The Russians had experimented with prototype instruments that applied two ligatures, but these did not reach clinical acceptance.

The logical next step has been taken and all of these instruments are now available in a totally disposable form, so that no maintenance is involved and the question of proper insertion of the cartridge, etc., does not arise.

To continue with the historical note, the skin staplers (SFS) that first appeared in this country in 1969 had no Russian counterpart at all. We find the skin stapler and the ligating and dividing stapler extremely convenient and use them routinely.

It is our ordinary expectation, in advance of any operation today, that visceral transection and suturing, and gastroenteric anastomoses will be made entirely with the staples unless special situations exist. The instruments of the TA series are used to divide and staple bronchi, pulmonary vessels, pulmonary parenchyma as in wedge biopsy, and division of incomplete fissures, or sublobar resections, for transection and stapling of all portions of the gastrointestinal tract, for excision and sta-

---

*United States Surgical Corporation, Norwalk, CT.
**I.L.S.-Ethicon, Inc., Somerville, NJ.

pling of Zenker's diverticula, Meckel's diverticula, or mural lesions treated by a tangential resection, and for closing the opening left after a GIA anastomosis. The pancreas is satisfactorily transected and stapled with the TA 55 instrument. Russian authors[41-44] express enthusiasm for stapling and dividing liver and kidney with their instruments of this type, up to the obvious limitations of thickness of the tissue to be divided and stapled, and we have anecdotal accounts of their use on the liver in this country.

The TA 30 instrument, in addition to the cartridge containing the 3.5 mm and the 4.8 mm staples, has a third cartridge and corresponding anvil for smaller, more closely spaced staples for closure of pulmonary vessels, patent ductus, Potts' aortopulmonary shunt, portal vein, etc. The staple cartridge for this purpose is coded TA 30-V, and the cartridge delivers 15 staples of .21 mm wire, 3 mm across the bar, 1.5 mm apart, and in two rows separated by 1.5 mm, compressing tissue to approximately 1.0 mm.

Figure 8 shows the basic applications of the TA instruments. Surgeons varying the applications of these instruments in ingenious ways have developed a broad range of procedures, particularly for reestablishing continuity in the gastrointestinal tract. In all its applications, however, certain principles must be observed.

1. One must bring the instrument down to the tissue to be stapled, rather than pulling the organ up to the instrument. Stapling tissue on stretch invites the staple hole to tear.

2. The tissue retaining pins must always be used, to keep the tissues from being squeezed beyond the staple line, and to guarantee alignment of upper and lower jaw—i.e., of staples and anvil grooves.

3. The tissues should be cut, as shown in Figure 8, on the edge of the stapler. This provides enough tissue for safety beyond the staple line, and no more. Cutting freehand after the stapler has been removed increases the risk of cutting into the staple line on the one hand or leaving an excessive stump of tissue on the other.

4. In the original steel TA instruments, one must close the jaws with the wing nut until the vernier markings are opposed. With the totally disposable instruments, and the steel Premium instruments, an automatic mechanism regulates jaw dis-

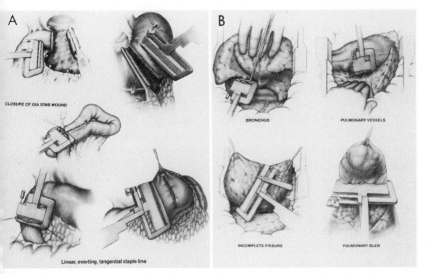

Fig 8.—A, TA^{TM} procedures in the gastrointestinal tract. The instruments provide 30-, 55-, or 90-mm, double-staggered staple lines for mucosa-to-mucosa closure of transected duodenum or stomach, as shown, or other portions of the GI tract, from the esophagus to the rectum. In performing anastomoses with the GIA^{TM} instrument *(middle)*, the single opening created is usually closed mucosa-to-mucosa with the TA^{TM} instruments. Linear incisions in the bowel, as in a duodenectomy for exposure of the ampulla of Vater *(lower left)*, are readily closed mucosa-to-mucosa with a TA^{TM} instrument. Portions of bowel wall containing mural lesions are slid through the jaws of the stapler; the bowel is then stapled and the specimen excised. *Lower right,* the result after excision of a posterior wall gastric ulcer.

B, TA^{TM} procedures in pulmonary surgery. *Upper left,* mucosa-to-mucosa closure with a TA 55^{TM} or TA 30^{TM} stapler. *Upper right,* stapling of the pulmonary vessels with the fine vascular cartridge in the TA 30^{TM} stapler. *Lower left,* bloodless division and closure of an incomplete fissure, e.g., between the upper and middle lobes in a right upper lobectomy, using a TA 90^{TM} or TA 55^{TM} instrument. *Lower right,* amputation of a pulmonary bulla, using a TA 90^{TM} or TA 55^{TM} stapler. (From Steichen F.M., Ravitch M.M.: *Stapling in Surgery.* Chicago, Year Book Medical Publishers. 1984.)

tance and tissue pressure when the lever is thrown, closing the jaw.

5. Do not include omentum or mesentery in the tissue to be stapled and divided. Bleeding will result.

6. In closing GIA stab wounds be certain the TA jaws are on serosa the full 360 degrees of the opening.

Entirely disposable TA instruments with cartridge and stapler combined into a compact unit duplicate the specifications of staple size, shape, alignment and length of suture lines of the standard instruments. They embody a hinge-like opening and closing mechanism for the upper, staple-cartridge jaw, as well as a tissue-retaining pin which moves into position automatically as the jaws are closed. The jaws are opened and closed by activating a lever in the vertical shaft of the instrument, obviating the annoying need for turning a wing nut. The staples are driven in by the familiar compression of the handles.

In using any of the TA instruments, the jaws are opened, the lower jaw slipped under the tissue to be stapled, the retention pin introduced, the jaws approximated, and the staples fired. The instrument is brought down to the tissues, avoiding traction upon them. The bronchus, vessel, or bowel is divided on the edge of the instrument before the instrument is removed. The bowel and bronchus closures are all mucosa-to-mucosa.

The GIA instrument consists of two interlocking halves which form a flat handle with two straight limbs. One limb accommodates the staple cartridge and the other accepts the anvil to form the two double-staggered rows of staples, 16 staples in each double row, thus one double row on each side of a central groove through which the knife blade will advance. To divide bowel, the instrument is partially assembled, the loop of bowel slid between the two jaws, and the instrument locked and activated. The knife divides the bowel, both ends of which are simultaneously closed mucosa-to-mucosa with a double-staggered row of staples. In anastomosing two portions of the gastrointestinal tract, one limb is inserted into the lumen of each loop. As the instrument halves are then matched, mated, and locked, the double thickness of bowel wall is grasped between the limbs of the instrument. Operating the instrument now drives home the four rows of staples at the same time, dividing the stapled tissue, so as to leave a double row of staples on either side of the division, the knife stopping one and one-half staples short of the end of the staple line. The assembly, which is driven home by the thumb, as in operating a piston-syringe, consists of three blades, the two outer ones drive in the staples, the central one, the knife, divides the tissues; each of the three blades slides in a separate channel of the cartridge. The instrument is scored at 1 cm intervals up to 5 cm so that one can control the size of an anastomosis.

Anastomoses done with the GIA instrument are serosa-to-serosa, but inconsequentially inverting. As the knife divides the stapled partition between the two loops, it converts the two stab wounds used for insertion of the instrument limbs into a single opening. This is then closed mucosa-to-mucosa with the TA instrument. The GIA stapler has been used by some surgeons for dividing the duodenum in gastrectomy, a practice we have not adopted. It serves very well for creating greater curvature gastric tubes, or Janeway gastrostomies. When, as in these procedures, both walls of the stomach are transected with the GIA instrument, because of the greater thickness of both gastric walls and the shorter GIA staples, we reinforce the staple suture lines, the only time when reinforcing sutures are routinely used by us. The GIA instrument serves very well for transection and stapling of pulmonary parenchyma, in many applications (Fig 9).

As with the TA instrument, certain principles must be adhered to in the use of the GIA instrument.

1. The two limbs must be correctly mated and locked. This does not require force. If force is required to drive in the staples, the instrument limbs have been improperly assembled.

2. Be certain the two staple drivers and the knife are each in their separate slots.

3. In dividing bowel or lung be sure the tissue to be divided is all within the graduations—i.e., in the staple-bearing portion of the jaws.

4. Do not attempt to include mesentery or omentum in the suture line. Bleeding will result.

5. Inspect anastomoses for bleeding. Reinforce with fine sutures if a bleeding point is seen.

The GIA instrument, too, is now provided in a totally disposable form, the basic instrument being already armed with staple-loaded cartridge, anvil, and knife staple-driver assembly. The staples are shorter, finer and closer together than in the prior GIA instrument. There are still four rows of staples but these are now of 0.20 mm wire, 3 mm bar, and 3.85 mm legs. The two sets of staple lines are approximately 3.5 mm apart. There are 26 staples in each double row which is 5.3 cm long. The two jaws, instead of being held together only at their base by a lock, are now additionally held by a small shoe above and below the knife shaft. The shoes fit into slots in the cartridge and anvil and hold the two limbs constantly compressed to the same degree while the staples are progressively driven home

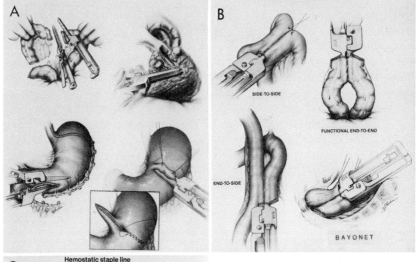

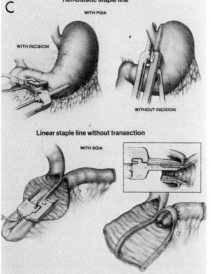

Fig 9.—Procedures that employ the GIA™ instrument. **A,** transection between two staple lines and simultaneous stapling of lung and bowel. The *upper left* shows the colon simultaneously transected and both ends stapled. Mesenteric vessels have been secured by the LDS™ instrument. Wedge resection of the lung is shown in the *upper right.* Note how the staple lines cross. The *lower left* shows the greater curvature gastric tube produced by repeated applications of the GIA™ stapler, which yields a 5-cm increment in the length of the tube with each application of the instrument. *Lower right,* a Janeway mucosa-lined gastrostomy produced with a single operation of the GIA™ instrument. As shown, we usually oversew GIA™ suture lines when two layers of stomach are involved. **B,** Intestinal anastomoses. These are all serosa-to-serosa and minimally inverted. In each case the two openings, one for each prong of the GIA™ instrument, are converted into one when the two loops are stapled together and the stapled tissue divided. The single opening that remains is usually closed mucosa-to-mucosa with the TA™ instrument. *Upper left:* side-to-side enteroenterostomy. *Upper right:* functional end-to-end colocolostomy. *Lower left:* end-to-side jejunojejunostomy. *Lower right:* bayonet anastomosis, as in low anterior resection. **C,** special uses of the GIA™ instrument. The *upper left* shows how gastrotomy with the PGIA™ (pediatric cartridge) avoids troublesome bleeding from the gastrotomy during the intragastric manipulation. The *upper right* shows application of the PGIA™ instrument *without* the knife blade to the anterior and pos-

the length of the instrument. It was thought that the original GIA stapler had not been as regularly hemostatic as desirable because of a tendency for the distal ends of the limbs to spread with repeated use. The new mechanism described, and the staple line changes, are aimed at better hemostasis. The newest steel instrument, GIA Premium, incorporates all the same features.

The EEA instrument is a tubular instrument looking not unlike a sigmoidoscope. At the distal end, the tubular shaft of the EEA instrument can be loaded with a disposable cartridge that consists of a cylinder containing two circular rows of staggered staples, the pushers to drive the staples and a circular knife just inside the inner ring of staples. A dome-shaped nose cone, carrying the anvils, screws onto the rod that passes through the center of the staple cartridge. Within the nose cone, just inside the inner row of anvil recesses, is a heavy plastic ring against which the circular knife cuts the bowel ends, purse-stringed around the central rod of the EEA instrument. The staples are of .28 mm wire, the bar 4 mm, and the limbs 4.8 mm. A wing nut in the handle separates or approximates the disposable staple and anvil portions of the instrument. The purse-stringed ends of the bowel segments to be anastomosed are slipped over the dome-shaped anvil and the cylindrical cartridge, respectively. The purse-strings are tied tightly around the central shaft, the anvil and cartridge approximated, and the handles compressed, creating an instantaneous, minimally inverting, end-to-end or end-to-side anastomosis. The instrument can be positioned three ways: (1) through a natural orifice, such as the anus in a low anterior resection of the rectum, or the mouth in special circumstances for high esophagogastric anastomoses; (2) through an opening made in the ordinary course of operation, as in the stomach for esophagogastrostomy, the small bowel for esophagojejunostomy, the terminal ileum for esophagocecostomy; and (3) through a special gastrotomy, enterotomy or colotomy made only for the purpose of inserting

---

terior walls of the cardia through a cardiotomy for control of esophageal varices. *Lower left:* all four rows of staples, without the knife (SGIA™), anastomosing the two loops in a Kock pouch. The *lower right* and the *insert* show the GIA™ instrument without the knife being used to staple the inverted nipple to reduce the likelihood of loss of the nipple in a Kock pouch. (From Steichen F.M., Ravitch M.M.: *Stapling in Surgery*. Chicago, Year Book Medical Publishers. 1984)

the EEA instrument (Fig 10). In all its uses, certain principles apply.

1. Forcing the use of too large a cartridge risks tearing the bowel.

2. Secure closure of the purse-string about the central rod is essential to security.

Fig 10.—Techniques for using the EEA™ instrument for end-to-end and end-to-side anastomoses. As the upper illustration shows, the instrument can be inserted through an anatomical opening—the anus in low rectal anastomoses and the mouth in esophageal reconstructions in the neck. The instrument can be inserted through a stab wound made for the purpose as in the end-to-end colocolostomy and the Billroth I operations pictured at the left. Finally, the instrument can be inserted through the open end of bowel divided in the normal course of the operation as in the end-to-side esophagojejunostomy or esophagocolostomy. The same technique can be employed in passing the instrument back into the stomach through the open antral end, performing the EEA™ gastroduodenostomy or gastroenterostomy before the stapled amputation of the stomach. In the two right-hand operations, the stumps of the jejunum, and of the terminal ileum, will be stapled and amputated once the anastomosis has been completed. (From Steichen F.M., Ravitch M.M: *Stapling in Surgery.* Chicago, Year Book Medical Publishers. 1984)

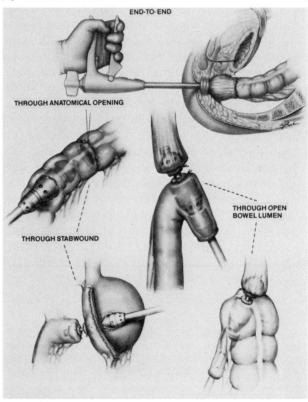

END-TO-END

THROUGH ANATOMICAL OPENING

THROUGH OPEN BOWEL LUMEN

THROUGH STABWOUND

3. Placing the purse-string back from the edge, or turning in a mass of fat, places more tissue in the capsule than can be held without tissue-destroying pressure.

4. The instrument must be opened before its gentle withdrawal.

5. The rings of tissue stamped out by the circular knife must be checked to see they are unbroken.

The EEA instrument is supplied with cartridges approximately 31, 28 and 25 mm in outside diameter, which produce anastomoses of 21, 18 and 15 mm internal diameter, respectively. The largest of these is designed for the adult rectum, although on occasion a smaller size is required. It is uncommon for the adult esophagus to accept the largest size. Ovoid sizers permit one to gauge the caliber of the bowel to assess which cartridge is to be employed, to avoid making the anastomosis smaller than required, or alternatively to prevent injuring the bowel in the attempt to stretch it over too large a cartridge.

The disposable EEA instrument comes fully assembled with any of the three cartridge sizes. As in the steel instrument, the nose cone is removable, for those procedures in which the instrument is passed into the lumen of a segment of the gastrointestinal tract, and the central rod, emerging through a puncture wound, then capped with the nose cone over which is slid the purse-stringed segment of bowel to be anastomosed. The staple sizes and staple line specifications are unchanged. There has not yet been time to acquire extensive experience with the new curved model of the totally disposable EEA instrument. The instrument is a response to our long-time request for a curved shaft that would more easily be introduced from the anus or from the mouth, and more comfortably placed deep in the chest or abdomen through thoracotomy and laparotomy incisions. The demonstrated need for a smaller diameter cartridge in some applications, particularly the esophagus, has been met by the 20.9 mm cartridge diameter and 11.4 mm knife diameter of the smallest cartridge, made for the curved disposable EEA instrument, in addition to the same three sizes previously available for the straight instruments.

Specific Use of the Instruments

Limitations of space preclude detailed discussion of the use of stapling instruments in all their applications. We have chosen to discuss their use in gastric and in pulmonary surgery, and to illustrate the variety of ways in which they may be employed in rectal resection (Figs 11–20).

A number of general principles are found to apply to the various gastric operations. As in all portions of the gastrointes-

Fig 11.—Low anterior resection through functional end-to-end anastomosis. **A,** with the GIA™ or TA™ instrument, the bowel has been transected and stapled at either end. **B,** the ends of the descending colon and rectum are held in shotgun fashion as shown. The GIA™ instrument is inserted through cutaway corners of the staple lines. The rectal stump need not be dissected out or delivered up into the wound. At this point, before removing the GIA™ instrument, we usually place a single suture at the lowest point of the approximation between the two loops, to protect against any possible tension at the close of the operative procedure. **C,** the anastomosis having been made, the GIA™ opening is stapled shut and the protruding tissue cut away using the edge of the TA™ instrument as a guide. **D,** the final result.

In the functional end-to-end anastomosis, although the anastomosis is made side-to-side, the effect is of an end-to-end anastomosis and, in fact, in follow-up endoscopy or barium enema it is not possible to discern that this was anything other than an end-to-end anastomosis.

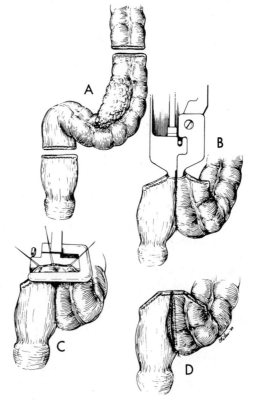

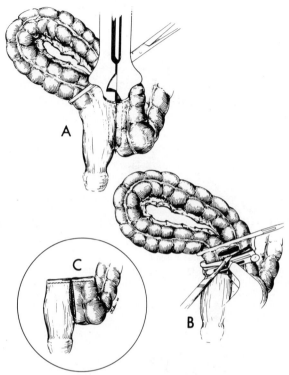

Fig 12.—Low anterior resection through modified functional end-to-end anastomosis. **A,** the bowel to be resected is devascularized in the usual fashion, the antimesenteric borders carefully matched, and the bowel cross-clamped with Kocher clamp. The limbs of the GIA™ instrument are inserted through symmetric orifices in the colon and rectum and the anastomosis formed. As shown in Figure 11, we often apply a single, tiny suture externally at the distal end of the anastomotic line before the GIA™ instrument is withdrawn. **B,** the two limbs are stapled together with the TA 55™ instrument so as to staple the two limbs together and exclude the now common orifice made by the use of the GIA™ instrument. **C,** the result is the conventional functional end-to-end anastomosis, but it employs two staple cartridges fewer and allows even less opportunity for contamination.

tinal tract, stapling and transection of the stomach and duodenum are carried out at the selected level, along the very edge of the viable portion of the remaining viscus. This closure and transection should be within the immediate proximity (literally millimeters) of the intact vascular supply and should not staple the vessels outside the stomach. The cut ends of the stomach and duodenum stapled mucosa-to-mucosa by the TA instruments are essentially never reinforced. A little bleeding from the cut edge coming through the staples is a reassuring sign of good blood supply up to the very cut edge. An occasional spurting vessel requires a single suture. Very rarely is there enough bleeding to suggest the need for reinforcing the suture line, and after closure of the abdomen, only on one occasion have we suspected bleeding, from the cut surface of a tangential gastric excision. There was a significant drop in hemoglobin concentration, no abdominal or systemic signs, and no intervention was required. If there is significant bleeding when the TA instrument has been removed from the duodenum or stomach, it will almost invariably be disclosed that the extragastric, omental

Fig 13.—Low anterior resection with GIA™ bayonet anastomosis. **A,** the bowel is divided at the appropriate points with the GIA™ instrument, or upon the edge of the TA™ instrument, and the end of the proximal bowel placed behind the rectal stump. For a very low anastomosis, as shown, the splenic flexure must usually be taken down for full mobilization of the left colon. **B,** one blade of the GIA™ instrument is inserted through the cutaway corner of the stapled rectum, while the other is inserted through a stab wound in the colon, placed some 6 cm (the length of the GIA™ blade) proximal to the colon closure. Operation of the GIA™ instrument leaves initially only a minimal distal pouch on the colonic side and subsequently, with contraction and healing, none at all. **C,** in very low anastomoses of this kind, it may not be feasible to close the GIA™ introduction site with the stapler.

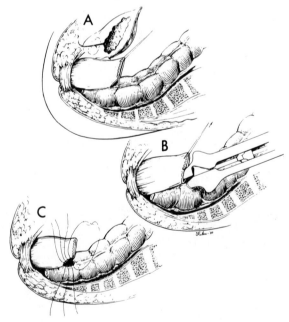

vessels to the residual stomach or duodenum have been included in the clamp. The TA instruments do not provide secure hemostasis of such vessels. Until the advent of the EEA instrument performing circular, minimally inverting anastomoses, we made all Billroth II anastomoses with the GIA instrument, one limb inserted into the stomach and one into the jejunum, the opening left after withdrawal of the GIA instrument being closed mucosa-to-mucosa with the TA instrument. It is possible to perform a Billroth II with the EEA instrument, either inserting it into the open and unstapled end of the stomach and thence through the gastric wall into the jejunum, in the manner analogous to the use of the EEA instrument for Billroth I anastomosis, or inserting the EEA instrument through a gastrotomy in the already amputated and stapled stomach by analogy with the Billroth I technique. We have been so satisfied with the GIA anastomosis that we have not ourselves employed this Billroth II technique, although we gather it is becoming popular.[30] Prior to the use of the EEA instrument, the anastomosis in the Billroth I operation was performed manually. The EEA instrument lends itself admirably to the performance of the Billroth I reconstruction by either of the two techniques. A hazard of dealing with the duodenal stump has been suggested by us and others. If the duodenum is transected and stapled proximal to the ulcer, it is possible that with the leverage of the long instrument, one may unwittingly separate the ulcer borders from the pancreas, inviting a duodenal leak, which in the postoperative period will be diagnosed as a "duodenal stump blow-out."[49] Similarly, it is conceivable that, if the staple line is made through the indurated tissue of the ulcer which has been mobilized, this thick and brittle tissue will be crushed through and will leak. In a single instance in one of our affiliated hospitals, there was a leak from a stapled Billroth II anastomosis. The stomach had been noted to be extremely thick and edematous and the explanation appears to be that under these circumstances the degree of tissue compression required to permit the staples to form correctly resulted in injury to the tissues, causing the leak and the resultant fistula.

It is occasionally useful to transect the stomach, or form tubes, with the GIA instrument, as in a Janeway gastrostomy or the greater curvature Beck-Jianu-Gavriliu tube. Because of the shorter length of the staples in the GIA instrument, we

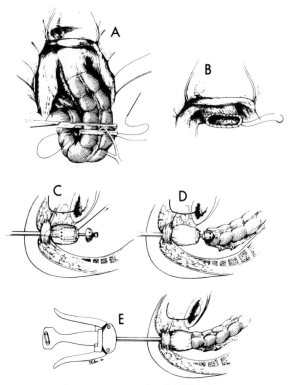

Fig 14.—Low rectal anastomosis with the EEA™ instrument inserted transanally.
A, the modified Furniss purse-string clamp, is shown applied to the descending colon.
The needle being passed through one channel and out the other completes the purse-string suture, and the bowel may then be divided along the distal face of the purse-string clamp.

B, particularly with a low anastomosis in a male pelvis, there may not be room for both the Furniss clamp and the long straight needle, and one then preferentially employs a manual purse-string suture that begins outside the bowel, whips around the circumference of the bowel, including all coats, and emerges once more outside the bowel. This technique takes a little longer than the use of the purse-string clamp, but even in situations in which there is room for the clamp purse-string suture technique, we are inclined to find this manually-placed whip-stitch, purse-string suture more secure and more satisfactory. In either case, 2–0 or heavier monofilament suture is employed to provide easy sliding for a tight and secure closure about the central rod.

C, the EEA™ instrument (here shown, the totally disposable model) is inserted through the rectum and, as the anvil-bearing nose cone emerges, the wing nut on the instrument is turned to separate the nose cone from the staple cartridge, allowing the purse-stringed end to slip down below the nose cone and to be tied tightly around the central rod. The EEA™ instrument may be inserted by an assistant working under the drapes or, as we prefer, the patient may have been initially placed in the lithotomy-Trendelenburg position with wide abduction and minimal flexion of the hips, the anus and perianal region draped out for easy manipulation. At times, we have performed

have insisted on reinforcing such suture lines involving both walls of the stomach, either with a continuous inverting suture or an over-and-over whipstitch placed behind the staples.

The use of the staples on the stomach and the duodenum, avoiding the necessity for clamps of various kinds dangling from the organs, permits one to perform the gastrojejunostomy immediately upon the transection of the stomach, providing a steady flow in the operation procedure—gastric transection, gastrojejunostomy, duodenal transection.

A number of surgeons have employed the LDS instrument in the serial division of the branches of the vagus nerve in parietal cell vagotomy. Engelke, Kamphausen and vom Rath,[50] of Krefeld, Germany, in the performance of parietal cell vagotomy in 216 cases, found the LDS instrument useful for the serial division of the vessels and vagal branches on the lesser curvature.

Our experiences in gastrointestinal surgery and the reported experiences from this country, from Western Europe, Japan and Australia have convinced us that the instruments currently in use permit the surgeon to divide and to anastomose at least as safely as by what were the traditional methods, with the advantages of a substantial saving in time and a decrease

---

the operation with a patient in the Sims's lateral decubitus position, which also makes it easy to insert the EEA™ instrument. As in many other situations, the curved model of the disposable EEA™ instrument very greatly facilitates the manipulation of the instrument, in this case, allowing it to curve upward into the pelvis.

D, the nose cone has been inserted into the proximal bowel and the proximal pursestring securely tied around the central rod.

E, the handle having been turned by the winged end until, as shown by the vernier marks, the bowel ends are approximated, the two handles are strongly closed, driving in the two rows of staples and the circular knife, which cuts out the abutting pursestringed ends. The anvil and the cartridge are separated by counterclockwise rotation of the central element of the handle, so the instrument can be withdrawn, by spiral twisting (not shown). It may be necessary to steady the proximal end with the fingers on a sponge or to place a traction suture through the bowel anteriorly, at the anastomosis, to steady the bowel. If the patient is in the lithotomy-Trendelenburg position, it is convenient for the operator to steady the anastomosis with one hand and to extract the instrument himself with the other. We do not ordinarily employ reinforcing or security sutures. The double rings of excised bowel still inside the cartridge must always be carefully inspected while their orientation is maintained. If there is a deficiency in either ring, sutures are placed at that point. We do not ordinarily employ oversewing or security sutures, nor do we test the anastomosis with saline, antiseptic solution or gas any more than we ever did in a manual anastomosis, although a number of authors report such techniques.

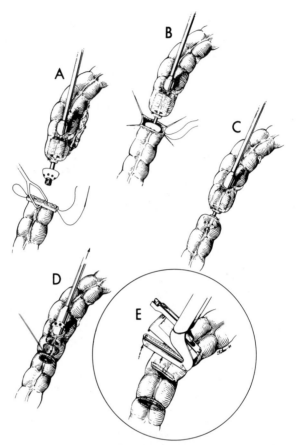

Fig 15.—EEA^{TM} instrument inserted through proximal colotomy. **A,** the purse-string is shown being placed on the distal rectum and the EEA^{TM} instrument inserted through a colotomy in the proximal colon, the purse-string already tied about the stem. **B,** the nose cone anvil is inserted into the distal lumen. **C,** the distal purse-string has been tied tightly around the spindle, and the ends are being approximated. **D,** the EEA^{TM} instrument, having been fired, is opened and withdrawn. A suture is shown across the anastomosis, to aid in withdrawal of the opened EEA^{TM} instrument. **E,** the procedure is completed by transverse TA 55^{TM} closure of the colotomy made for insertion of the EEA^{TM} instrument.

The proximal colotomy or enterotomy technique for insertion of the EEA^{TM} instrument obviously permits end-to-end or end-to-side anastomoses anywhere in the intestinal tract, and this technique has many advocates. In general, we prefer to employ a natural orifice, or an opening necessarily made in the bowel for purposes of the resection, rather than to make a proximal enterotomy with its additional suture line and perhaps increased opportunity for intraoperative soiling.

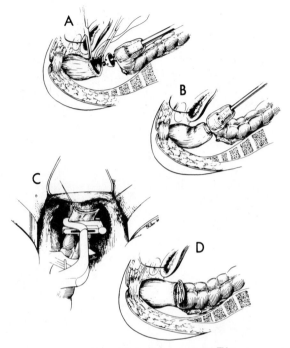

Fig 16.—Low anterior resection with insertion of EEA™ instrument through open end of proximal bowel. **A,** after resection of the specimen, the EEA™ instrument, without the nose cone, has been inserted through the open distal end of the proximal bowel, the central rod emerging through a purse-string in the antimesenteric border, and the nose cone-anvil then screwed on and passed into the distal segment through the purse-string suture, which will be tightly tied about the center rod. **B,** the anvil and cartridge are being approximated until the loops are firmly abutted. Activation of the instrument produces the usual minimally inverting anastomosis. **C,** the EEA™ instrument having been opened and withdrawn, the redundant stump of proximal bowel is stapled conveniently close to the anastomosis with the TA 55™ instrument and the excess cut away on the instrument edge. **D,** the end result is an end-to-end anastomosis that has been made from above, and without the necessity for a proximal colotomy, although there are indeed two suture lines.

in opportunity for bleeding and contamination. In three special circumstances—anastomoses to the esophagus, anastomoses to the lower rectum, and the resection of complicated lesions—the instruments clearly provide a degree of safety and precision, and an improvement of results, over prior methods. There is general agreement, and large experience, to testify that when the EEA instrument is used in esophageal anastomoses[51–57] and in low rectal anastomoses,[46, 58-66] the results produced are superior to those previously achieved. In uncommon and complicated situations, such as the takedown of prior anastomoses associated with inflammation, as in gastrocolic fistulas or as in the restoration of alimentary continuity in patients who have had jejunoileal shunts, the instruments provide a tidy and almost effortless solution to the problems, because each time the stapling instrument is operated the tissues are not only divided, but stapled closed and soiling does not occur. By the same token, in difficult pneumonectomies for inflammatory dis-

Fig 17.—Low anterior anastomosis via the Strasbourg technique (Adloff, Arnaud, Beeharry and Turbelin, 1980).[45] The Strasbourg technique combines the proximal enterotomy technique shown in Figure 15 with the introduction of the stapler through what is part of the specimen shown in Figure 16. The operation represents a simplification in that the TA 55™ application shown in **B** not only excludes the colotomy made for the introduction of the EEA™ instrument but serves for the amputation of the specimen.

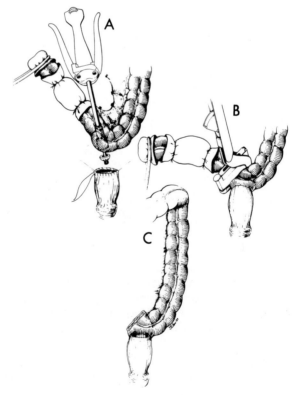

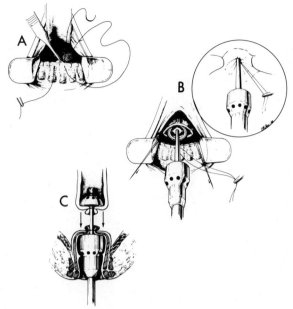

Fig 18.—Low rectal resection: the technique of J. C. Goligher (1979).[46] Goligher, after a large experience with the Russian stapling instruments, was even more enthusiastic about the American instruments. The illustrations show his technique of placing the distal purse-string through the anus for the extremely low resections. **A,** the over-and-over purse-string is placed over the distal transection of the rectum, in this case almost at the columns of Morgagni. **B,** the anvil-carrying nose cone is inserted into the proximal bowel from below and *(insert)* the proximal purse-string tied. **C,** the distal purse-string is then tied and the instrument activated in the usual fashion. Goligher's initial experience with such low anastomoses—always accompanied by transverse colostomy—suggested that increased frequency of stools resulted but that the initial incontinence was gradually overcome.

ease with large masses of hilar lymph nodes, if one can create a tunnel which will admit a clamp under any hilar structure, one can insert the lower jaw of the TA instrument and at once staple and then divide bronchus or vessel, opening up the remainder of the hilum for easy dissection.

The thoracic surgeons, in this country at least, were very quick to learn the advantages of the instruments and there is now ample evidence that the incidence of bronchial stump leaks has been reduced and the treatment of the hilar vessels made substantially safer.

The uses of the stapling instruments in stapling the bronchi and the pulmonary vessels are self-evident, and intrapericardial division of the vessels in pneumonectomy is made remarkably safe and simple. As important as any use in thoracic surgery, from the standpoint of advantage over manual surgery, is the use of the stapling instruments, whether the GIA instrument or the TA instrument, in the completion of incomplete fissures. The instruments have completely altered the manner

Fig 19.—Low anterior resection of the rectum using the EEA™ stapler: the technique of Knight and Griffen (1980).[47] **A,** after the rectosigmoid colon has been mobilized, the TA 55™ stapler is applied at the lower limit of the resection. **B,** the EEA™ stapler, with the anvil-nose cone removed, is introduced per anum into the rectal segment. The naked center rod is passed through a stab wound posterior to the staple line, and the anvil is fitted to the rod. A noncrushing clamp on the proximal colon prevents spillage. **C,** after the anvil has been attached to the spindle and fitted into the open sigmoid colon, the proximal purse-string is tied and the noncrushing clamp removed. **D,** the EEA™ stapler is closed and activated to make the circular end-to-end inverting anastomosis. In this technique, no attempt is made to include the entire circumference of the rectal segment, and the need for a distal purse-string is obviated. We had been hesitant to employ this technique, but animal experiments now in progress support its safety despite the fact that the EEA™ knife cuts the TA™ closure of the rectum at two points. Others have reported clinical use of this principle in various parts of the gastrointestinal tract and it is in routine use at the clinic of one of us.

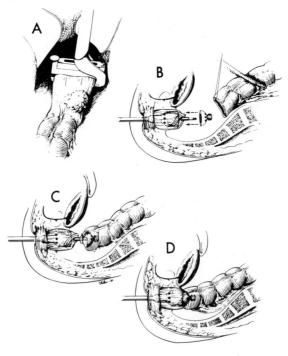

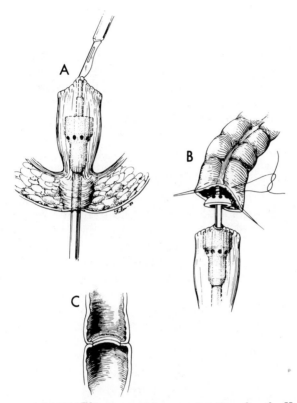

Fig 20.—Use of the EEA™ instrument in reconstruction after the Hartmann procedure: the technique of Robbins, Sohn, Weinstein, and Steichen, (1981).[48] The EEA™ instrument is passed up through the anus without the anvil-nose cone until the spindle presses against the upper end of the Hartmann pouch, which need not be dissected except to expose its surface. The spindle is passed through as small an incision as possible, the nose cone applied and slipped into the purse-stringed proximal bowel, and the anastomosis performed thereafter as in the other applications of the EEA™ instrument. This technique enormously simplifies the reconstruction after a Hartmann procedure and minimizes the need for dissection in the scarred pelvis. One must exercise some care to avoid perforation of the rectum by the spindle before it reaches the upper end of the rectal pouch.

of procuring lung biopsies, excising bullae and blebs, wedging out coin lesions, and have made feasible and reasonable the excision of multiple pulmonary metastases. In pulmonary surgery, the bronchial fistula and air leak rate has provided a ready means of evaluating the function of the instruments. Kirksey and colleagues[67] at the 1970 meeting of the Society of

Thoracic Surgeons reported their early experience with stapling in pulmonary resection. In 147 pulmonary resections, they had one bronchial fistula, an empyema after lobectomy, and two prolonged air leaks after lobectomy both resolving spontaneously. Takaro and associates from Oteen, North Carolina,[68] reported an experience with 407 pulmonary resections with the Russian instruments and 86 with the American instruments which became available later in their experience. The instruments were used on pulmonary vessels, bronchi, and pulmonary parenchyma. With the Russian instruments, they had eight bronchopleural fistulas and four persistent air leaks and stated that with the Russian instruments, improper staple closure ". . . could be attributed to inappropriate size of the staple for the tissue being approximated; or improper manual loading of the individual staples, allowing malposition or premature loss of staples to occur; or defective staples. . . No instances of technical failure and no bronchopleural fistulas were noted following 86 pulmonary resections using the American stapler."

At that same meeting of the Society of Thoracic Surgeons, Goldman[69] commented on the passage of vessels through the B staples.

Konrad and Tarbiat,[70] from Düsseldorf, reported with apparent pleasure the occurrence of bronchial fistulas in only four out of 80 bronchial closures with the American staplers. In 1973, before the Society of Thoracic Surgeons, Hood and associates[71] reported their experience with the American instruments in 349 cases, using the 30V cartridge for the pulmonary vessels, including intrapericardial division, and the instrument for stapling the bronchi and pulmonary parenchyma. In 60 pneumonectomies, there were two bronchopleural fistulas, and in their 136 lobectomies, none. There were five prolonged air leaks, three of them requiring reoperation.

The instruments have made the formal segmental resection obsolete; the stapler is utilized as seems appropriate to excise the diseased tissue, with or without separate dissection of the segmental bronchus or vessels. Such transsegmental resections spare pulmonary parenchyma which might be sacrificed by a formal segmentectomy. Kirsh,[72] of Ann Arbor, at the same 1973 meeting, stated that complications had decreased with the use of staplers even in irradiated patients and they had no bronchopleural fistulas. As we had pointed out, Kirsh indicated that a disadvantage of stapling the unopened bronchus was that it prevented inspection of the interior of the bronchus. Jensik,[73] of Chicago, reported 107 bronchial closures with the staplers with two fistulas, both in patients with severe, diffuse pulmonary infection, one of them previously irradiated. Cook and colleagues,[74] in 1974, reported 150 consecutive pulmonary resections with the use of the Auto Suture staplers, with three bronchial fistulas. Lawson and associates,[75] in Glasgow, reported 43 pulmonary resections with no complications and no deaths. Forrester-Wood,[76] of Cornwall, found that the staples decreased his bronchopleural fistula rate from 11% to 2.6%. Irlich and colleagues,[77] from Düsseldorf, in 1981, said that after abandoning closure of the bronchi with wire sutures and adopting the Auto Suture staplers, their empyema rate, taken as representing bronchial stump leak rate, had fallen from 4.2% to 2.1%, and in only one of these (0.3%) was a suture failure held responsible.

It has been the general experience of thoracic surgeons with a variety of manually inserted nonabsorbable bronchial sutures, that occasional patients develop chronic cough and are found to have sutures in granulations at the bronchial stump, which require bronchoscopic removal. Baumgartner and Mark,[78] of Stanford, in 1981, addressed themselves specifically to this point and said that such bronchoscopic extraction of sutures had been necessary in eight out of 180 patients in whom the bronchus had been closed with synthetic thread, whereas, in the immediately subsequent series of over 100 consecutive pulmonary resections with the Auto Suture staplers, there had been no bronchopleural fistulas and no granulomas.

The stapling instruments do not abrogate the general principles of surgery. Devascularized tissues will not heal, and tissues which are the seat of active disease—tuberculosis, cancer, inflammatory bowel disease, etc.—may not reliably be counted upon to heal. The instruments are sufficiently long so that powerful leverage can be applied with them and injury produced. The stapling instruments will not automatically convert the untrained surgeon into a brilliant virtuoso. They do provide precision, neatness, a decrease in trauma, a decrease in the opportunity for bleeding or for contamination and an important saving in time.

276 M. M. RAVITCH AND F. M. STEICHEN

REFERENCES

1. Gudov V.F.: A method for the application of vascular sutures by mechanical means. *Khirurgiia (Mosk.)* 12:58, 1950.
2. Steichen F.M., Ravitch M.M.: History of mechanical devices and instruments for suturing. *Curr. Probl. Surg.* 19:1, 1982.
3. Steichen F.M., Ravitch M.M.: *Stapling in Surgery.* Chicago, Year Book Medical Publishers, 1984.
4. Denans F.N.: Nouveau procédé pour la guérison des plaies des intestins. Recueil de la Société Royale dé Medecine de Marseille [Séance du 24 fev. 1826, rédigé par M. P. Roux], Imprimerie d'Archard, Marseille, Tome I:127, 1827.
5. Gross S.D.: An experimental and critical inquiry into the nature and treatment of wounds of the intestines. Prentice and Weissinger, Louisville, 1843.
6. Henroz J.H.F.: Dissertatio Inauguralis Critica Medico-Chirurgica de Methodis ad Sananda Intestina Divisa Adhibitis, In Qua Nova Sanationis Methodus Proponitur. Universitate Leondiensi, June 1826. P.J. Collardin, Typographi Academici, 1826.
7. Lembert A.: Mémoire sur l'entéroraphie. *Rep. Gen. Anat. Physiol. Pathol.* II:101, 1826.
8. Senn N.: Enterorrhaphy: Its history, technique and present status. *JAMA* 21:217, 1893.
9. Travers B.: An inquiry into the process of nature in repairing injuries of the intestines. London, Longman, 1812, pp. 121, 128–135, 180–189.
10. Dunn H., Robbins P., Decanini C., Goldberg S., Delaney J.P.: A comparison of stapled and hand-sewn colonic anastomoses. *Dis. Colon Rectum* 21:636, 1978.
11. Pimenta A.P.A.: Personal communication. September 20, 1981.
12. Pimenta A.P.A., Cardoso V., Rodrigues J.S.: A mechanical suturing method for the gastrointestinal tract: Experimental and clinical experience with a new stapling instrument. 6th World Congress of the Collegium Internationale Chirurgiae Digestivae, Lisbon, Portugal, September 1980.
13. Pimenta A.P.A., Cardosa V., Rodrigues J.S.: Un nouvel instrument pour agrafage mécanique en chirurgie gastro-intestinale. Etude expérimentale préliminaire. *Ann. Chir.* 35:469, 1981.
14. Pimenta A.P.A., Cardosa V.M.B., Rodrigues J.S.: A mechanical suturing method for the gastrointestinal tract: Clinical experience with a new stapling instrument. *World J. Surg.* 6:786, 1982.
15. Amat C.: Les appareils à sutures: les viroles de Denans; les pointes de Bonnier; les boutons de Murphy. *Arch. Med. Pharm. Milit.* XXV:273, 1895.
16. Murphy J.B.: Cholecysto-intestinal, gastro-intestinal, entero-intestinal anastomosis, and approximation without sutures (original research). Medical Record, New York 42:665, 1892, and Chicago Medical Record XIII:803, 1892.
17. Halsted W.S.: Circular suture of the intestine—An experimental study. *Am. J. Med.Sci.* XCIV:436, 1887.

18. Meyer W.: Murphy's Knopf in der Chirurgie des Magen Darm-Kanales und der Gallenblase. *Zentralbl. Chir.* XXI:866, 1894.
19. Marwedel G.: Ueber Enteroanastomose nebst experimentellen Beiträgen zur Frage des Murphyschen Darmknopfes. *Beitr. Klin. Chir.* XIII:605, 1895.
20. Czerny V.: Ueber die Verwendung des Murphyknopfes als Ersatz für die Darmnaht. Verhandlungen der Deutsch. Gesellschaft für Chirurgie, Berlin, XXV Congress, p. 94, 1896.
21. Ramaugé A.: Entéroplexie: Considérations preliminaires. Mémoire presenté et couronné au concours de Médicine International Sud-Américain. pp. 5–32, 20 January 1893.
22. Ramaugé A.: Enteroplexis. Consideraciones preliminares. Memoria presentada al jurado del concurso de Medicine International Sudamericano. pp. 7–41. (ed.) Jacobo Peuser, 1893.
23. Ramaugé A.: Enteroplexo. *Rev. Soc. Med. Argentina* 2:667, 1902.
24. Boerema I.: The technique of our method of transabdominal total gastrectomy in cases of gastric cancer. *Arch. Chir. Neerl.* 6:95, 1954.
25. Boerema I., Klopper P.J., Holscher A.A.: Transabdominal ligation-resection of the esophagus in cases of bleeding esophageal varices. *Surgery* 67:409, 1970.
26. Prioton J.-B.: La ligature de l'oesophage sur bouton de Murphy dans les hemorragies par rupture de varices oesophagiennes. *Ann. Chir.* 27:343, 1973.
27. Ton J.G., Boelens W.C., Gallas: Resection of the rectum with preservation of the anal sphincter. *Arch. Chir. Neerl.* XXV–II:179, 1973.
28. Halsted W.S.: End-to-end suture of the intestine by a bulkhead method. Transactions of the American Surgical Association 28:256, 1910.
29. Halsted W.S.: Blind-end circular suture of the intestine, closed ends abutted and the double diaphragm punctured with a knife introduced per rectum. *Ann. Surg.* 75:356, 1922.
30. Nance F.C.: New techniques of gastrointestinal anastomoses with the EEA stapler. *Ann. Surg.* 189:587, 1979.
31. Sugarbaker E.D., Wiley H.M.: Rectocolic anastomosis. A simplified method. *Surg. Gynecol. Obstet.* 93:597, 1951.
32. Hallenbeck G.A., Judd E.S., David C.: An instrument for colorectal anastomosis without sutures. *Dis. Colon Rectum* 4:98, 1963.
33. Brummelkamp R.: The rectoresector: A new instrument for resection of the rectum and colorectal anastomosis without sutures. *Dis. Colon Rectum* 8:49, 1965.
34. Jansen A., Becker A.E., Brummelkamp W.H., Keeman J.N., Klopper, P.J.: The importance of the apposition of the submocosal intestinal layers for primary wound healing of intestinal anatomosis. *Surg. Gynecol. Obstet.* 152:51, 1981.
35. Jansen A., Brummelkamp W.H., Davies G.A.G., Klopper P.J., Keeman J.N.: Clinical applications of magnetic rings in colorectal anastomosis. *Surg. Gynecol. Obstet.* 153:537, 1981.
36. Hültl H.: II Kongress der Ungarischen Gesellschaft für Chirurgie, Budapest, May 1908. *Pester Med.-Chir. Presse* 45:108–110, 121–122, 1909.
37. Meyer W.: Extrathoracic and intrathoracic esophagoplasty in connection

with resection of the thoracic portion of the esophagus for carcinoma. *JAMA* 62:100, 1914.

38. von Petz A.: Zur Technik der Magenresektion. Ein neuer Magen-Darm-nähpparat. *Zentralbl. Chir.* 51:179, 1924.

39. von Petz A.: Aseptic technique of stomach resections. *Ann. Surg.* 86:388, 1927.

40. Friedrich H.: Ein neuer Magen-Darm-Nähapparat. *Zentralbl. Chir.* 61:504, 1934.

41. Kulish N.I., Burakov I.: Liver resection with stapling apparatus. *Klin. Khir.* 7:56, 1973.

42. Vinogradov V.V., Ryneisky S.V., Zenonos A.: Application of a mechanical suture in operations on the liver and bile ducts. *Vestn. Khir.* 114:40, 1975.

43. Rustamov I.R., Shalimov S.A., Zemskov V.S., Diachuk I.S., Radzikovsky A.P.: Liver resection using mechanical suturing by means of the UKL and UAP apparatus. *Klin. Khir.* 9:50, 1979.

44. Khalid M.: Mechanical tantalum suture in kidney resection. *Urol. Nefrol. (Mosk.)* 3:49, 1981.

45. Adloff M., Arnaud J.P., Beeharry S., Turbelin J.M.: Side-to-end anastomosis in low anterior resection with the EEA stapler. *Dis. Colon Rectum* 23:456, 1980.

46. Goligher J.C.: Use of circular stapling gun with peranal insertion of anorectal purse-string suture for construction of very low colorectal or colo-anal anastomoses. *Br. J. Surg.* 66:501, 1979.

47. Knight C.D., Griffen F.D.: An improved technique for low anterior resection of the rectum using the EEA stapler. *Surgery* 88:710, 1980.

48. Robbins R.D., Sohn N., Weinstein M.A., Steichen F.: A simplified technique utilizing the EEA suture device for re-establishing intestinal continuity following Hartmann's operation. *Colo-Proctol.* III(4):266, 1981.

49. Hinchey E.J.: In discussion of Reiling R.B., et al. *Am. J. Surg.* 139:147, 1980.

50. Engelke B., Kamphausen U., vom Rath E.W.: Selektive proximale vagotomie (SPV). Erfahrungen und technik mit dem LDS-Gerät. *Chirurg.* 48:728, 1977.

51. Akiyama H.: Personal communication, June 17, 1981.

52. Féketé F.: Personal communication. June 17, 1981.

53. Féketé F., Breil Ph., Ronsse H.: Anastomoses mécaniques à la pince EEA en chirurgie oesophagienne. *Chirurg.* 106:659, 1980.

54. Féketé F., Breil Ph., Ronsse H., Tossen J.C., Langonnet F.: EEA^R stapler and omental graft in esophagogastrectomy. *Ann. Surg.* 193:825, 1981.

55. Griffen W.O., Jr., Daugherty M.E., McGee E.M., Utley J.R.: Unified approach to carcinoma of the esophagus. *Ann. Surg.* 183:511, 1976.

56. Molina J.E., Lawton B.R., Avance D.: Use of circumferential stapler in reconstruction following resections for carcinoma of the cardia. *Ann. Thorac. Surg.* 31:325, 1981.

57. Molina J.E., Lawton B.R., Meyers W.O., Humphrey E.W.: Esophagogastrectomy for adenocarcinoma of the cardia. *Ann. Surg.* 195:146, 1982.

58. Goligher J.C.: Recent trends in the practice of sphincter-saving excision for rectal cancer. *Ann. R. Coll. Surg. Engl.* 61:169, 1979.

59. Goligher J.C., Lee P.W.R., Macfie J., Simpkins K.C., Lintott D.J.: Experience with the Russian Model 249 suture gun for anastomosis of the rectum. *Surg. Gynecol. Obstet.* 148:517, 1979.
60. Polglase A.L., Hughes E.S.R., McDermott F.T.: Improved techniques in EEA stapling for ultra low colorectal and colo-anal anastomosis. *Aust. NZ J. Surg.* 51:211, 1981.
61. Wheeless C.R., Jr.: Avoidance of permanent colostomy in pelvic malignancy using the surgical stapler. *Obstet. Gynecol.* 54:501, 1979.
62. Wheeless C.R., Jr.: Personal communication, July 7, 1981.
63. Wheeless C.R., Jr.: Personal communication, July 30, 1982.
64. Heald R.J.: Towards fewer colostomies—the impact of circular stapling devices on the surgery of rectal cancer in a district hospital. *Br. J. Surg.* 67:198, 1980.
65. Heald R.J., Leicester R.J.: The low stapled anastomosis. *Dis. Colon Rectum* 24:437, 1981.
66. Fiala J.-M., Marti M.-C., Meyer P., Rohner A.: L'agrafeuse EEA en chirurgie colique. *Helv. Chir. Acta* 47:639, 1980.
67. Kirksey T.D., Arnold H.S., Calhoon J.H., Hood R.M.: Techniques of pulmonary resection. Tradition and travail. *Ann. Thorac. Surg.* 9:525, 1970.
68. Dart C.H., Jr., Scott S.M., Takaro T.: Six-year clinical experience using automatic stapling device for lung resections. *Ann. Thorac. Surg.* 9:535, 1970.
69. Goldman A.: In discussion of dart C.H., Jr., Scott S.M., Takaro T. *Ann. Thorac. Surg.* 9:535, 1970.
70. Konrad R.M., Tarbiat S.: Die Insuffizienzquote nach Verwendung des Klammernaht-Gerätes beim Bronchusverschluss. *Thoraxchir. Vask. Chir.* 19:179, 1971.
71. Hood R.M., Kirksey T.D., Calhoon J.H., Arnold H.S., Tate R.S.: The use of automatic stapling devices in pulmonary resection. *Ann. Thorac. Surg.* 16:85, 1973.
72. Kirsh M.M.: In discussion of Hood R.M., Kirksey T.D., Calhoon H.H., Arnold H.S., Tate R.S. *Ann. Thorac. Surg.* 16:85, 1973.
73. Jensik R.J.: In discussion of Hood R.M., Kirksey T.D., Calhoon J.H., Arnold H.S., Tate R.S. *Ann. Thorac. Surg.* 16:85, 1973.
74. Cook W.A., Lee C.W., You K.D., Santos G.H.: Pulmonary resection. Autosuture technique. *NY State J. Med.* 74:967, 1974.
75. Lawson W.R., Hutchinson J., Longland C.J., Haque M.A.: Mechanical suture methods in thoracic and abdominal surgery. *Br. J. Surg.* 64:115, 1977.
76. Forrester-Wood, C.P.: Bronchopleural fistula following pneumonectomy for carcinoma of the bronchus. Mechanical stapling versus hand suturing. *J. Thorac. Cardiovasc. Surg.* 80:406, 1980.
77. Irlich G., Schulte H.D., Koch J.: Klammernahtgeräte an der Lunge und am Bronchus. Abstract. 98th Kongress, Deutsche Gesellschaft für Chirurgie, Munich, April 22–25, 1981.
78. Baumgartner W.A., Mark J.B.D.: Bronchoscopic diagnosis and treatment of bronchial stump suture granulomas. *J. Thorac. Cardiovasc. Surg.* 81:553, 1981.

The Evaluation and Management of Pheochromocytomas

STEVEN N. LEVINE, M.D.* AND JOHN C.
McDONALD, M.D.†

*Section of Endocrinology and †Department of Surgery, Louisiana State
University Medical Center, Shreveport, Louisiana

PHEOCHROMOCYTOMAS are catecholamine-secreting neoplasms
that most frequently arise in the adrenal medulla, although
they may be found in any location from the neck to the pelvic
floor. Although these endocrine tumors are relatively uncommon, they have always fascinated clinicians. This interest
stems from a number of unique features, including (1) the curable nature of the hypertension, (2) the rather dramatic paroxysms produced by catecholamine excess, (3) the highly lethal
potential of undiagnosed or untreated pheochromocytomas, and
(4) the association of pheochromocytomas with other endocrine
neoplasms.

A clear understanding of the metabolism and physiologic effects of catecholamines is required in order to appropriately diagnose and manage patients with pheochromocytomas. Perti-
nent aspects of the anatomy, biochemistry, and physiology of
the sympathoadrenal system are reviewed below.

Sympathoadrenal System

ANATOMY AND EMBRYOLOGY

The cells of the adrenal medulla are frequently referred to as
chromaffin cells due to the dark color produced when their

281

0065-3411/84/0017-0281-0314-$04.00

large stores of catecholamines are oxidized in the presence of dichromate salts. In adults, the majority of chromaffin cells are located in the adrenal medulla, although groups of these cells exist in the sympathetic ganglia, in the carotid body, and along the branches of the vagus nerves. In young children groups of extra-adrenal chromaffin cells are more conspicuous—the largest lies anterior to the aorta, below the origin of the inferior mesenteric artery (the organ of Zuckerkandl).[1] Later in life these extra-adrenal chromaffin cells regress but remnants persist that may be the future locus for a pheochromocytoma.

The cells of the adrenal medulla are derived from primitive precursor cells that migrate from the neural crest to the sympathetic ganglia and the regions of the developing adrenal glands. This is the same embryologic origin as the origin of the calcitonin-secreting C cells of the thyroid, the pancreatic islet cells, and the argentaffin cells of the foregut.[2] The common origin of these varied cell types may help to explain why tumors of several endocrine tissues can arise in the same individual or in members of the same family.

BIOSYNTHESIS AND SECRETION OF CATECHOLAMINES

The initial substrate for the biosynthesis of catecholamines is tyrosine, which may be of dietary origin or synthesized in vivo by hydroxylation of phenylalanine (Fig 1). Tyrosine is converted to levodopa by the enzyme tyrosine hydroxylase, the rate-limiting enzyme of catecholamine biosynthesis. Levodopa is subsequently converted to dopamine and then to norepinephrine. The last enzyme, phenylethanolamine-N-methyltransferase, which metabolizes norepinephrine to epinephrine, is present only in the adrenal medulla and a few neurons of the CNS. This explains the presence of high concentrations of epinephrine in the adrenal medulla, while norepinephrine remains the neurotransmitter at the sympathetic nerve endings. Of interest, the activity of phenylethanolamine-N-methyltransferase is increased by high concentrations of glucocorticoids. This may account for the anatomical positioning of the adrenal medulla surrounded by the adrenal cortex, and the presence of a portal system bathing the medullary cells in blood containing high concentrations of adrenocortical hormones.[3]

Knowledge of this biosynthetic pathway has enabled chem-

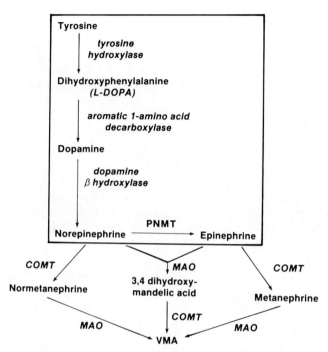

Fig 1.—Biosynthesis and metabolism of catecholamines. Biosynthetic pathways are enclosed within the square. PNMT, phenylethanolamine-N-methyl transferase; MAO, monoamine oxidase; COMT, catechol-O-methyl transferase; VMA, vanillylmandelic acid.

ists to synthesize a compound that functions as an antagonist of tyrosine hydroxylase and thus inhibits catecholamine production. α-Methyl-para-tyrosine (metyrosine) is now commercially available and has proved to be a useful adjunct in the management of selected patients with pheochromocytomas.

Norepinephrine and epinephrine are stored within specific membrane-bound electron-dense granules. Figure 2 shows an electron micrograph of a pheochromocytoma that contained such granules. This tumor appeared to contain norepinephrine. Following appropriate physiologic stimuli, exocytosis occurs, with release of the soluble components of the granule. An interesting observation has been that stimulation of α receptors on the presynaptic membrane diminishes the further release of norepinephrine by neural stimuli; conversely, β stimulation enhances the release of this neurotransmitter.[3]

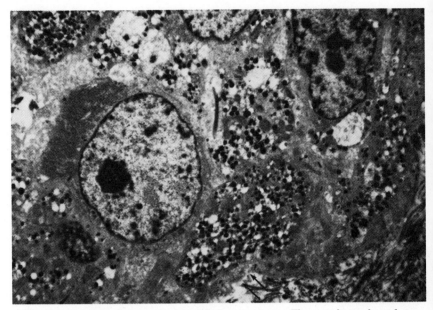

Fig 2.—Electron micrograph of a pheochromocytoma. The membrane-bound granules within the cytoplasm were of the dense-core variety. The tumor cells abutted prominent perivascular spaces *(arrows)*. The dense-core vesicles have been described by Coupland to contain norepinephrine.[1] Section was fixed in glutaraldehyde and embedded in Epon. (Uranyl acetate lead citrate; ×17,125.) (Micrograph courtesy of Michael S. Rohr, M.D. Ph.D.)

METABOLISM OF CATECHOLAMINES

The onset of the biologic effects of the catecholamines is extremely rapid but short-lived. Termination occurs by reuptake at the sympathetic nerve endings and metabolic transformation, primarily involving oxidative deamination and O-methylation (see Fig 1). Catechol-O-methyl transferase (COMT) transfers a methyl group to either epinephrine or norepinephrine, producing metanephrine or normetanephrine, respectively. The other major enzyme, monoamine oxidase (MAO), catalyzes oxidative deamination of epinephrine and norepinephrine to 3,4-dihydroxymandelic acid. This product can be further metabolized by COMT to vanillylmandelic acid (VMA). MAO also catalyzes the reaction that produces VMA from both metanephrine and normetanephrine.[4]

These metabolites, as well as small quantities of unmetabolized epinephrine and norepinephrine, are excreted in the urine. Further details on urinary catecholamines and their metabolites are presented in a later section describing the tests used to diagnose pheochromocytomas.

PHYSIOLOGIC EFFECTS OF CATECHOLAMINES

The physiologic effects of catecholamines are numerous, as most tissues can be demonstrated to have characteristic responses (Table 1). It is generally acknowledged that catecholamines function by binding to specific receptors located on the cell surface and do not require intracellular uptake to produce an effect. This binding is specific, reversible, and saturable. In 1948, Ahlquist, based on his observations of different adrenergic agonists, postulated the existence of two distinct populations of receptors.[5] The development of selective adrenergic antagonists confirmed this hypothesis, and the recognition of α- and β-adrenergic receptors is now common knowledge. In addition, more recent experimental data confirm that these major types of receptors can be further subdivided into α_1, α_2 and β_1, β_2 receptors.

A detailed analysis of the numerous effects of the catecholamines is beyond the scope of this review, but some general comments are appropriate. Catecholamine secretion is a rapid and predictable response to a wide variety of stresses. The effects on the cardiovascular system are designed to preserve cerebral and myocardial blood flow. Vasoconstriction (an α effect) occurs in the splanchnic, subcutaneous, and renal vessels, while alterations in blood flow to the heart and brain are minimized. β stimulation increases cardiac output by accelerating the heart rate, increasing conduction velocity, and increasing cardiac contractility.[6]

TABLE 1.—PHYSIOLOGIC EFFECTS OF CATECHOLAMINES

α	β
Vasoconstriction	Vasodilation
	Increased heart rate
	Increased cardiac contractility
	Bronchodilation
Intestinal relaxation	Intestinal relaxation
Uterine contraction	Uterine relaxation
	Increased glycogenolysis
	Increased lipolysis

Catecholamines regulate metabolic pathways to promote catabolism of stored fuels so that caloric needs can be met from endogenous sources. Glycogenolysis, gluconeogenesis, lipolysis, and ketogenesis are all enhanced. In addition, glucagon secretion is increased but insulin secretion is inhibited—a set of circumstances that promotes the catabolism and utilization of stored fuels. Catecholamines are known to influence these alterations of hormonal secretion.[6]

Pheochromocytoma

INCIDENCE

Estimates of the incidence of pheochromocytomas vary from 0.1% to 2% of patients with sustained diastolic hypertension. However, most authorities favor an incidence toward the lower end of this range.[7-9] Since only 50% of patients with pheochromocytomas have persistent hypertension, an equal number of patients with pheochromocytomas will be found in the population without classic (sustained) hypertension. In a review of 40,078 consecutive autopsies performed at the Mayo Clinic, the incidence of pheochromocytomas was 0.13%.[10] This rather high incidence may have been biased by several features, such as patterns of patient referral and the circumstances surrounding a death more likely to result in an autopsy. For example, a patient who dies during induction of anesthesia is more likely to undergo an autopsy than one who has been previously diagnosed as having metastatic carcinoma. While pheochromocytomas can occur in all age groups, the peak incidence is in the third to fifth decades. In most series approximately 10% of all cases are reported in children.[9, 11]

PATHOLOGY AND LOCALIZATION

Macroscopically, pheochromocytomas are of variable size, most frequently in the range of 50–200 gm, but tumors have been resected that have been as small as several hundred milligrams and as large as several kilograms.[10] Catecholamine-secreting tumors that are situated outside the confines of the adrenal medulla have been referred to by a number of terms, including chromaffinoma, paraganglioma, extra-adrenal pheochromocytoma, and pheochromocytoma of the organ of Zucker-kandl (if located below the origin of the inferior mesenteric artery). However, it seems more appropriate simply to refer to pheochromocytomas as being of either intra- or extra-adrenal origin.

The tumors are usually encapsulated. In familial pheochromocytomas they are typically bilateral and multicentric. In sporadic cases, while they may appear to be composed of several individual tumor masses, on pathologic sectioning these "nodules" are usually projections extending from a single neoplasm.[12] Pheochromocytomas tend to be highly vascular, often with areas of cystic necrosis from previous hemorrhage into portions of the tumor.[11] Figure 3 shows a pheochromocytoma shortly after excision. Note the characteristic thin but well-developed capsule. The darker areas represent some hemorrhage into areas of necrosis and are typical.

Microscopically, the cells are generally polygonal in shape and larger than normal pheochromocytes. There is often considerable variation in the size and shape of the individual cells and occasionally multinucleated giant cells are evident. The staining characteristics of the cytoplasm may vary from basophilic to acidophilic, but the secretory granules containing

Fig 3.—A bisected pheochromocytoma, recently excised. The fleshy tumor measured 2.5 × 4 cm and contained numerous areas of necrosis and hemorrhage.

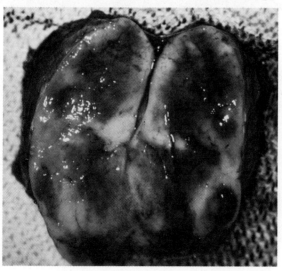

catecholamines stain a characteristic brown when reacted with chromate salts. The nuclear morphology can be quite variable. Nuclei may be multiple, hyperchromatic, and degenerating, with large prominent nucleoli.[9, 11] Yet despite these features, which usually suggest malignancy, approximately 90% follow a benign clinical course.[8] Figure 4 illustrates most of these findings. Pathologically it is thus extremely difficult to assign such a tumor to a benign or malignant category. Not infrequently tumors with obvious capsular invasion or blood vessel penetration act in a benign fashion. In general, invasion of adjacent tissues or distant metastasis is required to establish the diagnosis of a malignant pheochromocytoma.

Pheochromocytomas (often bilateral) are frequently observed in individuals from families with multiple endocrine neoplasia (MEN) type IIA and IIB syndromes. In these cases (but not with sporadic pheochromocytomas) pathologic lesions that are

Fig 4.—Light micrograph of pheochromocytoma. The tumor was composed of sheets of cells. Mitotic figures were absent. The tumor contained large vascular spaces and the cytoplasm of the tumor cells was finely granular. Despite the rather monotonous appearance of the cell configuration and cytoplasm, there was considerable variation of nuclear structure. Section was embedded in paraffin. (Hematoxylin-eosin; ×940.) (Courtesy of Michael S. Rohr, M.D., Ph.D.)

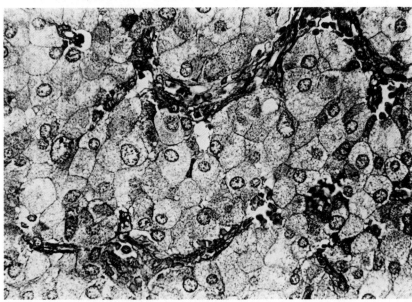

precursors to actual tumor formation have been demonstrated. Both diffuse and nodular hyperplasia of the adrenal medulla have been identified in these patients.[12-14] Often, at the time of abdominal exploration for a pheochromocytoma evident on one side, the contralateral gland is found to be hyperplastic. Clinical experience has taught that if it is left in situ, the hyperplastic gland will eventually be the locus of a future pheochromocytoma.

While 85%–90% of pheochromocytomas originate within the adrenal medulla, they can be located anywhere from the neck to the bladder. In adults approximately 8%–15% of pheochromocytomas are multiple, 10%–15% are extra-adrenal, and 10%–20% are malignant.[3, 7, 9, 15-19] These percentages tend to vary in different series. However, the variation depends largely on the proportion of familial and pediatric cases that make up the entire group of patients. As previously noted, familial pheochromocytomas are typically bilateral but rarely extra-adrenal. In children the incidence of multiple and extra-adrenal tumors is approximately 25%–35% for each category.[3, 9, 19]

The most frequent location for extra-adrenal pheochromocytomas is along the sympathetic chain, often below the origin of the inferior mesenteric artery (the organ of Zuckerkandl). Figure 5 shows a pheochromocytoma of the organ of Zuckerkandl. This tumor was located at the aortic bifurcation. The patient became pregnant, and whenever she lay on her back she became severely hypertensive and symptomatic. After appropriate preparation she had a cesarean section and excision of the tumor, with recovery of baby and mother. Van Heerden et al. recently reported that 40% of extra-adrenal tumors proved to be malignant.[18] Only 1%–2% of tumors are situated outside the abdomen, almost always in the posterior mediastinum in a paravertebral location. Chest x-rays, particularly lateral and oblique views, will usually demonstrate such tumors.[7]

CLINICAL FEATURES

The signs and symptoms of pheochromocytomas are quite numerous but in many respects quite nonspecific. Hypertension, headaches, palpitations, anxiety, and excessive perspiration are all common complaints or physical findings in patients with no demonstrable abnormality of adrenal medullary function.

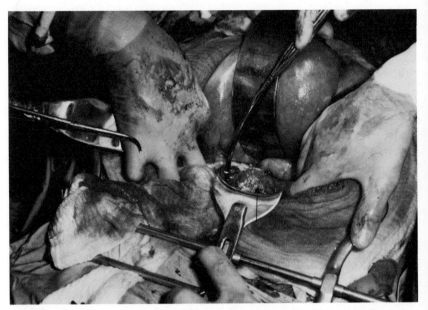

Fig 5.—Operative photograph looking into the pelvis of a woman with a pheochromocytoma of the organ of Zuckerkandl. The recently evacuated uterus is retracted anteriorly with the Deaver retractor. The tumor *(arrow)* was found at the bifurcation of the aorta.

However, a physician who never considers the diagnosis of a pheochromocytoma or who feels it is so rare that it is not worth the diagnostic evaluation will never diagnose one—sometimes with lethal consequences.

In a report from the Mayo Clinic, only 24% of the 50 patients found to have a pheochromocytoma at autopsy had the diagnosis made during life. Of those in whom the diagnosis was made post mortem, a careful review of the clinical record demonstrated that most had signs or symptoms suggestive of catecholamine excess. In this undiagnosed group, 27% died during a surgical procedure (one following minor surgery on a finger and one during anesthesia for an episiotomy) and 44% died from myocardial infarctions or hemorrhagic strokes.[10]

The most frequent manifestation of pheochromocytomas is hypertension. The majority of patients (50%–60%) have sustained hypertension while the remainder have elevated blood pressures only during the paroxysms.[3, 7] Even in patients with sustained hypertension the blood pressure tends to be more variable than in patients with essential hypertension, and these patients often experience further increases of blood pressure during a paroxysm. Unexplained hypertension or hypotension during induction of anesthesia or surgery should always make one suspicious of the diagnosis. It is noteworthy that 70% of untreated patients with pheochromocytomas have orthostatic hypotension. Although the pathophysiologic basis for this finding is not settled, two mechanisms have been proposed. Brunjes et al. reported a reduction of blood volume caused by chronic vascular constriction resulting from the increased sympathetic tone.[20] More recently, it has been proposed that the high levels of catecholamines produce a state of autonomic dysfunction simulating ganglionic blockade.[7] Independent of the mechanism, adequate preoperative adrenergic blockade reverses these abnormalities and reduces operative risk.

More specific than hypertension, and found in the great majority of patients with pheochromocytomas, are the paroxysmal symptoms caused by catecholamine excess. These begin abruptly, last from a few minutes to several hours, and then gradually subside. Twenty-five percent of the patients experience paroxysms daily; almost all the rest have symptoms at least at weekly intervals.[9] While paroxysms often occur without provocation, a variety of situations have commonly been noted to precipitate a paroxysm: pressure in the region of the tumor, lying in certain positions, bending, vigorous exercise, anxiety, trauma, increases in intra-abdominal pressure, certain foods (especially those of high tyramine content), micturition, intercourse, angiography, intubation and induction of anesthesia, and surgical procedures.

The more common symptoms of pheochromocytomas are listed in Table 2 and include headaches, sweating, palpitations, anxiety, pallor, chest or abdominal pain, paresthesias, and weakness. Ninety-five percent of patients have headaches, palpitations, or increased sweating, either alone or in combination. Moreover, with recurrent attacks patients often experience the same symptoms in a rather stereotyped manner.[15, 16, 21]

Patients with pheochromocytomas may experience a number of other adverse consequences of catecholamine excess. Hypermetabolism, manifested by an elevated basal metabolic rate

TABLE 2.—SYMPTOMS OF
PHEOCHROMOCYTOMA

SYMPTOM	%
Headache	78
Sweating	70
Palpitations	63
Pallor	43
Tremor	34
Nausea	37
Weakness	27
Significant weight loss	14

and weight loss, is common. These signs are secondary to the mobilization of free fatty acids by catecholamines. Abnormal glucose tolerance is commonly diagnosed and is often reversed following successful surgery. Myocardial disease is frequently observed. This can include infarctions, ventricular hypertrophy typical of that seen in essential hypertension, or congestive heart failure due to a specific cardiomyopathy resulting from catecholamine excess. Pathologically a focal myocarditis is evident with degeneration of myocardial fibers and foci of inflammatory cells. Compared to its frequency in the general population, cholelithiasis occurs with an increased frequency in patients with pheochromocytoma—a clinical observation that remains without explanation. In addition, patients at times present with abdominal pain and distention, reflecting the effects of both α and β stimuli on decreasing gastrointestinal motility.[7]

DISORDERS THAT MAY COEXIST WITH PHEOCHROMOCYTOMAS

The familial occurrence of pheochromocytomas has been recognized for over 20 years; estimates are that 10%–20% of these tumors are familial. It may be inherited without other associated endocrinopathies or as part of a MEN syndrome (Table 3). In the MEN IIA and IIB syndromes, the pheochromocytomas are almost universally intra-adrenal, bilateral, and multicentric.[22–25] Therefore, in affected patients bilateral adrenalectomy is generally recommended. In addition, a state of diffuse or nodular adrenal medullary hyperplasia frequently precedes actual tumor formation.[13, 14] Pheochromocytomas in these syn-

TABLE 3.—FAMILIAL SYNDROMES ASSOCIATED WITH
PHEOCHROMOCYTOMAS

Simple familial pheochromocytoma	Pheochromocytoma
Multiple endocrine neoplasia IIA	Pheochromocytoma Medullary carcinoma of thyroid Parathyroid hyperplasia
Multiple endocrine neoplasia IIB (III)	Pheochromocytoma Medullary carcinoma of thyroid Mucosal neuromas Marfanoid appearance Ganglioneuromas of GI tract
Neurofibromatosis	Pheochromocytoma Neurofibromas
von Hippel-Landau disease	Pheochromocytoma Cerebellar hemangioblastoma Retinal angiomas

dromes may secrete epinephrine predominantly, and specific measurement of urine or plasma epinephrine levels may be required to substantiate a diagnosis.[3] It should be emphasized that in a patient suspected of having MEN IIA or IIB, any consideration of neck exploration should be delayed until the possibility of a pheochromocytoma has been excluded. Neck surgery in a patient with an unsuspected pheochromocytoma could well prove fatal. A comprehensive discussion of the other features of these syndromes is beyond the scope of this review but a number of excellent articles are available to the interested reader.[22, 23, 25]

While it has been reported that 5% of patients with pheochromocytomas have features of neurofibromatosis, only 1% of patients with neurofibromas are found to have a pheochromocytoma. Finally, an increased incidence of pheochromocytomas has been noted in patients with von Hippel-Landau disease.

DIFFERENTIAL DIAGNOSIS

Due to the protean manifestations of pheochromocytomas, this tumor is often considered in the differential diagnosis of many disorders, including essential hypertension, hyperthyroidism, paroxysmal tachycardia, anxiety states, hyperventilation, psychoses, migraine, menopausal symptoms, toxemia of pregnancy, hypertensive crises induced by MAO inhibitors, and use of sympathomimetic drugs, to mention only the most common. Screening all such patients for catecholamine excess would therefore represent a massive undertaking and would be extremely inefficient from a cost-effective point of view.

It is a difficult task to set strict criteria for selection of patients to screen for a pheochromocytoma. If loose criteria are accepted, hundreds, if not thousands, of patients will be screened before one with a pheochromocytoma is diagnosed. On the other hand, overly restrictive criteria may allow significant numbers of patients with such tumors to go undiagnosed. Recommendations for appropriate populations of patients to screen are given in Table 4.

Diagnosis of Pheochromocytoma

Three major categories of diagnostic tests are available to help evaluate patients with suspected pheochromocytomas: (1) pharmacologic tests, consisting of provocative tests (glucagon, histamine, and tyramine) and adrenolytic tests (phentolamine and clonidine); (2) biochemical tests of urine and plasma; and (3) anatomical localization, consisting of intravenous pyelography with nephrotomograms, arteriography, venography and ve-

TABLE 4.—RECOMMENDATIONS FOR
PHEOCHROMOCYTOMA SCREENING

Hypertension with symptoms of pheochromocytoma
Hypertension resistant to conventional therapy
Hypertension with orthostatic hypotension off medication
Hypertension in children
Hypertension in patients with neurofibromas
Paroxysmal hypertension
Unexplained hypertension or hypotension during
  induction of anesthesia or surgery
Hyperparathyroidism with hypertension or symptoms of
  pheochromocytoma
Symptoms highly suggestive of pheochromocytoma in a
  normotensive patient
Hypermetabolism without evidence of hyperthyroidism
Familial history of pheochromocytoma or endocrine
  tumors
Undiagnosed suprarenal or para-aortic mass

nous sampling, CT scans, adrenal imaging, and sonography. Recently, pharmacologic testing done in conjunction with measurements of plasma catecholamines has been employed to aid in the diagnosis of more difficult cases.

Appropriate utilization of a modern clinical chemistry laboratory and sophisticated radiologic techniques now allow physicians to diagnoses virtually all cases of pheochromocytomas preoperatively. Therefore, surgical exploration for a suspected pheochromocytoma can rarely be justified in the absence of biochemical or radiologic evidence of such a tumor.

Pharmacologic Tests

The introduction of reliable methods of measuring catecholamines in the urine and plasma or catecholamine metabolites in the urine has largely eliminated the need for pharmacologic testing. Besides the inherent danger in both the provocative and adrenolytic tests, each is hampered by a significant percentage of both false positive and false negative results. Provocative testing with glucagon, histamine, or tyramine should be considered only in a normotensive individual with intermittent catecholamine release and long asymptomatic periods between attacks and in whom urine and plasma determinations have been nondiagnostic. Following administration of histamine or glucagon, an increase in blood pressure of at least 60/40 mm Hg is considered positive. After tyramine administration, a systolic increase of 20 mm Hg is suggestive of the diagnosis.[7] Each test yields a 25% incidence of false positive and negative results and is accompanied by the danger of precipitating a serious paroxysm. Deaths from vascular complications (myocardial infarctions or strokes) have been observed.

Measurement of urine and/or plasma catecholamines before and after a provocative stimulus improves diagnostic accuracy. In a recent report, glucagon produced a significant elevation of the blood pressure and plasma catecholamines in six patients with pheochromocytomas.[26] In four of these patients the diagnosis was obvious from the data provided by the baseline urine or plasma determinations. In the other two patients the baseline VMA or metanephrine level was slightly increased but glucagon stimulation confirmed the diagnosis.

Adrenolytic tests have traditionally been done with phentolamine (Regitine), a rapidly acting α antagonist: 1–5 mg is injected intravenously (IV). A positive response is indicated by a decrease in blood pressure of at least 35/25 mm Hg within 3 minutes that lasts for more than 10 minutes. This test is beneficial only in patients with hypertension at the time of the study, and as might be anticipated, significant hypotension with shock may be the end result. While false negative tests are uncommon, false positive responses are frequently observed in hypertensive patients without a pheochromocytoma.[3]

Bravo et al. recently reported the use of oral clonidine in conjunction with quantitation of plasma catecholamines as a test of high diagnostic accuracy for pheochromocytomas.[27] Clonidine suppressed plasma catecholamine levels in normal individuals and in those with essential hypertension but had no inhibitory effect on the plasma concentrations in patients with pheochromocytomas.

BIOCHEMICAL TESTS

For the past two decades the principal methods of diagnosing pheochromocytomas have been based on measurements of catecholamines or their metabolites in timed urine collections. These have included total catecholamines, fractionation of catecholamines into epinephrine and norepinephrine, VMA, and metanephrines (metanephrine + normetanephrine). In patients with sustained hypertension, a single 24-hour urine sample provides a diagnosis in the vast majority of cases.[7, 18, 28, 29] In individuals with paroxysmal hypertension and evidence of only intermittent catecholamine secretion, a collection beginning with the onset of symptoms and continuing for 24 hours is indicated. While several investigators have reported that spot urine collections provide reliable diagnostic information, an appropriately collected 24-hour urine specimen is probably preferable.[19, 30]

The urine should be collected into a special container with 6N HCl. Collection should be avoided after a recent severe stress, such as a myocardial infarction, which may give false positive results. While the patient need not be at bed rest, strenuous activity should be avoided. One must always be familiar with the various drugs that may interfere with the individual tests and avoid their administration before and during the collection.[19, 31] Table 5 lists the normal values for these tests as well as some of the more frequent interfering substances.

It should be noted that some tests for VMA are quite nonspecific and measure a variety of phenolic acids. These test results are often affected by a variety of foods and can be recognized because the upper limits of normal are in the range of 10–12 mg/24 hours. More specific assays that actually measure quantitatively the amount of vanillin converted from VMA are preferred.[29, 32] The upper limit of normal by this method is usually 6.5 mg/24 hours.

The question often arises as to which single test provides the most reliable data. A number of investigators favor the use of urinary metanephrines; however, individual reports differ, and each test, if done appropriately, will usually provide the necessary diagnostic information.[18, 19, 28, 29]

Fractionation of urinary catecholamines into epinephrine and norepinephrine may provide additional useful information. Most pheochromocytomas, even those of adrenal origin, secrete

TABLE 5.—BIOCHEMICAL TESTS FOR PHEOCHROMOCYTOMA AND INTERFERING SUBSTANCES

	VMA	METANEPHRINES	CATECHOLAMINES
Normal values	<6.5 mg/24 hours	<1.3 mg/24 hours	<100 μg/24 hours E <20 μg/24 hours NE <80 μg/24 hours

Increase	Catecholamines
	Drugs containing
	    catecholamines
	Amphetamines
	Methyldopa
	Levodopa
	Clonidine withdrawal
	
	Methocarbamol
	Glyceryl guaiacolate
	Nalidixic acid
		Catecholamines
		Drugs containing
		    catecholamines
		Amphetamines
		Methyldopa
		
		Clonidine withdrawal
		Ethanol
		Diatrizoate
		MAO inhibitors
			Catecholamines
			Drugs containing
			    catecholamines
			Amphetamines
			
			Clonidine withdrawal
			Ethanol
			Erythromycin
			Tetracycline
			Chlorpromazine
			Quinine
			Quinidine

Decrease	Metyrosine Reserpine Guanethidine MAO inhibitors Clofibrate Disulfiram Ethanol	Metyrosine Reserpine Guanethidine	Metyrosine Reserpine Guanethidine

E, epinephrine; NE, norepinephrine.

primarily norepinephrine.[3] However, if a significant fraction of the urinary catecholamines is epinephrine (>10%), the tumor most likely resides within the adrenal gland. As with most rules, exceptions have been noted, and predominantly epinephrine-secreting extra-adrenal pheochromocytomas have been reported.[7] In addition, some members of families with MEN type IIA or IIB have had epinephrine-secreting pheochromocytomas in which elevation of the urine or plasma epinephrine level was the only biochemical abnormality detectable.[3]

A recent study made use of the suppression of catecholamine production that normally occurs during sleep.[33] Patients voided prior to going to sleep and then collected all urine excreted during the night plus the first voided morning specimen. All six patients with a pheochromocytoma had elevated overnight norepinephrine excretion expressed in micrograms per hour. However, all had increased norepinephrine excretion during the daytime as well. Thus, in most patients, the overnight collection does not enhance diagnostic accuracy.

As in most areas of endocrinology, in recent years a greater emphasis has been placed on the measurement of plasma hormone levels in the diagnosis of pheochromocytomas. In the past, quantitation of plasma epinephrine and norepinephrine concentrations by fluorometric techniques did not provide sufficient sensitivity to be reliable. However, the recent development of radioenzymatic assays for catecholamines has overcome this problem. These assays are based on the conversion of epinephrine and norepinephrine, in the presence of COMT and labeled S-adenosylmethionine, to their respectively labeled 3–O derivative.[34]

Several precautionary comments deserve emphasis. The plasma half-life of circulating catecholamines is less than 1 minute. Some patients with intermittent catecholamine secretion may therefore be missed with plasma measurements. In addition, any stress, even that of venipuncture, will acutely elevate the plasma epinephrine and norepinephrine concentrations. The sample must be drawn with the patient supine (preferably in the morning before arising) and through an indwelling venous line that has been inserted at least 20 minutes prior to sampling. Measurement of plasma catecholamines is therefore not well suited for outpatient screening.

As with many new diagnostic tests, early reports measuring

plasma catecholamines claimed 100% accuracy in differentiating patients with from those without pheochromocytomas.[35] However, a careful review of the literature reveals occasional patients with documented tumors in whom the plasma catecholamine levels are normal while urinary levels are elevated. To be fair, the converse also holds true; some patients have normal urinary catecholamine, VMA, and metanephrine levels but elevated plasma norepinephrine or epinephrine concentrations. A survey of a number of studies demonstrates that plasma catecholamine determinations are attended by approximately the same rate of false negative results as carefully performed urines for catecholamines or their metabolites.[18, 19, 26, 36] If urinary levels prove normal in a patient suspected of having a pheochromocytoma, measurement of plasma norepinephrine or epinephrine levels will occasionally be diagnostic.

As mentioned previously, measurement of plasma catecholamines prior to and following administration of an oral dose of clonidine has proved to be an effective diagnostic test.[27] If the clinical suspicion of a pheochromocytoma is high and the routine studies are inconclusive, then a clonidine suppression test is advisable.

Zweifler and Julius recently reported that platelet catecholamine levels are increased in patients with pheochromocytomas and provide more reliable data than plasma measurements.[37] These studies were undertaken with the knowledge that catecholamines are concentrated by platelets. At present this test must still be considered investigational and not readily available to most practicing physicians. Other diagnostic tests, including quantitation of plasma or urinary dopamine or plasma dopamine β-hydroxylase, have not proved sufficiently sensitive to be of practical value.[3]

ANATOMICAL LOCALIZATION

In general, the primary care physician is faced with a patient in whom the diagnosis of a pheochromocytoma is suspected on the basis of the clinical data provided by the history and physical examination. Less commonly the patient presents with an undiagnosed mass that later proves to be a pheochromocytoma. This latter circumstance is more common in the surgical and urologic experience.

In the absence of a demonstrated mass, anatomical studies attempting to locate a pheochromocytoma should not be initiated before the presence of such a tumor is confirmed by biochemical (urine or plasma) determinations. Two good reasons can be given to support this contention. First, appropriate biochemical tests should be able to detect virtually all patients with a pheochromocytoma. These tests are relatively inexpensive and without complication. Second, arteriography and venography carry significant risks unless the patient is properly pretreated with adrenergic blocking agents (see below).

Intravenous pyelograms with nephrotomograms can generally be done in patients with a pheochromocytoma at little risk of a significant complication. Some 40%–70% of intra-adrenal tumors are localized by this technique.[9, 18, 19, 35]

In the past arteriography was the principal radiologic procedure employed to localize pheochromocytomas preoperatively. Aortography and/or selective arteriography should be done only in a patient suspected of having a pheochromocytoma who has previously been blocked with phenoxybenzamine (a long-acting α-receptor antagonist). In addition, parenteral phentolamine (a short-acting α blocker) and propranolol should always be available in case a severe paroxysm is induced during the procedure. Nonselective aortography is frequently diagnostic and less likely to result in complications than selective arteriography. If the former study is nondiagnostic, selective injection of vessels should be undertaken. Subtraction films enhance the diagnostic accuracy and may allow visualization of smaller lesions missed on the original films. Some 85%–95% of pheochromocytomas can be demonstrated by these techniques.[16, 33, 35] Because 10%–15% of patients with pheochromocytomas have multiple lesions, the films should be carefully reviewed for more than a single abnormality. Figure 6 demonstrates a left para-aortic pheochromocytoma as seen on the arterial and venous phases of an arteriogram.

Recently CT scans have proved quite successful in preoperative localization of pheochromocytomas. Figure 7 shows such a CT scan that demonstrates a pheochromocytoma. The noninvasive nature of this test (as compared to angiography) has great appeal. Several studies report an 80%–95% ability to localize pheochromocytomas with CT scans, while in the recent experience at the Mayo Clinic, 96% of these tumors were iden-

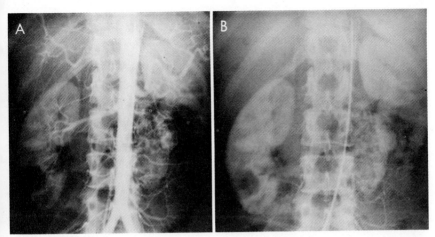

Fig 6.—Arteriogram of a left paraaortic pheochromocytoma. A, arterial phase; B, venous phase.

tified by this technique.[18, 33, 35] As greater experience with this diagnostic tool is accumulated, the need for angiography may be eliminated in the majority of patients. At present it is difficult to give firm recommendations. The choice of CT scan or arteriography should be based on the experience and expertise of the radiologists at each individual hospital.

Venography, with or without venous sampling at different

Fig 7.—CT scan demonstrating a large mass (p) associated with the left kidney that proved to be a pheochromocytoma.

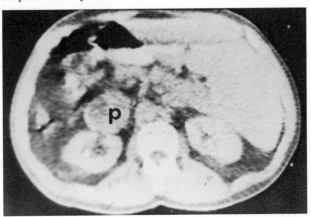

levels of the vena cava, is, in general, not a routine preoperative procedure.[38] This diagnostic approach should be considered when localization by less invasive techniques is nondiagnostic or when patients have persisting catecholamine excess after surgery.

Sonography has also been employed to localize pheochromocytomas.[39] While this technique has appeal as a noninvasive procedure, most clinicians would desire the more thorough anatomical definition of the pathology as provided by a CT scan or arteriogram before proceeding to the operating room.

Most recently, visualization of pheochromocytomas with nuclear imaging techniques has been reported using iodinated derivatives of guanidine. ^{131}I-metaiodobenzylguanidine is taken up by chromaffin tissue and incorporated into the storage granule.[40-42] Initial results suggest this could be a valuable diagnostic test, although at present its availability is limited to a small number of medical centers. Finally, chest x-ray films, including oblique views, should be carefully examined for intrathoracic lesions before abdominal exploration is performed.

As yet, no reports have appeared on the use of digital subtraction angiography to localize pheochromocytomas. This newly available radiologic technique may prove quite valuable as experience with it is accumulated.

Always bear in mind that because of the significant incidence of multiple pheochromocytomas, surgical exploration remains the definitive diagnostic as well as therapeutic procedure. Following removal of all the previously localized tumors a thorough exploration of any remaining adrenal tissue and the entire sympathetic chain is essential.

Management

While the ultimate therapy of patients with pheochromocytomas is surgical, complications will be minimized if management is handled cooperatively by a surgeon, internist, and anesthesiologist all experienced in dealing with such patients. Before adrenergic antagonists became available, the surgical mortality in patients with a preoperative diagnosis of a pheochromocytoma was 24%, but it was 50% in patients with an unsuspected pheochromocytoma operated on for other reasons.[43] Presently, even in expert hands, the perioperative mortality is still 2%–3%.[11, 16, 18, 44, 45]

Management can be divided into several specific areas:
1. Preoperative preparation. The comments below concerning the use of adrenergic blocking agents apply not only to preparing the patient for surgery but also to preparing the patient with a pheochromocytoma for invasive procedures such as angiography.
2. Anesthetic and operative technique.
3. Postoperative care.

PREOPERATIVE MANAGEMENT

Clinicians now have at their disposal a number of pharmacologic agents that function as specific α- or β-adrenergic antagonists. Proper administration of these drugs in the preoperative period ameliorates the signs and symptoms that patients with pheochromocytoma experience and generally reduces the incidence and severity of hypertension during surgery. Not only will these drugs lower the blood pressure and prevent paroxysms, but they also reverse the intravascular volume depletion that in the past was largely responsible for intraoperative and postoperative hypotension.

Despite these seemingly obvious advantages, some physicians avoid the routine administration of adrenergic blockade in the preoperative period. They contend that such therapy blunts the intraoperative rises in blood pressure during manipulation of the tumor that help the surgeon localize and remove all abnormal tissue.[9] However, adrenergic blockade is rarely complete. Even in patients pretreated with α- and/or β-adrenergic antagonists, rises in blood pressure are typically observed during manipulation of the tumor.[18, 36] The magnitude of such rises, however, is generally not as great as in patients who have not been treated with adrenergic blockade. We would not consider operating on a patient with a pheochromocytoma without preoperative blockade.

The agent of choice for initiating adrenergic blockade is phenoxybenzamine (Dibenzyline), a long-acting α-receptor antagonist. The initial dose is 20–40 mg/day in 2 or 3 divided doses. The dose is gradually increased until the blood pressure is controlled and paroxysms disappear or show a significant reduction in frequency. In patients with only intermittent hypertension the goal is to terminate the occurrence of paroxysmal symptoms. Most patients require between 20 and 100 mg/day, although occasionally doses as high as 300 mg/day may be necessary. Side effects include lethargy, nasal congestion, and tachycardia. Phentolamine (Regitine) is a short-acting α antagonist. Due to its short duration of action, its use is generally limited to IV administration for rapid reversal of hypertension during a spontaneous paroxysm or one induced during an invasive radiologic procedure or surgery. One to five milligrams can be given as an IV bolus or the drug may be administered by continuous IV infusion.

β blockade is generally reserved for patients with tachyarrhythmias, and then only after effective α blockade has been established. The administration of propranolol (or other β blockers) in the absence of adequate α blockade to a patient with a pheochromocytoma may precipitate severe hypertension. This results from inhibition of β-receptor-mediated vasodilation in a patient with catecholamine excess in whom α-receptor-mediated vasoconstriction remains unopposed. If propranolol is needed, an initial dose of 10 mg 4 times a day is gradually increased until tachyarrhythmias are controlled. β-Adrenergic antagonists should be avoided, or used with extreme caution, if there is evidence of congestive heart failure, cardiomyopathy, cardiac conduction defects, or asthma. Use of other α- or β-adrenergic antagonists or labetolol (a combined α and β antagonist) in patients with pheochromocytomas has been reported, but at present experience with these drugs is quite limited.[46, 47]

An alternative therapeutic agent for use in patients with pheochromocytomas is α-methyl-para-tyrosine (metyrosine), an inhibitor of tyrosine hydroxylase, the rate-limiting enzyme in the synthesis of catecholamines. Doses of 1–4 gm/day result in a 50%–80% decrease in catecholamine production as well as symptomatic improvement. Side effects are relatively common and include sedation, extrapyramidal signs, psychic disturbances, and diarrhea. α-Methyl-para-tyrosine has been used successfully to prepare patients with pheochromocytomas for surgery. It can also be administered on a long-term basis to those patients with pheochromocytomas who are inoperable.[7, 48]

The obvious aim of preoperative adrenergic blockade or inhibition of catecholamine synthesis is to prevent significant elevations of the blood pressure during arteriography and surgery. Of equal importance is the effect of such blockade on the intravascular volume. As noted previously, many patients with pheochromocytomas have intravascular volume depletion from chronic vasoconstriction.[20] Several weeks of α blockade or reduction in catecholamine levels allows restoration of a normal blood volume (often reflected in a decrease in the hematocrit of approximately 5%).[3] Attention to this particular detail of care will decrease the incidence and severity of hypotension during surgery and in the postoperative period. While adequate α blockade or inhibition of catecholamine synthesis will usually restore the depleted intravascular volume, some authorities also recommend IV administration of fluids or even blood prior to surgery to ensure a normal circulating blood volume.[49]

If bilateral adrenalectomy is anticipated (as in a patient with MEN syndrome or radiologic evidence of bilateral adrenal involvement), administration of corticosteroids should be initiated the evening prior to surgery. Hydrocortisone, 100 mg given IV every 8 hours, will prevent the development of adrenal insufficiency. The rapidity with which the steroids can be tapered in the postoperative period will depend on individual circumstances.

ANESTHETIC AND OPERATIVE TECHNIQUE

Careful attention to all details of care is absolutely essential if morbidity and mortality are to be minimized. During and immediately following surgery the hemodynamic status of the patient must be monitored continuously. Electrocardiographic monitoring, direct measurement of central venous and arterial pressures, and meticulous attention to fluid balance are all essential. In patients with evidence of cardiopulmonary disease, monitoring of the pulmonary capillary wedge pressure is advisable.

Parenteral preparations of propranolol, sodium nitroprusside, lidocaine, and norepinephrine or phenylephrine must be immediately available in case a need for their administration should arise. Indirectly acting sympathomimetic amines such as methoxamine (Aramine) do not give predictable responses in patients with pheochromocytomas and are best avoided. Induction of anesthesia is apt to provoke a paroxysm, so all the equipment for hemodynamic monitoring must be functioning and all drugs must be available before induction is attempted.

Many drugs and anesthetic agents can produce adverse effects on the cardiovascular system, particularly in patients with catecholamine excess. Drugs for induction and maintenance of anesthesia must therefore be selected with utmost care. Preoperative administration of atropine should be avoided, as this is apt to result in tachycardia and elevation of the blood pressure.[19, 50] Induction with thiopental is generally smooth and is currently recommended by many groups.[8, 44, 50, 51]

The choice of anesthetic agent remains somewhat controversial. Cyclopropane should not be used since it can potentiate catecholamine-induced arrhythmias. Methoxyflurane was found to be quite satisfactory, but the significant risk of nephrotoxicity has sharply curtailed its use. Either halothane or enflurane is the anesthetic generally considered for patients with pheochromocytomas. However, in one report most patients that received halothane developed ventricular arrhythmias.[52] Most recent surgical series favor the administration of enflurane with or without the addition of nitrous oxide.[9, 18, 19, 51, 53] Recently neuroleptanalgesia has been advocated, but most anesthesiologists still prefer enflurane.[18, 54]

Exacerbations of hypertension are most likely to occur during induction of anesthesia and manipulation of the tumor. A report by Feldman et al. documented that these hypertensive episodes are associated with dramatic increases in the plasma concentration of norepinephrine, often to values in excess of 100,000 pg/ml.[53] For several decades these episodes have been treated with IV phentolamine, but recently sodium nitroprusside has proved to be an effective and reliable alternative. Phentolamine is administered in an IV bolus of 1–5 mg; however, the effect dissipates rapidly, within 5 minutes. If a more prolonged effect is required, phentolamine can be given as a continuous IV infusion. Therapy can be initiated at a rate of 1 mg/minute and the dose titrated to control the blood pressure. Sodium nitroprusside, a potent vasodilator, is generally given by continuous IV infusion. The initial rate of infusion should be approximately 200 μg/minute with adjustments as required to prevent significant hypertension. Its onset of action is extremely rapid, and effects terminate within 3 minutes of discontinuing the infusion.[55] Both phentolamine and sodium nitroprusside are effective agents with few side effects if administered with appropriate care. The individual preference and experience of the anesthesiologist should probably dictate which drug should be chosen to treat intraoperative hypertension.

Ventricular ectopy is best managed with lidocaine. Fifty to one hundred milligrams are given as an IV bolus, and if required, a constant infusion of 2–4 mg/minute can be employed. Propranolol given IV is used for treatment of tachyarrhythmias. A bolus of 0.1–0.5 mg is administered to control heart rates greater than 120 beats/minute and is repeated if necessary.[55]

The other major intraoperative complication is a precipitous decline in the blood pressure, most frequently observed following excision of the pheochromocytoma. As previously noted, two mechanisms have been proposed to explain this phenomenon: a reduced blood volume and an autonomic dysfunction simulating adrenergic blockade.[7, 20] Independent of the pathophysiologic basis of the hypotension, careful attention to the patient's volume status will minimize this complication. The patient should not be considered for surgery until the physician feels certain that the blood volume is normal. In addition, some recommend IV fluids or even blood transfusions the evening prior to surgery.[43] If hypotension develops during surgery, initial treatment is the infusion of liberal quantities of volume expanders. Blood, plasma, albumin, or 0.9% saline can be chosen, depending on the severity of the hypotension. Volume expansion is generally sufficient to correct this complication and the need for pressor agents can usually be eliminated.[3, 7, 19, 50] If this approach to reversing the hypotension is unsuccessful, directly acting vasopressors such as norepinephrine or phenylephrine can be given IV. However, administration of vasopressors is best avoided. High infusion rates are often required to maintain the blood pressure and their use will only serve to perpetuate the autonomic abnormalities produced by the longstanding catecholamine excess.

We have used the midline abdominal incision for pheochromocytomas because of its flexibility. Careful exploration of the entire abdominal cavity is mandatory. The surgeon must exclude additional pheochromocytomas other than the one known to be present. The extent of dissection required to accomplish this will depend on the body habitus of the patient. Psychologically it is probably best to do the exploration prior to approaching the known tumor. If removal of the known tumor is difficult and time-consuming, the surgeon has a tendency to become less diligent with the search for a second lesion.

These tumors are quite vascular and very little progress is made in their removal without encountering substantial bleeding. It seems to make little difference where the dissection starts, since small vessels enter and leave the tumor from all over its surface. At some point along its circumference the dissection is started. We use the cautery extensively and divide adventitial tissues with the coagulating current. Smaller, visible vessels are controlled with small clips and larger vessels are ligated. The most important factors are patience and meticulous care. The tumor should be manipulated as little as possible.

Communication among the surgeon, anesthesiologist, and internist during the operation is essential. Changes in cardiovascular stability can be so rapid and severe that the surgeon should not attempt to be primarily responsible for treating them while simultaneously performing the demanding dissection.

POSTOPERATIVE CARE

Following surgery, close observation in the recovery room and then in an intensive care unit is imperative. Frequent monitoring of the cardiac rhythm, central venous pressure, arterial pressure, and fluid balance is required until the patient's status has unequivocally stabilized.

Postoperative hypotension is best managed by IV administration of fluids, particularly if the central venous pressure is low. The same principles of treating hypotension apply at this time as during surgery. Vasopressor agents should be held in reserve, to be used only for severe, refractory hypotension unresponsive to volume expansion.

Postoperative hypertension is a relatively frequent observation and may result from a number of potential etiologies, including overexpansion of the intravascular volume, residual pheochromocytoma tissue left in situ, or inadvertent injury to a renal artery. A trial of diuretics, particularly if the central venous pressure is elevated, will frequently lower the blood pressure to normal if overhydration is the etiology. If residual pheochromocytoma is suspected, caution needs to be exercised in interpreting laboratory data. Even with complete resection of all functioning pheochromocytoma tissue, levels of plasma and urinary catecholamines and their metabolites may not return to normal until the fourth or fifth postoperative day.[7, 26] Therefore, a decision to reoperate in the early postoperative period should not be based on these biochemical determinations. However, a significant lowering of the blood pressure following IV phentolamine administration implies persistent catecholamine excess. In addition, approximately 25% of patients will have persistent hypertension despite a surgical cure.[16, 56]

In recent years there has been an increased awareness of hypoglycemia following resection of pheochromocytomas. This complication, which is usually transient, may result from a sudden reduction in circulating catecholamine levels with continued, increased secretion of insulin. Alternatively, α-adrenergic blockade may play a role by stimulating insulin secretion.

Prior to discharge, repeat measurements of plasma or urinary catecholamines or their metabolites is advisable to ascertain whether surgery has been curative. If there is no evidence of residual tumor, follow-up studies are recommended every 6 months. After several years, if catecholamine levels remain normal, annual determinations are sufficient.

Patients with benign pheochromocytomas have excellent long-term survival—96% at 5 years. The 5-year survival in malignant disease, on the other hand, is reported to be 44%.[56] However, Gittes and Mahoney reported an improved survival rate for malignant pheochromocytoma when an aggressive surgical approach was judiciously applied in selected patients.[8] Most attempts at treating these patients with chemotherapy or radiotherapy have met with very limited success, although radiotherapy may provide substantial palliation to bone metastases.[17, 57]

Patients who are inoperable because of other complicating medical illnesses, who refuse surgery, or who have malignant pheochromocytoma should be treated long-term with adrenergic blocking agents or α-methyl-para-tyrosine. In an interesting case report, therapeutic embolization of lymph nodes infiltrated with malignant pheochromocytoma was successfully achieved without complications in a patient pretreated with adrenergic blockade.[58]

Summary

Despite the relative infrequency of pheochromocytomas, they remain a potentially curable yet lethal etiology of hypertension. Appropriate utilization of a modern clinical chemistry laboratory and sophisticated radiologic techniques should allow a suspecting physician to establish the presence or absence of such a catecholamine-secreting tumor. The treatment of pheochromocytoma remains surgical; however, strict attention to preoperative details is crucial if mortality is to be minimized. Judicious use of adrenergic blocking agents and measures to ensure a normal circulating blood volume are of utmost importance during the preoperative period. Surgery remains the ultimate diagnostic and therapeutic maneuver. A thorough and meticulous exploration of the entire abdominal cavity and both adrenal beds is essential in all patients with pheochromocytoma. Monitoring of electrocardiographic and hemodynamic parameters is critical during surgery and postoperatively, since changes in cardiovascular stability can be dramatic and rapid. Appropriate measures must be taken to reverse such changes but must be made based on a thorough understanding of the effects of catecholamines, the drugs available to alter these effects, and the potential problems that patients with pheochromocytomas are likely to experience.

Acknowledgments

The authors thank Ms. Teresa Bays for her excellent secretarial assistance in preparing this manuscript and Michael S. Rohr, M.D., Ph.D., for his help in providing the graphic materials.

REFERENCES

1. Coupland R.E.: *The Natural History of the Chromaffin Cell.* London, Longmans, Green & Co., Ltd., 1965.
2. Pearse A.G.E.: The APUD cell concept and its implications in pathology. *Pathol. Annu.* 9:27, 1974.
3. Landsberg L., Young J.B.: Catecholamines and the adrenal medulla, in

Bondy P.K., Rosenberg L.E. (eds.): *Metabolic Control and Disease*. Philadelphia, W.B. Saunders Co., 1980.
4. Sharman D.F.: The catabolism of catecholamines. *Br. Med. Bull.* 29:110, 1973.
5. Ahlquist R.P.: A study of the adrenotropic receptors. *Am. J. Physiol.* 153:586, 1948.
6. Cryer P.E.: Physiology and pathophysiology of the human sympathoadrenal neuroendocrine system. *N. Engl. J. Med.* 303:436, 1980.
7. Engelman K.: Phaeochromocytoma. *Clin. Endocrinol. Metab.* 6:769, 1977.
8. Gittes R.F., Mahoney E.M.: Pheochromocytoma. *Urol. Clin. North Am.* 4:239, 1977.
9. Manger W.M., Gifford R.W. Jr.: *Pheochromocytoma*. New York, Springer-Verlag, 1977.
10. St. John Sutton M.G., Sheps S.G., Lie J.T.: Prevalence of clinically unsuspected pheochromocytoma: Review of a 50-year autopsy series. *Mayo Clin. Proc.* 56:354, 1981.
11. Melicow M.M.: One hundred cases of pheochromocytoma (107 tumors) at the Columbia-Presbyterian Medical Center, 1926–1976. *Cancer* 40:1987, 1977.
12. Webb T.A., Sheps S.G., Carney J.A.: Differences between sporadic pheochromocytoma and pheochromocytoma in multiple endocrine neoplasia, type 2. *Am. J. Surg. Pathol.* 4:121, 1980.
13. Carney J.A., Sizemore G.W., Sheps S.G.: Adrenal medullary disease in multiple endocrine neoplasia, type 2: Pheochromocytoma and its precursors. *Am. J. Clin. Pathol.* 66:279, 1976.
14. DeLellis R.A., Wolfe H.J., Gagel R.F., et al.: Adrenal medullary hyperplasia: A morphometric analysis in patients with familial medullary thyroid carcinoma. *Am. J. Pathol.* 83:177, 1976.
15. Gifford R.W.J., Kvale W.F., Maher F.T., et al.: Clinical features, diagnosis and treatment of pheochromocytoma: A review of 76 cases. *Mayo Clin. Proc.* 39:281, 1964.
16. Öhman U., Granberg P., Lindvall N., et al.: Pheochromocytoma: Critical review of experiences with diagnosis and treatment. *Prog. Clin. Cancer* 7:135, 1978.
17. Scott H.W. Jr., Reynolds V., Green N., et al.: Clinical experience with malignant pheochromocytomas. *Surg. Gynecol. Obstet.* 154:801, 1982.
18. van Heerden J.A., Sheps S.G., Hamberger B., et al.: Pheochromocytoma: Current status and changing trends. *Surgery* 91:367, 1982.
19. Falterman C.J., Kreisberg R.: Pheochromocytoma: Clinical diagnosis and management. *South. Med. J.* 75:321, 1982.
20. Brunjes S., Johns V.J., Crane M.G.: Pheochromocytoma, postoperative shock and blood volume. *N. Engl. J. Med.* 262:393, 1960.
21. Thomas J.E., Rooke E.D., Kvale W.F.: The neurologist's experience with pheochromocytoma: A review of 100 cases. *JAMA* 197:754, 1966.
22. Khairi M.R., Dexter R.N., Burzynski N.J., et al.: Mucosal neuroma, pheochromocytoma and medullary thyroid carcinoma: Multiple endocrine neoplasia type 3. *Medicine* 54:89, 1975.
23. Lips K.J.M., Van Der Sluys Veer J., Struyvenberg A., et al.: Bilateral occurrence of pheochromocytoma in patients with multiple endocrine

312   S. N. LEVINE AND J. C. MCDONALD

neoplasia syndrome type 2A (Sipple's syndrome). *Am. J. Med.* 70:1051, 1981.
24. Sipple J.H.: The association of pheochromocytoma with carcinoma of the thyroid gland. *Am. J. Med.* 31:163, 1961.
25. Steiner A.L., Goodman A.D., Powers S.R.: Study of a kindred with pheo-chromocytoma, medullary thyroid carcinoma, hyperparathyroidism, and Cushing's disease: Multiple endocrine neoplasia, type 2. *Medicine* 47:371, 1968.
26. Bravo E.L., Tarazi R.C., Gifford R.W., et al.: Circulating and urinary catecholamines in pheochromocytoma. *N. Engl. J. Med.* 301:682, 1979.
27. Bravo E.L., Tarazi R.C., Fouad F.M., et al.: Clonidine-suppression test: A useful aid in the diagnosis of pheochromocytoma. *N. Engl. J. Med.* 305:623, 1981.
28. Sjoerdsma A., Engelman K., Waldmann T.A., et al.: Pheochromocytoma: Current concepts of diagnosis and treatment. *Ann. Intern. Med.* 65:1302, 1966.
29. Gitlow S.E., Mendlowitz M., Bertani L.M.: The biochemical techniques for detecting and establishing the presence of a pheochromocytoma. *Am. J. Cardiol.* 26:270, 1970.
30. Kaplan N.M., Kramer N.J., Holland O.B., et al.: Single-voided urine me-tanephrine assays in screening for pheochromocytoma. *Arch. Intern. Med.* 137:190, 1977.
31. Cryer P.E.: The adrenergic nervous system, in Cryer P.E. (ed.): *Diagnostic Endocrinology.* New York, Oxford University Press, 1979.
32. Rayfield E.J., Cain J.P., Casey M.P., et al.: Influence of diet on urinary VMA excretion. *JAMA* 221:704, 1972.
33. Ganguly A., Henry D.P., Yune H.Y., et al.: Diagnosis and localization of pheochromocytoma: Detection by measurement of urinary norepineph-rine excretion during sleep, plasma norepinephrine concentration and computerized axial tomography (CT-scan). *Am. J. Med.* 67:21, 1979.
34. Cryer P.E.: Isotope-derivative measurements of plasma norepinephrine and epinephrine in man. *Diabetes* 25:1071, 1976.
35. Stewart B.H., Bravo E.L., Meany T.F.: A new simplified approach to the diagnosis of pheochromocytoma. *J. Urol.* 122:579, 1979.
36. Plouin P.F., Duclos J.M., Menard J., et al.: Biochemical tests for diagno-sis of pheochromocytoma: Urinary versus plasma determinations. *Br. Med. J.* 282:853, 1981.
37. Zweifler A.J., Julius S.: Increased platelet catecholamine content in pheo-chromocytoma: A diagnostic test in patients with elevated plasma cate-cholamines. *N. Engl. J. Med.* 306:890, 1982.
38. Georgi M., Cordes U., Günther R., et al.: Phlebographic diagnosis of pheochromocytomas. *Fortschr. Geb. Roentgenstr. Nuklearmed.* 128:727, 1978.
39. Bowerman R.A., Silver T.M., Jaffe M.H., et al.: Sonography of adrenal pheochromocytomas. *AJR* 137:1227, 1981.
40. Valk T.W., Frager M.S., Gross M.D., et al.: Spectrum of pheochromocy-toma in multiple endocrine neoplasia: A scintigraphic portrayal using ^{131}I-metaiodobenzylguanidine. *Ann. Intern. Med.* 94:762, 1981.
41. Sisson J.C., Frager M.S., Valk T.W., et al.: Scintigraphic localization of pheochromocytoma. *N. Engl. J. Med.* 305:12, 1981.

42. Wieland D.M., Swanson D.P., Brown L.E., et al.: Imaging the adrenal medulla with an I-131-labeled antiadrenergic agent. *J. Nucl. Med.* 20:155, 1979.
43. Apgar V., Papper E.M.: Pheochromocytoma: Anesthetic management during surgical treatment. *Arch. Surg.* 62:634, 1951.
44. Scott H.W. Jr., Dean R.H., Oates J.A., et al.: Surgical management of pheochromocytoma. *Am. Surg.* 47:8, 1981.
45. Freier D.T., Eckhauser F.E., Harrison T.S.: Pheochromocytoma: A persistently problematic and still potentially lethal disease. *Arch. Surg.* 115:388, 1980.
46. Cubeddu L.X., Zarate N.A., Rosales C.B., et al.: Prazosin and propranolol in preoperative management of pheochromocytoma. *Clin. Pharmacol. Ther.* 32:156, 1982.
47. Russell W.J., Kaines A.H., Hooper M.J., et al.: Labetolol in the preoperative management of pheochromocytoma. *Anaesth. Intensive Care* 10:160, 1982.
48. Karasov R.S., Sheps S.G., Carney J.A., et al.: Paragangliomatosis with numerous catecholamine-producing tumors. *Mayo Clin. Proc.* 57:590, 1982.
49. Deoreo G.A., Stewart B.H., Tarazi R.C., et al.: Preoperative blood transfusion in the safe surgical management of pheochromocytoma: A review of 46 cases. *J. Urol.* 111:715, 1974.
50. Sever P.S., Roberts J.C., Snell M.E.: Phaeochromocytoma. *Clin. Endocrinol. Metab.* 9:543, 1980.
51. Ellis D., Gartner J.C.: The intraoperative medical management of childhood pheochromocytoma. *J. Pediatr. Surg.* 35:655, 1980.
52. Cooperman L.H., Engelman K., Mann P.E.G.: Anesthetic management of pheochromocytoma employing halothane and beta adrenergic blockade: A report of fourteen cases. *Anesthesiology* 28:575, 1967.
53. Feldman J.M., Blalock J.A., Fagraeus L., et al.: Alterations in plasma norepinephrine concentration during surgical resection of pheochromocytoma. *Ann. Surg.* 188:758, 1978.
54. Stamenković L., Spierdijk J.: Anaesthesia in patients with phaeochromocytoma. *Anaesthesia* 31:941, 1976.
55. Juan D.: Pharmacologic agents in the management of pheochromocytoma. *South. Med. J.* 75:211, 1982.
56. Remine W.H., Chong G.C., van Heerden J.A., et al.: Current management of pheochromocytoma. *Ann. Surg.* 179:740, 1974.
57. Hamilton B.P.M., Cheikh I.E., Rivera L.E.: Attempted treatment of inoperable pheochromocytoma with streptozocin. *Arch. Intern. Med.* 137:762, 1977.
58. Timmis J.B., Brown M.J., Allison I.J.: Therapeutic embolization of phaeochromocytoma. *Br. J. Radiol.* 54:420, 1981.

Subject Index

A

Abdomen
  abscess, CT of, 186–187
  CT of, 171–196
  fluid collections, CT of, 186–187
  paracentesis, 140
Abscess
  abdomen, CT of, 186–187
  diverticulum, CT of, 184
  liver, pyogenic, CT of, 174
  pancreas, CT of, 181
  subphrenic, CT of, 187
Adenocarcinoma
  omentum, metastatic, CT of, 186
  stomach, CT of, 183
Adrenals
  CT of, 190–192
  hyperplasia of, CT of, 191
  sympathoadrenal system (*see*
      Sympathoadrenal system)
Allograft (*see* Transplantation)
Amino acid(s)
  essential, in kidney failure, 26
  losses during dialysis, 24
  solutions
    protein after, 27
    in total parenteral nutrition, 26–28
Anabolic agent: postoperative, insulin as,
    28–29
Anastomosis
  colorectal, Sugarbaker technique, 247
  EEA™ instrument for, 260
  end-to-end, functional
    GIA™ and TA™ instruments for,
    262
    modified, 263
  GIA™ bayonet, 264
  Murphy's button for, 245
  rectum, with EEA™ instrument,
    266–267
  by Strasbourg technique, 270

Anesthesia
  for arthroscopy, 210
  for liver resection, 148–149
  for pheochromocytoma, 305–308
Aneurysm
  aortic, abdominal, CT of, 190
  iliac artery, CT of, 190
Angiomyolipoma: renal, CT of, 193
Ankle defect: reconstruction, 92
Antibiotic prophylaxis: after
    splenectomy, 62–63
Antibody production: by spleen, 51–52
Aorta, abdominal
  aneurysm, CT of, 190
  CT of, 189–190
Arm: right, replantation of, 80
Arteries: iliac, CT of aneurysm of, 190
Arteriography
  of liver hematoma, 148
  of pheochromocytoma, 301
Arthritis: degenerative, arthroscopy in,
    235-236
Arthroscopes, 206–207
  examples of, 203
  operating, skills for, 202
  television camera attached to, 208
Arthroscopy, 197–240
  advantages, 204–205
  anesthesia for, 210
  in arthritis, degenerative, 235–236
  cost of, 204
  diagnostic
    skills for, 199
    technique, 212–217
  disadvantages, 205–206
  future developments of, 237
  history, 197–198
  indications for, 202–204
  instruments for, 206–212
    arthroscopes (*see* Arthroscopes)
    cutting, 200
    expense of, 205

GIA™ procedures, 258–259
Glucose
  in kidney failure, 26
  protein after, 27
Goligher technique: in rectal resection,
    271
Graft: jejunal, for esophageal
    reconstruction, 86

H

Hamartoma: hepatic fatty, CT of, 193
Hand: toe-to-hand transfer, 93–94
Hartmann procedure: reconstruction
    after, 273
Head reconstruction, 84–88
  omentum in, 87–88
Heart
  surgery, total parenteral nutrition
    after, 26
  transplantation, cyclosporin A in, 113
    (in rat), 102–103
Hemangioma: of liver, CT of, 173
Hematoma
  of liver, 149
    arteriography of, 148
  spleen, CT of, 176
Hemihepatectomy
  extended, 134
  left, 134
    extended, technique, 153–154
    technique, 153–154
  right, 134
    extended, 134
    extended, technique, 151–153
    technique, 151–153
Hemostasis: by collagen in avulsion of
    spleen, 58
Henroz' technique, 244
Hepatic (see Liver)
Hepatoma: multicentric, CT of, 174
Hernia
  hiatal, CT of, 185
  inguinal, CT of, 185
Hültl stapler, 249
Hypernephroma: CT of, 193
Hyperplasia: adrenal, CT of, 191

I

Ileal-vesical fistula: CT of, 184
Ileo-ileal intussusception: CT of, 185
Iliac artery aneurysm: CT of, 190
Imaging: after liver injury, 142

Indian-file rows of staples, 250
Inguinal hernia: CT of, 185
Instrument(s)
  arthroscopy (see Arthroscopy,
    instruments for)
  EEA™ (see EEA™ instrument)
  GIA™, for anastomosis, 262
  for liver resection, 134–137
  TA™, for anastomosis, 262
Insulin: as postoperative anabolic agent,
    28–29
Intestine (see Gastrointestinal)
Intussusception: ileo-ileal, CT of, 185

J

Jejunal graft: for esophageal
    reconstruction, 86

K

Kidney
  angiomyolipoma, CT of, 193
  CT of, 192–195
  failure, amino acids and glucose in, 26
  insufficiency, total parenteral nutrition
    in, 23–26
  transplantation, cyclosporin A in,
    108–112
    (in rat), 100–102
Knee
  arthroscopy (see Arthroscopy, knee)
  injury, acute, 236
  model in learning endoscopic skills,
    206
Knight and Griffin technique: for rectal
    resection, 272

L

Lavage: peritoneal, 140–141
Light micrograph: of pheochromocytoma,
    288
Limb (see Extremities)
Liver
  abscess, CT of, 174
  anatomy, 132–134
  clamp
    atraumatic atraugrip jaw vascular,
      137, 138
    hemostatic, long, 137, 138
    hemostatic, small, 137
  CT of, 172–175
  ducts, obstruction of, 179